MEDICAL RADIATION PHYSICS

Medical
Radiation Physics

ROENTGENOLOGY, NUCLEAR MEDICINE & ULTRASOUND

WILLIAM R. HENDEE, PH.D.

Professor of Radiology
University of Colorado Medical Center
Denver, Colorado

SECOND EDITION

YEAR BOOK MEDICAL PUBLISHERS, INC.
CHICAGO • LONDON

Library of Congress Cataloging in Publication Data
Hendee, William R 1938-
    Medical radiation physics.
    Includes index.
    1. Radiology, Medical. I. Title.
[DNLM: 1. Biophysics. 2. Radiobiology.
WN610.3 H495m]
R895.H4 1979   616.07'57   78-10300
ISBN 0-8151-4240-4

To my wife *Jeannie*
and children
Mikal, Shonn, Eric, Gareth, Gregory,
Lara and *Karel*

Preface to the Second Edition

MANY CHANGES have occurred in radiology since publication of the first edition of this text nine years ago. These changes not only make a new edition of the text necessary, but also necessitate the addition of a number of new topics and the revision of a considerable portion of the original text. To accommodate the required changes, most of the material on the physics of radiation therapy has been deleted in the revised edition. The deleted material, with considerable updating and expansion, is in preparation as a separate text on the physics of radiation therapy. The second edition of *Medical Radiation Physics* is confined to the principles of radiologic physics and their applications to the principal modalities of diagnostic imaging.

In this revised edition, four chapters have been added on the principles of diagnostic ultrasound, and one new chapter is devoted exclusively to computed tomography. To accommodate an audience with varying mathematical backgrounds, all calculus has been removed from the text. The chapters on x-ray tubes, nuclear medicine imaging, roentgenography, fluoroscopy and special imaging procedures have been rewritten extensively to include new information. The chapters on image quality, external radiation protection and internal radiation protection have been approached differently in an effort to make the topics more comprehensible.

So many persons have helped in this revision that I can thank them only collectively rather than individually. One person has contributed so much, however, that to omit her name from the preface would be too great an oversight. I am indebted deeply to Ms. Carolyn Yandle for her diligence and patience in keeping the entire manuscript intact and well organized during the revision process.

WILLIAM R. HENDEE

Preface to the First Edition

THIS TEXT was compiled and edited from tape recordings of lectures in medical radiation physics at the University of Colorado School of Medicine. The lectures are attended by resident physicians in radiology, by radiologic technologists and by students beginning graduate study in medical physics and in radiation biology. The text is intended for a similar audience.

Many of the more recent developments in medical radiation physics are discussed in the text. However, innovations are frequent in radiology, and the reader should supplement the book with perusal of the current literature. References at the end of each chapter may be used as a guide to additional sources of information.

Mathematical prerequisites for understanding the text are minimal. In the few sections where calculus is introduced in the derivation of an equation, a description of symbols and procedures is provided with the hope that the use of the equation is intelligible even if the derivation is obscure.

Problem solving is the most effective way to understand physics in general and medical radiation physics in particular. Problems are included at the end of each chapter, with answers at the end of the book. Students are encouraged to explore, discuss and solve these problems. Example problems with solutions are scattered throughout the text.

Acknowledgments

Few textbooks would be written without the inspiration provided by colleagues, students and friends. I am grateful to all of my associates who have contributed in so many ways toward the completion of this text. The original lectures were recorded by Carlos Garciga, M.D., and typed by Mrs. Marilyn Seckler and Mrs. Carolyn McCain. Parts of the book have been reviewed in unfinished form by: Martin Bischoff, M.D., Winston Boone, B.S., Donald Brown, M.D., Frank Brunstetter, M.D., Duncan Burdick, M.D., Lawrence Coleman, Ph.D., Walter Croft, Ph.D., Marvin Daves, M.D., Neal Goodman, M.D., Albert Hazle, B.S., Donald Herbert, Ph.D., F. Bing Johnson, M.D., Gordon Kenney, M.S., Jack Krohmer, Ph.D., John Pettigrew, M.D., Robert Siek, M.P.H., John Taubman, M.D., Richard Trow, B.S., and Marvin Williams, Ph.D. I appreciate the comments offered by these reviewers. Edward Chaney, Ph.D., reviewed the entire manuscript and furnished many helpful suggestions. Robert Cadigan, B.S., assisted with the proofreading and worked many of the problems. Geoffrey Ibbott, Kenneth Crusha, Lyle Lindsey, R.T., and Charles Ahrens, R.T., obtained much of the experimental data included in the book.

Mrs. Josephine Ibbott prepared most of the line drawings for the book, and I am grateful for her diligence and cooperation. Mrs. Suzan Ibbott and Mr. Billie Wheeler helped with some of the illustrations, and Miss Lynn Wisehart typed the appendixes. Mr. David Kuhner of the John Crerar Library in Chicago located many of the references to early work. Representatives of various instrument companies have helped in many ways. I thank Year Book Medical Publishers for encouragement and patience and Marvin Daves, M.D., for his understanding and support.

I am indebted deeply to Miss Carolyn Yandle for typing each chapter many times, and for contributing in many other ways toward the completion of the book.

Finally, I wish to recognize my former teachers for all they have contributed so unselfishly. In particular, I wish to thank Fred Bonte, M.D., and Jack Krohmer, Ph.D., for their guidance during my years as a graduate student. I wish also to recognize my indebtedness to Elda E. Anderson, Ph.D., and to William Zebrun, Ph.D. I shall not forget their encouragement during my early years of graduate study.

WILLIAM R. HENDEE

Contents

1 / Structure of Matter

THE ATOM

History of the Concept of the Atom

Matter composed of small, indivisible particles is not a new concept. Demokritos and the Epicurean school (400–300 B.C.) in Greece postulated that "the only existing things are atoms and empty space."[1] During the Middle Ages and Renaissance period, however, the continuum of matter philosophy of Aristotle and the Stoic philosophers prevailed over the philosophy of atomism. Not until 1802, when John Dalton developed the principle of multiple proportions,[2] was the atomic theory of matter revived. The concept of the atom was strengthened by results of studies by Gay-Lussac (law of gas volumes, 1809),[3] Avogadro (Avogadro's hypothesis, 1811),[4] Prout (multiple hydrogen atom hypothesis, 1815),[5] Faraday (law of electrolysis, 1833),[6] Cannizzaro (determination of atomic weights, 1858),[7] Meyer and Mendeleev (periodic table, 1869–70),[8] and Perrin (studies of Brownian motion, 1908).[9] Few skeptics of the atomic composition of matter remained after publication of Perrin's results.

Studies by J. J. Thomson in 1897 established the ratio of charge to mass for cathode rays, identified later as *electrons*.[10] The electrical charge possessed by electrons, now accepted as -1.6×10^{-19} coulomb, was measured in 1909 by Robert Millikan.[11] J. J. Thomson advanced a "plum pudding" model for the atom, in which electrons were distributed randomly within a heavy matrix of positive charge.[12] Experiments performed in 1911 by Ernest Rutherford suggested that Thomson's model of the atom was invalid.[13]

Bohr's Model of the Atom

Results of Rutherford's experiments implied that the positive charge and most of the mass of an atom are located in a central core or *nucleus* that is much smaller than the atom. The diameter of the nucleus was estimated to be about 10^{-4} Å (10^{-14} m). Diameters of atoms were thought to average about 1 Å (10^{-10} m). Electrons surround the nucleus and are bound to it by the electrostatic force of attraction between particles with opposite charge. Why electrons are not pulled into the nucleus by the electrostatic force was a question puzzling to many physicists.

In 1913, Niels Bohr suggested that electrons remain outside the nucleus because they move at high velocity in circular orbits.[14] The centripetal electrostatic force exerted by the nucleus prevents the electrons from leaving the atom in a direction tangent to their orbits. The electrostatic force exerted by the nucleus may be pictured as acting similar to the centripetal force exerted by a string attached to a small steel ball revolving in a plane containing the string.

According to classical physics, electrons revolving in circular orbits should radiate energy and spiral into the nucleus. To justify his atomic model, Bohr advanced two postulates that contradict principles of classical physics:

1. Electrons revolve about the nucleus only in orbits with radii that satisfy the relationship

$$p_\phi = \frac{nh}{2\pi}$$

where p_ϕ = angular momentum of electron, h = Planck's constant [6.62 × 10^{-34} joule-second (J-sec)], n = integer (1, 2, 3 . . .), and π = 3.1416. . . .

2. Electrons lose or gain energy only when they "jump" from one orbit to another. No change in energy occurs so long as the electrons remain in specified orbits.

With these axioms, Bohr constructed an atomic model for hydrogen, a simple atom consisting of a nucleus and one electron. Normally, the electron in hydrogen occupies the innermost electron orbit, for which n = 1 in the preceding equation. The innermost electron orbit of an atom is termed the K shell. A hydrogen atom is said to be in its ground state when the electron is in the K shell. The atom may be excited by raising the electron to the n = 2 orbit (L shell), to the n = 3 orbit (M shell), or to other shells farther from the nucleus. Energy from an external source (e.g., electromagnetic radiation) must be supplied to raise an electron to a higher shell, because work must be done against the attractive force of the nucleus. Energy is released as the electron returns to a lower shell.

Measurements of the energy radiated from excited atoms of hydrogen confirmed the applicability of Bohr's model of the atom to hydrogen. However, spectral distributions of energy radiated from excited atoms more complex than hydrogen were not predictable from Bohr's model. To secure better correlation between model and experiment, Bohr's simple model was modified by several physicists, including Arnold Sommerfeld,[15] William Wilson,[16] E. C. Stoner,[17] Wolfgang Pauli[18] and George Uhlenbeck and Samuel Goudsmit.[19] The result was a model for multielectron atoms which is used today to explain many aspects of atomic physics.

Atoms in their normal state are neutral, because the number of electrons outside the nucleus equals the positive charge of the nucleus, assuming 1 unit of positive charge is $+1.6 \times 10^{-19}$ coulomb. The positive charge of the nucleus (or the number of electrons in a neutral atom) is termed the atomic number Z and defines the element under which a particular atom is classified. Elements with atomic numbers ranging from 1 to 105 either exist in nature or can be synthesized in the laboratory. Elements with atomic numbers greater than 105 may be produced in the future.[20]

Electrons are positioned in shells or energy levels that surround the nucleus. The first ($n = 1$) or K shell contains no more than 2 electrons, the second ($n = 2$) or L shell no more than 8 electrons, and the third ($n = 3$) or M shell no more than 18 electrons (Fig 1-1). The outermost electron shell of an atom, no matter which shell it is, never contains more than 8 electrons. Electrons in the outermost shell are termed *valence* electrons and determine to a large degree the chemical properties of an atom. Atoms with an outer shell filled with electrons seldom react chemically. These atoms constitute elements known as the *inert gases* (helium, neon, argon, krypton, xenon and radon).

Energy levels for electrons are divided into sublevels separated slightly from each other. To describe the position of an electron in the extranuclear structure of an atom, the electron is assigned four quantum num-

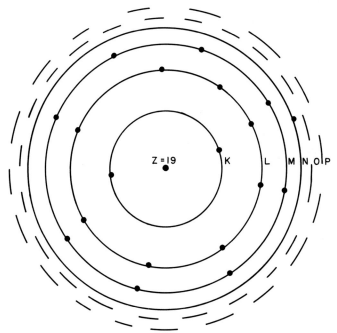

Fig 1-1. — Electron orbits in potassium ($Z = 19$).

TABLE 1-1.—QUANTUM NUMBERS FOR
ELECTRONS IN HELIUM, CARBON
AND SODIUM

ELEMENT	n	ℓ	m_ℓ	m_S
Helium (Z = 2)	1	0	0	$-\frac{1}{2}$
	1	0	0	$+\frac{1}{2}$
Carbon (Z = 6)	1	0	0	$-\frac{1}{2}$
	1	0	0	$+\frac{1}{2}$
	2	0	0	$-\frac{1}{2}$
	2	0	0	$+\frac{1}{2}$
	2	1	-1	$-\frac{1}{2}$
	2	1	-1	$+\frac{1}{2}$
Sodium (Z = 11)	1	0	0	$-\frac{1}{2}$
	1	0	0	$+\frac{1}{2}$
	2	0	0	$-\frac{1}{2}$
	2	0	0	$+\frac{1}{2}$
	2	1	-1	$-\frac{1}{2}$
	2	1	-1	$+\frac{1}{2}$
	2	1	0	$-\frac{1}{2}$
	2	1	0	$+\frac{1}{2}$
	2	1	1	$-\frac{1}{2}$
	2	1	1	$+\frac{1}{2}$
	3	0	0	$-\frac{1}{2}$

bers. The principal quantum number n defines the main energy level or shell within which the electron resides ($n = 1$ for the K shell, $n = 2$ for the L shell, etc.). The azimuthal quantum number ℓ describes the electron's angular momentum ($\ell = 0, 1, 2, . . . , n - 1$). The orientation of the electron's magnetic moment in a magnetic field is defined by the magnetic quantum number m_ℓ ($m_\ell = -\ell, -\ell + 1, . . . , 0, . . . , \ell - 1, \ell$). The direction of the electron's spin upon its own axis is specified by the spin quantum number m_S ($m_S = + \frac{1}{2}$ or $- \frac{1}{2}$). The Pauli exclusion principle states that no two electrons in the same atomic system may be assigned identical values for all four quantum numbers. Illustrated in Table 1-1 are quantum numbers for electrons in a few atoms with low atomic numbers.

Wave-Mechanical Model

Results of many experiments have been explained with the modified Bohr model for multielectron atoms. Unfortunately, a number of discrepancies between model and experiment also have been found. In 1925 and 1926, Max Born,[21] Werner Heisenberg[22] and Erwin Schroedinger[23] introduced the wave- or quantum-mechanical model of the atom. The Schroedinger wave equation defines space- and time-dependent probability density functions for electrons. From these probability density functions, a model for the atom may be constructed. Experimental results have been predicted more successfully with the wave-mechanical model than with other atomic models yet developed. Fortunately, the

Bohr model of the atom may be used without embarrassment to explain most aspects of medical radiation physics. We shall not need to evoke the wave-mechanical model with its specter of sophisticated mathematics.

Electron Binding Energy and Energy Levels

An electron in an inner shell of an atom is attracted to the nucleus by a force greater than that which the nucleus exerts upon an electron farther away. An electron may be moved from one shell to another farther from the nucleus only if energy is supplied by an external energy source. The energy required to remove an electron completely from an atom is termed the *binding energy* (E_B) for the electron. Binding energies are negative, because they represent amounts of energy that must be sup-

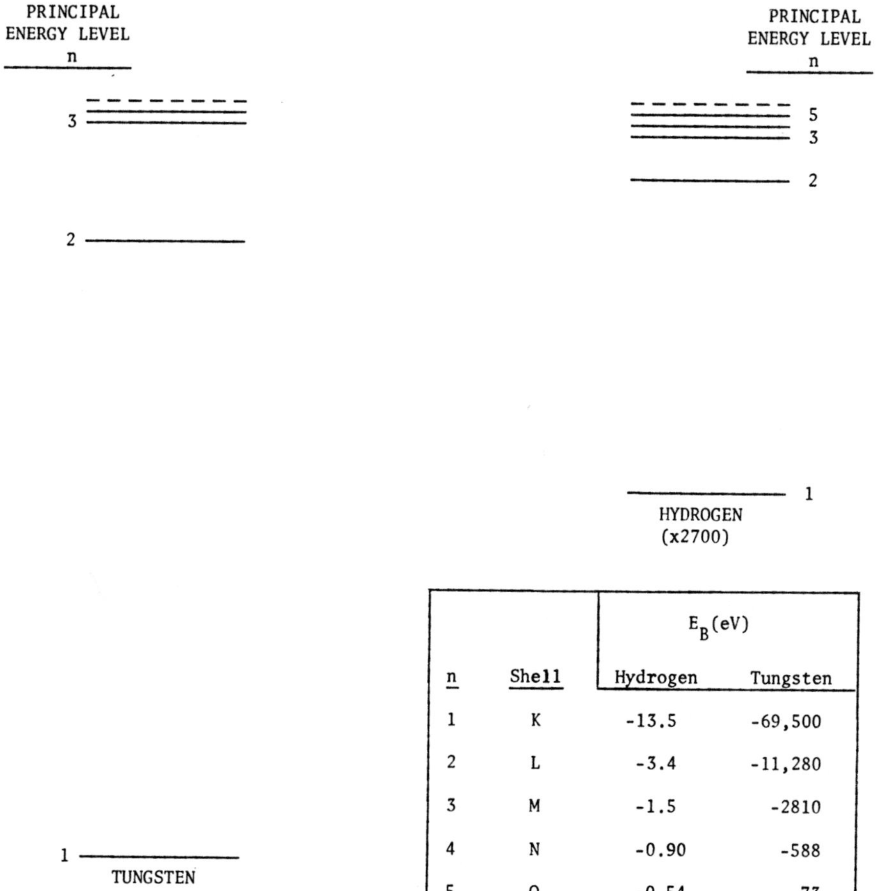

n	Shell	E_B (eV) Hydrogen	Tungsten
1	K	-13.5	-69,500
2	L	-3.4	-11,280
3	M	-1.5	-2810
4	N	-0.90	-588
5	O	-0.54	-73

Fig 1-2. — Average binding energies for electrons in hydrogen ($Z = 1$) and tungsten ($Z = 74$).

plied to remove electrons from atoms. Electron shells often are described in terms of the binding energy of electrons occupying the shells. For example, the binding energy is -13.5 eV* for an electron in the K shell of hydrogen. The binding energy for an electron in the L shell of hydrogen is -3.4 eV. The energy required to move an electron from the K to the L shell in hydrogen is $(-3.4 \text{ eV}) - (-13.5 \text{ eV}) = 10.1$ eV.

Electrons in inner energy levels of high-Z atoms are near nuclei with high positive charge. Inner electrons are bound to these nuclei with a force much greater than that exerted upon the solitary electron in hydrogen. Binding energies of electrons in high- and low-Z atoms are compared in Figure 1-2.

Electron Transitions and Characteristic Radiation

Vacancies or "holes" exist in electron shells from which electrons have been removed. These vacancies are filled promptly by electrons cascading from energy levels farther from the nucleus. As the vacancies are filled, energy is released, usually in the form of electromagnetic radiation. During the transition of a particular electron, the energy released equals the difference in binding energy between the original and the final energy levels for the electron. For example, an electron moving from the M to the K shell of tungsten is accompanied by the release of $[(-69,500)-(-2810)]$ eV $= -66,690$ eV or -66.69 keV, where the negative sign indicates that the energy is released. In most cases, the energy is released as a *photon* or packet of electromagnetic radiation. Occasionally, especially in low-Z atoms, the energy may be used to eject a second electron, usually from the same shell as the cascading electron. The ejected electron is termed an *Auger electron*. Photons emitted during electron transitions are considered x rays if they are sufficiently energetic (>100 eV). Photons with energy less than 100 eV are classified as ultraviolet, visible, infrared or other electromagnetic radiation. Electromagnetic radiation released during electron transitions is termed *characteristic radiation* because the photon energies are characteristic of differences in binding energies of electrons in a specific atom. The radiation may be described as K-characteristic radiation or K-fluorescence, L-characteristic radiation or L-fluorescence, etc., denoting the destination of the cascading electron.

THE NUCLEUS

Models of the Nucleus and Nuclear Energy Levels

For most purposes, a nucleus may be considered to consist of two types of particles, referred to collectively as *nucleons*. The positive

---

*An electron volt (eV) is a unit of energy defined as the kinetic energy of an electron accelerated through a potential difference of 1 volt; 1 eV = 1.6×10^{-19} joule; 1 keV = 10^3 eV; 1 MeV = 10^6 eV.

charge and roughly one-half the mass of the nucleus are contributed by *protons*. Each proton possesses a positive charge of 1.6×10^{-19} coulomb, equal in magnitude but opposite in sign to the charge of an electron. The number of protons (or positive charges) in the nucleus is the atomic number for the atom. The mass of a proton is 1.6724×10^{-27} kg. *Neutrons,*[*] the second type of nucleon, are uncharged particles with a mass of 1.6747×10^{-27} kg. Neutrons and protons sometimes are considered to be two forms of a single particle, the nucleon. Outside the nucleus, neutrons are unstable, dividing into protons, electrons and antineutrinos (see chap. 2). The half-life[†] of this transition is 12.8 minutes. Neutrons usually are stable inside nuclei. The number of neutrons in a nucleus is the neutron number N for the nucleus. The mass number A of the nucleus is the number of nucleons (neutrons and protons) in the nucleus. The mass number $A = Z + N$.

Expressing the mass of atomic particles in kilograms is unwieldy. The atomic mass unit (amu) is a more convenient unit of mass for atomic particles: 1 amu is defined as $1/12$ the mass of the carbon atom with 6 protons, 6 neutrons and 6 electrons. Also,

$$1 \text{ amu} = 1.6605 + 10^{-27} \text{ kg}$$

Masses of atomic particles in amu's are:

Electron = 0.00055 amu
Proton = 1.00727 amu
Neutron = 1.00866 amu

Many models for the nucleus have been proposed. Niels Bohr suggested that a nucleus may be considered as a droplet of liquid.[25] Bohr's model is known as the "liquid drop" model of the nucleus, and has been used to explain phenomena such as nuclear binding energy and nuclear fission. According to the liquid drop model, a nucleus is composed of closely packed nucleons that are in constant motion. Particles are emitted from nuclei in ways analogous to the evaporation of molecules from a droplet of liquid. Experimental data suggest that discrete energy levels exist within nuclei. Since Bohr's liquid drop model does not include discrete intranuclear energy levels, it is not useful for explaining all properties of nuclei.

The shell model of the nucleus was introduced to explain the existence of discrete nuclear energy states. In this model, nucleons are arranged in shells similar to those available to electrons in the extranuclear structure of an atom. Nuclei are extraordinarily stable if they contain 2, 8, 20, 82 or 126 protons or similar numbers of neutrons. These numbers are

---

[*] The neutron was discovered by Chadwick in 1932.[24]

[†] For the moment, the half-life may be defined as $\ln 2/\lambda$, where λ is a decay constant in the equation $P = e^{-\lambda t}$, and P is the probability that the neutron will not decay in time t.

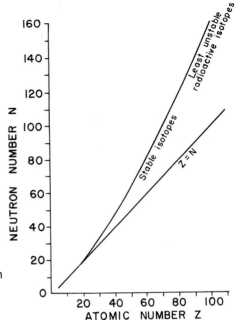

Fig 1-3.—Number of neutrons in stable (or least unstable) nuclei plotted as a function of the number of protons.

termed *magic numbers*, and may reflect full occupancy of nuclear shells. Nuclei with odd numbers of neutrons or protons tend to be less stable than nuclei with even numbers of neutrons or protons. Apparently, the pairing of similar nucleons increases the stability of the nucleus. Data tabulated below support this hypothesis:

NO. OF PROTONS	NO. OF NEUTRONS	NO. OF STABLE NUCLEI
Even	Even	165
Even	Odd	57
Odd	Even	53
Odd	Odd	6

The number of neutrons is about equal to the number of protons in stable nuclei with low atomic numbers. As the atomic number increases, the number of neutrons in stable nuclei increases more rapidly than the number of protons. This differential rate of increase provides n/p ratios greater than 1 for stable nuclei with intermediate and high atomic numbers. The shell model of the nucleus explains the higher n/p ratios for heavier stable nuclei by suggesting that for nuclei with more than a few nucleons, the energy difference between levels for neutrons is slightly less than the energy difference between levels for protons.

Ratios of neutrons to protons in stable nuclei are illustrated in Figure 1-3.

A number of other models of the nucleus have been proposed. However, most aspects of medical radiation physics can be explained with the liquid drop and shell models.

Nuclear Binding Energy and the Nuclear Force

Electrostatic repulsive forces exist between particles of similar charge. Hence, protons repel each other when separated by a distance greater than the diameter of the nucleus. However, if the distance between protons is less than the diameter of the nucleus, then they remain together. The existence of a *nuclear force* has been postulated to explain this apparent contradiction.[26] This force is stronger than the electrostatic repulsive force and binds neutrons and protons together within the nucleus. The nuclear force (sometimes referred to as the *strong* force) is effective only when nucleons are separated by a distance smaller than the diameter of the nucleus. With a strength of 1 assigned to the nuclear force, relative strengths of other forces may be compared:

TYPE OF FORCE	RELATIVE STRENGTH
Nuclear	1
Electrostatic	10^{-2}
Weak	10^{-13}
Gravitational	10^{-39}

Only the first two forces are important in most discussions of atomic particles. No forces other than those listed above are known to exist in nature.

The mass of a nucleus is less than the sum of the masses of the nucleons in the nucleus. The mass difference is termed the *mass defect* and represents an amount of energy that must be supplied to separate the nucleus into individual nucleons. This amount of energy is the *binding energy of the nucleus*. The relationship between mass and energy is described by the formula for mass-energy equivalence postulated in 1905 by Einstein:[27]

$$E = mc^2$$

In this equation, E represents an amount of energy equivalent to a mass m, and c is a conversion coefficient equal to the speed of light *in vacuo* (3×10^8 m/sec). One kilogram of mass is equivalent to 9×10^{16} joule, an amount of energy equal roughly to that released during detonation of 30 million tons of TNT. The energy equivalent to 1 amu is:

$$\frac{(1 \text{ amu})(1.66 \times 10^{-27} \text{ kg/amu})(3 \times 10^8 \text{ m/sec})^2}{(1.6 \times 10^{-13} \text{ J/MeV})} = 931 \text{ MeV}$$

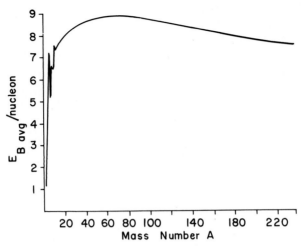

Fig 1-4. — Average binding energy per nucleon versus mass number.

The binding energy of the carbon nucleus with six protons and six neutrons (denoted as $^{12}_{6}C$) is calculated in Example 1-1.

Example 1-1

Mass 6 protons = 6 (1.00727 amu)	=	6.04362 amu
Mass 6 neutrons = 6 (1.00866 amu)	=	6.05196 amu
Mass 6 electrons = 6 (0.00055 amu)	=	0.00330 amu
Mass of components of $^{12}_{6}C$	=	12.09888 amu
Mass of $^{12}_{6}C$ atom	=	12.00000 amu
Mass defect	=	0.09888 amu

Binding energy of $^{12}_{6}C$ atom = (0.09888 amu)(931 MeV/amu)
= 92.0 MeV

Almost all of this binding energy is associated with the $^{12}_{6}C$ nucleus.

Average binding energy per nucleon of $^{12}_{6}C$ = (92.0 MeV) per 12 nucleons
= 7.67 MeV per nucleon

In Figure 1-4, the average binding energy per nucleon is plotted as a function of the mass number A for nuclei with mass numbers up to 240.

Nuclear Fission and Fusion

Energy is released if a nucleus with a high mass number separates or fissions into two parts, each with average binding energy per nucleon greater than that of the original nucleus. Certain high-A nuclei (e.g., ^{235}U, ^{239}Pu and ^{233}U) fission spontaneously after absorbing a slowly moving neutron. For ^{235}U, a typical fission reaction is:

$$^{235}_{92}U + \text{neutron} \rightarrow \, ^{236}_{92}U \rightarrow \, ^{92}_{36}Kr + \, ^{141}_{56}Ba + 3 \text{ neutrons} + Q$$

The energy released is designated as Q and averages more than 200 MeV per fission. The energy is liberated primarily as gamma radiation and kinetic energy of fission products and neutrons. Products such as ^{92}Kr and ^{141}Ba are termed *fission by-products* and are radioactive. Many different by-products are produced during fission. Neutrons released during fission may interact with other ^{235}U nuclei, creating the possibility of a chain reaction, provided sufficient mass (a critical mass) of fissionable material is contained within a small volume. The rate at which a material fissions may be regulated by controlling the number of neutrons available each instant to interact with fissionable nuclei. Fission reactions within a nuclear reactor are controlled in this way. Uncontrolled nuclear fission results in an "atomic explosion."

Nuclear fission was observed first in 1934 during an experiment conducted by Enrico Fermi.[28] However, the process was not described correctly until publication in 1939 of analyses by Hahn and Strassmann[29] and by Meitner and Frisch.[30] The first controlled chain reaction was achieved in 1942 at the University of Chicago. The first atomic bomb was exploded in 1945 at Alamogordo, New Mexico.

Certain low-mass nuclei may be combined to produce one nucleus with an average binding energy per nucleon greater than that for either of the original nuclei. This process is termed *nuclear fusion*, and is accompanied by the release of large amounts of energy. A typical reaction is:

$$^2_1H + ^3_1H \rightarrow ^4_2He + neutron + Q$$

In this particular reaction $Q = 18$ MeV.

Nuclei forming products with higher average binding energy per nucleon must be brought sufficiently near one another that the nuclear force can initiate fusion. As two nuclei approach each other, the strong electrostatic force of repulsion must be overcome. Nuclei moving at very high velocity possess enough momentum to overcome this repulsive force. Adequate velocities may be attained by heating a sample containing low-Z nuclei to a temperature greater than 12×10^6 K, roughly equivalent to the temperature in the inner region of the sun. Temperatures this high are attained on earth only in the center of a fission explosion. Consequently, fusion (hydrogen) bombs must be "triggered" with an atomic bomb. Controlled nuclear fusion has not yet been achieved, although much effort has been expended in the attempt.

Nuclear Reactors

Nuclear fission is controlled in a nuclear reactor. The nuclear fuel (e.g., ^{235}U or ^{239}Pu) is arranged as cylinders (fuel rods or elements) in a defined geometry within the reactor core. Fuel elements of ^{235}U fission most efficiently when bombarded by slow (thermal) neutrons with a kinetic energy of about 0.025 eV. Neutrons released during fission are fast neutrons, and are slowed to thermal energy (i.e., low velocity) during interactions with low-Z nuclei. Moderators composed of low-Z nuclei are positioned within the reactor core to decrease the velocity of the fast neutrons released during fission. A good moderator does not absorb a significant fraction of the neutrons. Typical moderators include graphite, water, heavy water and beryllium.

The number of neutrons available to initiate fission in a reactor is governed by the position of control rods in the reactor core. Control rods are composed of materials with a high efficiency (i.e., high cross section) for absorbing neutrons. Boron and cadmium often are used for control rods.

Heat generated during controlled fission is removed by cooling the reactor core with water, heavy water, various gases or liquid metals.

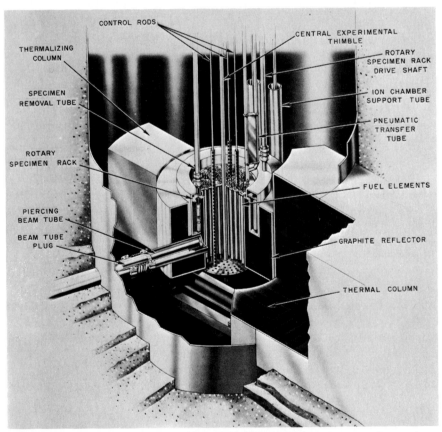

Fig 1-5.—Cross section of the core of a Triga pool-type research reactor. (Courtesy of Gulf General Atomic Incorporated.)

Reactors have many uses, including the production of nuclear power (power reactors), production of radioactive atoms (isotope-production reactors), production of nuclear fuel (breeder or plutonium-production reactors), testing of materials exposed to large quantities of radiation (materials-testing reactors) and education and research (research reactors). One type of reactor is illustrated in Figure 1-5.

Nuclear Nomenclature

Isotopes of a particular element are atoms that possess the same number of protons but a varying number of neutrons. For example, ^1_1H (protium), ^2_1H (deuterium) and ^3_1H (tritium) are isotopes of the element hydrogen, and ^9_6C, $^{10}_6C$, $^{11}_6C$, $^{12}_6C$, $^{13}_6C$, $^{14}_6C$, $^{15}_6C$ and $^{16}_6C$ are isotopes of carbon. An isotope is specified by its chemical symbol together with its mass number as a left superscript. The atomic number sometimes is added as a left subscript. An isotope often is referred to as a *nuclide*.

Isotones are atoms that possess the same number of neutrons but a different number of protons. For example, ^5_2He, ^6_3Li, ^7_4Be, ^8_5B and ^9_6C are isotones, because each isotope contains three neutrons. *Isobars* are atoms with the same number of nucleons but a different number of protons and a different number of neutrons. For example, ^6_2He, ^6_3Li and ^6_4Be are isobars ($A = 6$). *Isomers* represent different energy states for nuclei with the same number of neutrons and protons. Differences between isotopes, isotones, isobars and isomers are illustrated below:

	ATOMIC NO. Z	NEUTRON NO. N	MASS NO. A
Isotopes	Same	Different	Different
Isotones	Different	Same	Different
Isobars	Different	Different	Same
Isomers	Same	Same	Same (different nuclear energy states)

PROBLEMS

°1. What are the atomic and mass numbers of the oxygen isotope with 16 nucleons? Calculate the mass defect, binding energy, and binding energy per nucleon for this nuclide, with the assumption that the entire mass defect is associated with the nucleus. The mass of the atom is 15.9949 amu.

°2. Natural oxygen contains three isotopes with atomic masses of 15.9949, 16.9991 and 17.9992, and relative abundances of 2,500:1:5, respectively. Determine to three decimal places the average atomic mass of oxygen.

3. Using Table 1-1 as an example, write the quantum numbers for electrons in boron ($Z = 5$), oxygen ($Z = 8$) and phosphorus ($Z = 15$).

°4. Calculate the energy required for the transition of an electron from the K

°For those problems marked with an asterisk, answers are provided on the pages following the appendixes (see pp. 487–488).

shell to the L shell in tungsten. Compare the result to the energy necessary for a similar transition in hydrogen. Explain the difference.

°5. What is the energy equivalent to the mass of an electron? Since the mass of a particle increases with velocity, assume that the electron is at rest.

°6. The energy released during the atomic explosion at Hiroshima was estimated to be equal to that released by 20,000 tons of TNT. Assume that a total energy of 200 MeV is released during fission of a ^{235}U nucleus and that a total energy of 3.8×10^9 J is released during detonation of 1 ton of TNT. Find the number of fissions that occurred in the Hiroshima explosion and the total decrease in mass.

°7. A "4-megaton thermonuclear shot" means that a nuclear explosion releases as much energy as that liberated during detonation of 4 million tons of TNT. Using 3.8×10^9 J/ton as the heat of detonation for TNT, calculate the total energy in joules and in kilocalories released during the nuclear explosion (1 k-cal = 4,186 J).

8. Group the following atoms as isotopes, isotones and isobars:

$$^{131}_{54}Xe, \quad ^{132}_{54}Xe, \quad ^{130}_{53}I, \quad ^{133}_{54}Xe, \quad ^{131}_{53}I, \quad ^{129}_{52}Te, \quad ^{132}_{53}I, \quad ^{130}_{52}Te, \quad ^{131}_{52}Te.$$

REFERENCES

1. Lucretius: *On the Nature of Things* (Baltimore: Penguin Press, 1951), Latham translation; Bailey, C.: *The Greek Atomists and Epicurus* (New York: Oxford University Press, 1928).
2. Dalton, J.: Experimental enquiry into the proportions of the several gases or elastic fluids constituting the atmosphere, Mem. Literary Philosophical Soc. Manchester (2) 1:244, 1805.
3. Gay-Lussac, J.: Sur la combinaison des substances gazeuses, les unes avec les autres, Mem. Soc. d'Arcoeil 2:207, 1809.
4. Avogadro, A.: D'une manière de déterminer les masses relatives des molécules élémentaires des corps, et les proportions selon lesquelles elles entrent dans ces combinaisons, J. Phys. 73:58, 1811.
5. Anonymous: On the relation between the specific gravities of bodies in their gaseous state and the weights of their atoms, Ann. Phil. 6:321, 1815.
6. Faraday, M.: Identity of electricities derived from different sources, Philosophical Transactions, 1833, p. 23.
7. Cannizzaro, S.: An abridgement of a course of chemical philosophy given in the Royal University of Genoa, Nuovo Cimento 7:321, 1858.
8. Meyer, J.: Die Natur der chemischen Elemente als Funktion ihrer Atomgewichte, Ann. Chem., Supp., 7:354, 1870; Mendeleev, D.: The relation between the properties and atomic weights of the elements, J. Russ. Chem. Soc. 1:60, 1869.
9. Perrin, J.: *Atoms* (London: Constable, 1923).
10. Thomson, J.: Cathode rays, Phil. Mag., 5th series, 44:293, 1897.
11. Millikan, R.: A new modification of the cloud method of determining the elementary electrical charge and the most probable value of that charge, Phil. Mag. 19:209, 1910.
12. Thomson, J.: Papers on positive rays and isotopes, Phil. Mag., 6th series, 13: 561, 1907.
13. Rutherford, E.: The scattering of alpha and beta particles by matter and the structure of the atom, Phil. Mag. 21:669, 1911.

14. Bohr, N.: On the constitution of atoms and molecules, Phil. Mag. 26:1, 476, 875, 1913.
15. Sommerfeld, A.: Zur Quantentheorie der Spektrallinien, Ann. Phys. 1:125, 1916.
16. Wilson, W.: The quantum-theory of radiation and line spectra, Phil. Mag. 29: 795, 1915.
17. Stoner, E.: The distribution of electrons among atomic levels, Phil. Mag. 48: 719, 1924.
18. Pauli, W.: Über den Zusammenhang des Abschlusses der Elektronengruppen im Atom mit der Komplexstruktur der Spektren, Z. Phys. 31:765, 1925.
19. Uhlenbeck, G., and Goudsmit, S.: Ersetzung der Hypothese vom unmechanischen Zwang durch eine Forderung bezüglich des inneren Verhaltens jedes einzelnen Elektrons, Naturwissenschaften 13:953, 1925.
20. Seaborg, G., and Bloom, J.: The synthetic elements: IV, Sci. Am. 220:57, 1969.
21. Born, M.: Quantenmechanik der Stossvorgänge, Z. Phys. 38:803, 1926.
22. Heisenberg, W.: *The Physical Principles of the Quantum Theory* (Chicago: University of Chicago Press, 1929).
23. Schroedinger, E.: *Collected Papers on Wave Mechanics* (Glasgow: Blackie and Son, Ltd., 1928).
24. Chadwick, J.: Possible existence of a neutron, Proc. R. Soc. Lond. A 136: 696, 1932.
25. Bohr, N.: Neutron capture and nuclear constitution, Nature 137:344, 1936.
26. Marshak, R.: The nuclear force, Sci. Am. 202:98, 1960.
27. Einstein, A.: Über einen die Erzeugung and Verwandlung des Lichtes betreffenden heuristischen Gesichtspunkt, Ann. Phys. 17:132, 1905.
28. Fermi, E.: Radioactivity induced by neutron bombardment, Nature 133:757, 1934; Fermi, E.: Possible production of elements of atomic number higher than 92, Nature 133:898, 1934.
29. Hahn, O., and Strassmann, F.: Über den Nachweis und das Verhalten der bei der Bestrahlung des Urans mittels Neutronen entstehenden Erdalkalimetalle, Naturwissenschaften 27:11, 89, 1939.
30. Meitner, L., and Frisch, O.: Disintegration of uranium by neutrons: A new type of nuclear reaction, Nature 143:239, 1939.

2 / Radioactive Decay

WITH THE EXCEPTION of $^{209}_{83}$Bi, all nuclei with atomic numbers greater than 82 are unstable. Many nuclei with atomic numbers less than 82 also are unstable. Unstable nuclei undergo transitions such as nuclear fission or, far more frequently, radioactive decay. Energy is released during these transitions. The modes of radioactive decay available to a particular radioactive nuclide may be determined by identifying the radiation emitted during decay and the products remaining after decay.

ALPHA DECAY

Radioactive decay by emission of *alpha particles* was described in 1899 by Ernest Rutherford.[1] In 1911, Boltwood and Rutherford[2] identified alpha (α) particles as helium nuclei, two protons and two neutrons bound together in an exceptionally stable configuration. Many nuclei with high atomic number decay by alpha emission. A typical alpha transition is:

$$^{226}_{88}\text{Ra} \rightarrow \, ^{222}_{86}\text{Rn} + \, ^{4}_{2}\text{He}$$

The sum of the mass numbers of the alpha particle and the product or daughter nuclide equals the mass number of the parent nuclide. Similarly, the sum of the atomic numbers of the alpha particle and the daughter nuclide equals the atomic number of the parent.

The total energy released during the radioactive decay of a nucleus is

Fig 2-1. — Radioactive decay scheme for alpha decay of ^{226}Ra.

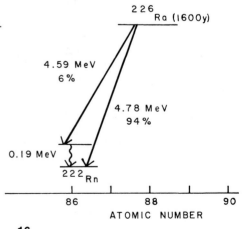

16

termed the *transition* or *disintegration energy*. During alpha decay, energy is released as kinetic energy of the alpha particle. Energy also may be released as gamma radiation. Alpha particles from a specific nuclide are ejected with discrete energies.

Radioactive decay processes are described by decay schemes. The decay scheme for ^{226}Ra is diagramed in Figure 2-1. A 4.78-MeV alpha particle is released during 94% of ^{226}Ra transitions. In the remaining transitions, a 4.59-MeV alpha is accompanied by a gamma ray of 0.19 MeV. The percent of nuclei that decay by a particular path is termed the *branching ratio* for the path. The transition energy (4.78 MeV) is the same for all transitions of ^{226}Ra nuclei.

NEGATRON DECAY AND SPECTRA

In 1896 Henri Becquerel[3] discovered the emission of energetic electrons from salts of uranium. This mode of radioactive decay usually is termed *beta decay*. Beta decay also refers to the emission of positive electrons from certain nuclei. These two decay processes are distinguished more readily if one is termed *negatron* (negative electron) *decay* and the other *positron* (positive electron) *decay*.

The ratio of neutrons to protons (n/p or N/Z ratio) in negatron-emitting nuclides is greater than that required for maximum stability of the nucleus (see Fig 1-3). During negatron decay, the n/p ratio of these nuclides is reduced by transition of a nucleon from one form to another. The transition may be written:

$$_{0}^{1}n \rightarrow {}_{1}^{1}p + {}_{-1}^{0}e + \tilde{\nu}$$

or

$$_{0}^{1}n \rightarrow {}_{1}^{1}p + {}_{-1}^{0}\beta + \tilde{\nu}$$

in which $_{-1}^{0}e$ represents an electron ejected from the nucleus and $_{-1}^{0}\beta$ designates the nuclear origin of the ejected electron. The symbol $\tilde{\nu}$ represents a second particle, the *antineutrino*, which is discussed later in

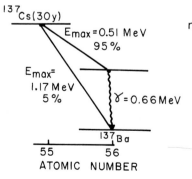

Fig 2-2. — Radioactive decay scheme for negatron decay of ^{137}Cs.

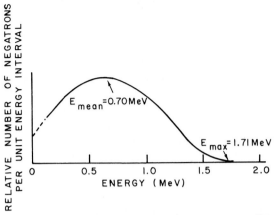

Fig 2-3. — Energy spectrum for negatrons from ^{32}P.

this section. The daughter nucleus possesses one proton more than the parent nucleus, and both nuclei possess the same number of nucleons. Therefore, negatron decay results in an increase in Z and a constant A. A representative negatron transition is:

$$^{137}_{55}\text{Cs} \rightarrow {}^{137}_{56}\text{Ba} + {}^{0}_{-1}\beta + \bar{\nu} + \gamma$$

A decay scheme for ^{137}Cs is presented in Figure 2-2. A negatron with a maximum energy E_{max} of 1.17 MeV is released during 5% of all decays of ^{137}Cs. In the remaining 95%, a negatron with $E_{max} = 0.51$ MeV is accompanied by a gamma (γ) of 0.66 MeV or by an electron ejected by internal conversion. The transition energy equals 1.17 MeV for the decay of ^{137}Cs.

Although negatrons emitted by a particular nuclide have discrete maximum energies, most negatrons are ejected with energies lower than these maxima. The mean energy E_{mean} of negatrons emitted during a particular transition is approximately $E_{max}/3$. Negatron spectra for a particular radioactive nuclide depict the relative frequency of emission of negatrons with different energies. A negatron spectrum exists for each value of E_{max} in the decay scheme. The shape of the spectra and the values for E_{max} are characteristic of the particular nuclide. Illustrated in Figure 2-3 is the negatron spectrum for ^{32}P, a nuclide that emits negatrons with a single maximum energy.

During the decay of a particular nucleus, the transition energy almost always exceeds the sum of the energy released as gamma radiation and the kinetic energy of the ejected negatron. To explain this difference in energy, Wolfgang Pauli suggested in 1933 that a second particle accompanies each negatron emitted from the nucleus.[4] The energy unaccounted for during each transition is possessed by the second particle, termed a *neutrino* by Fermi. The energy E_ν of the neutrino is

$$E_\nu = E_{max} - E_k$$

where E_k represents the kinetic energy of the negatron. Pauli proposed that neutrinos are uncharged particles with undetectably small mass, and suggested that these particles interact only rarely with matter. Refinements of the theory of beta decay led to designation of two forms for the neutrino. One form, the neutrino (ν), describes particles ejected during positron decay. The second form, the antineutrino ($\bar{\nu}$), designates particles that accompany negatrons. Existence of the antineutrino was verified experimentally in 1953 during experiments by Reines and Cowan.[5]

GAMMA EMISSION

Often during radioactive decay the daughter nucleus is formed in an excited, unstable state. Electromagnetic radiation is released during the transition of the daughter nucleus from the excited state to the ground energy level (i.e., from one isomeric state to another isomeric state of lower energy). The electromagnetic radiation is termed *gamma radiation* and was described first by Villard in 1900.[6] The position of gamma radiation within the electromagnetic spectrum is shown in Figure 2-4. Gamma rays and x rays occupy the same region within the spectrum. These two types of electromagnetic radiation are distinguishable only by their origin; γ rays result from nuclear transitions, x rays from interactions of electrons outside the nucleus.

Often it is convenient to assign wavelike properties to x and γ rays. At other times it is useful to regard these radiations as discrete bundles of energy termed *photons* or *quanta*.[7] The two interpretations of electromagnetic radiation are united by the equation

$$E = h\nu \tag{2-1}$$

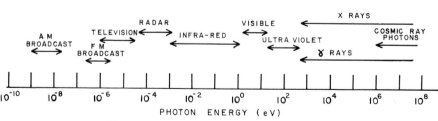

Fig 2-4. — The electromagnetic spectrum.

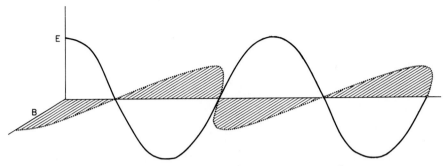

Fig 2-5.—Simplified diagram of an electromagnetic wave.

In equation (2-1), E represents the energy of a photon and ν represents the frequency of the electromagnetic wave. (Use of the symbol ν for frequency should not be confused with its use to designate a neutrino.) The symbol h represents Planck's constant, 6.62×10^{-34} J-sec. Electromagnetic radiation travels *in vacuo* at a constant speed c of 3×10^8 m/sec. The speed c is the product of the frequency ν and wavelength λ of the electromagnetic wave

$$c = \nu\lambda \qquad (2\text{-}2)$$

The wavelength is the distance between adjacent crests in the simplified diagram of an electromagnetic wave shown in Figure 2-5. In this diagram, an electromagnetic wave is represented by an oscillating electric field E and an oscillating magnetic field B. The wave is moving from left to right in the diagram. The frequency ν (cycles/sec or hertz) specifies

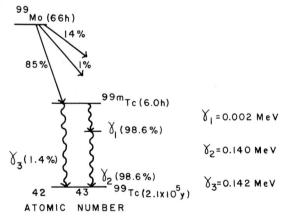

Fig 2-6.—Simplified radioactive decay scheme for ^{99}Mo.

the number of complete oscillations of either the electric or the magnetic field in 1 second. The frequency ν is:

$$\nu = \frac{c}{\lambda}$$

and the photon energy may be written as:

$$E = \frac{hc}{\lambda} \tag{2-3}$$

The energy in keV possessed by a photon of wavelength λ in angstroms may be computed with equation (2-4):

$$E = \frac{12.4}{\lambda} \tag{2-4}$$

Example 2-1

Derive equation (2-4) and calculate the energy of a gamma ray with a wavelength of 0.01 Å.

$$E = \frac{hc}{\lambda}$$

$$E \text{ (keV)} = \frac{(6.62 \times 10^{-34} \text{ J-sec})(3 \times 10^8 \text{ m/sec})}{\lambda(\text{Å})(10^{-10} \text{ m/Å})(1.6 \times 10^{-16} \text{ J/keV})}$$

$$= \frac{12.4}{\lambda(\text{Å})}$$

$$E = \frac{12.4}{0.01 \text{ Å}}$$

$$= 1{,}240 \text{ keV}$$

No radioactive isotope decays solely by gamma emission. Every gamma transition is preceded either by electron capture or by emission of an

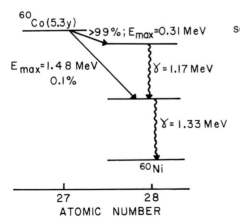

Fig 2-7. — Radioactive decay scheme for ^{60}Co.

alpha particle, negatron or positron. Often, gammas are ejected during the decay process. Sometimes one or more of the excited states of the daughter may exhibit a finite lifetime. An excited state is termed a *metastable state* if its half-life exceeds 10^{-6} seconds. For example, the decay scheme for ^{99}Mo (Fig 2-6) displays a metastable energy state, ^{99m}Tc, that has a half-life of 6.0 hr.

Nuclides emit gamma rays with characteristic energies. For example, photons of 142 and 140 keV are emitted by ^{99m}Tc. Photons of 1.17 and 1.33 MeV are emitted during the decay of ^{60}Co (Fig 2-7). The photons emitted during the decay of ^{60}Co actually are released during cascade transitions of daughter ^{60}Ni nuclei from excited to ground energy states.

POSITRON DECAY AND ELECTRON CAPTURE

Emission of positive electrons from radioactive nuclei was discovered in 1934 by Curie and Joliot[8] during their investigation of artificial radioactivity. Two years previously, Anderson[9] had discovered positrons in cosmic-ray showers. Positron decay results from the nuclear change

$$^1_1p \rightarrow {}^1_0n + {}^0_{+1}e + \nu$$

or

$$^1_1p \rightarrow {}^1_0n + {}^0_{+1}\beta + \nu$$

in which $_{+1}^0\beta$ designates the nuclear origin of the ejected positron. The n/p ratio of the nucleus is increased by this mode of decay. Hence, positron-emitting nuclides possess n/p (N/Z) ratios lower than those required for maximum stability. Positron decay is accompanied by a decrease in Z and no change in A. A representative positron transition is:

$$^{30}_{15}P \rightarrow {}^{30}_{14}Si + {}^0_{+1}\beta + \nu$$

The n/p ratio of a nucleus also may be increased by electron capture.

Fig 2-8. — Radioactive decay scheme for positron decay of ^{22}Na.

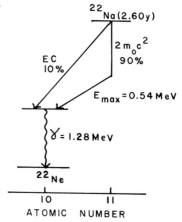

In this process, an electron captured from an electron shell results in the nuclear transition

$$\ ^1_1p + \ ^0_{-1}e \rightarrow \ ^1_0n + \nu$$

Most electrons are captured from the K shell, although an electron may be captured occasionally from the L shell or from a shell farther from the nucleus. During electron capture, a hole is created in an electron shell deep within the atom. This vacancy is filled by an electron cascading from an energy level farther from the nucleus. Energy released during this transition appears as x radiation or as kinetic energy of an Auger electron reduced by the binding energy of the Auger electron.

Many nuclei decay by both electron capture and positron emission, as illustrated in the decay scheme for $^{22}_{11}$Na in Figure 2-8. The decay of ^{22}Na may be written

$$^{22}_{11}\mathrm{Na} \begin{cases} \ ^0_{-1}e \ \xrightarrow{\ (10\%)\ } \ ^{22}_{10}\mathrm{Ne} + \nu - \\[2ex] \xrightarrow{\ (90\%)\ } \ ^0_{+1}\beta \ \ + \ ^{22}_{10}\mathrm{Ne} + \nu \end{cases}$$

The electron capture branching ratio for a particular radioactive nuclide reveals the probability of electron capture per disintegration of the

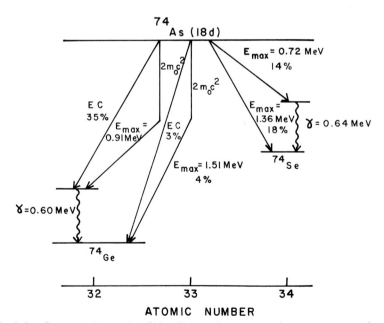

Fig 2-9.—Decay scheme for ^{74}As, illustrating competing processes of negatron emission, positron emission and electron capture.

nucleus. Generally, positron emission prevails over electron capture when both modes of decay occur. In Figure 2-8, the electron capture branching ratio is 10% for ^{22}Na; therefore, 90% of all decays occur with the emission of a positron.

In Figure 2-8, the 2 m_0c^2 listed alongside the vertical portion of the positron decay pathway represents the energy equivalent of the additional mass of the products of positron decay. This additional mass includes the greater mass of the neutron compared to the proton, together with the mass of the ejected positron. The energy equivalent of this additional mass is 1.02 MeV or 2 m_0c^2, where m_0 is the rest mass of the electron. This amount of energy must be supplied by the transition energy during positron decay. Nuclei that cannot furnish at least 1.02 MeV for the transition do not decay by positron emission. Those nuclei increase their n/p ratios solely by electron capture.

A few nuclides may decay by negatron emission, positron emission or electron capture. For example, the decay scheme for ^{74}As (Fig 2-9) indicates that this nuclide decays by negatron emission (32%), positron emission (30%) and electron capture (38%). All modes of decay result in transformation of the "odd-odd" ^{74}As nucleus (Z = 33, N = 41) into a daughter with even Z and even N, a more stable configuration for the nucleus.

INTERNAL CONVERSION

Usually, a daughter nucleus releases its excess energy by emitting gamma radiation. However, this release is achieved occasionally by *internal conversion*, during which the nucleus interacts with an inner electron. The electron is ejected with kinetic energy equal to the energy released by the nucleus, reduced by the binding energy of the electron. During internal conversion, no gamma ray is emitted. Instead, an energetic conversion electron is ejected, together with x rays and Auger electrons produced as the extranuclear structure of the atom resumes a stable configuration.

The internal conversion coefficient for a particular electron shell is the ratio of the number of conversion electrons from the shell to the number of γ rays emitted by the nucleus. The probability of internal conversion increases rapidly with increasing atomic number and with the lifetime of the excited state of the nucleus.

MATHEMATICS OF RADIOACTIVE DECAY

The decay of a sample of radioactive atoms may be described mathematically. The rate of decay is referred to as the *activity* of the sample. The unit of activity is the curie (Ci), defined as

$$1 \text{ Ci} = 3.7 \times 10^{10} \text{ disintegrations per second (dps)}$$

The millicurie (mCi), microcurie (μCi), nanocurie (nCi) and picocurie (pCi) are useful divisions of the curie:

$$1 \text{ mCi} = 10^{-3} \text{ Ci} = 3.7 \times 10^7 \text{ dps}$$
$$1 \text{ } \mu\text{Ci} = 10^{-6} \text{ Ci} = 3.7 \times 10^4 \text{ dps}$$
$$1 \text{ nCi} = 10^{-9} \text{ Ci} = 3.7 \times 10^1 \text{ dps}$$
$$1 \text{ pCi} = 10^{-12} \text{ Ci} = 3.7 \times 10^{-2} \text{ dps}$$

A common multiple of the curie is the kilocurie (kCi):

$$1 \text{ kCi} = 10^3 \text{ Ci} = 3.7 \times 10^{13} \text{ dps}$$

One curie was defined originally as the rate of decay of 1 gm of radium. Although recent measurements have established the decay rate as 3.61×10^{10} dps for radium, the curie has retained its original numerical definition.

Recently, the becquerel (Bq) has been proposed as a unit of activity.[10] The becquerel is defined as

$$1 \text{ Bq} = 1 \text{ dps} = 2.7 \times 10^{-11} \text{ Ci}$$

Decay Equations and Half-Life

The dependence of the activity A of a radioactive sample upon the number N of radioactive atoms in the sample may be expressed as

$$A = \lambda N \tag{2-5}$$

where λ represents the decay or disintegration constant for the sample. Every radioactive nuclide has a characteristic decay constant, defined as the fractional rate of decay of the particular nuclide in units of inverse time (sec^{-1}, min^{-1}, etc.). From this equation, the number of radioactive atoms remaining in the sample after a period of time t has elapsed can be shown to be

$$N = N_0 e^{-\lambda t} \tag{2-6}$$

where N_0 is the number of atoms originally present, and e is the exponential quantity 2.7183. This expression can be written also as

$$A = A_0 e^{-\lambda t} \tag{2-7}$$

where A is the activity remaining after time t, and A_0 is the original activity. This relationship often is referred to as the *equation for radioactive decay*.

The number of atoms N^* decaying in an interval t is $N_0 - N$ or

$$N^* = N_0 (1 - e^{-\lambda t}) \tag{2-8}$$

The probability that any particular atom will not decay during time t is N/N_0 or

$$P \text{ (no decay)} = e^{-\lambda t} \tag{2-9}$$

and the probability that a particular atom will decay during time t is

$$P \text{ (decay)} = 1 - e^{-\lambda t} \qquad (2\text{-}10)$$

For small values of λt, the probability of decay can be approximated as

$$P \text{ (decay)} \approx \lambda t$$

or, expressed per unit time, P (decay per unit time) $\approx \lambda$. That is, under certain circumstances (small values of λt) the decay constant λ can be thought of as approximating the probability of decay per unit time. In general, however, the probability of decay is $(1 - e^{-\lambda t})$, and the decay constant should be thought of as a fractional rate of decay rather than as a probability of decay.

The physical half-life $T_{1/2}$ of a radioactive nuclide is the time required for the decay of half of the atoms in a sample of the nuclide. In equation (2-6), $N = \frac{1}{2} N_0$ when $t = T_{1/2}$, if $N = N_0$ when $t = 0$. By substitution in equation (2-6),

$$\left(\frac{1}{2}\right)\left(\frac{N_0}{N_0}\right) = e^{-\lambda T_{1/2}}$$

$$\frac{1}{2} = e^{-\lambda T_{1/2}}$$

From the table in the Appendix for the exponential quantity e raised to selected powers:

$$\lambda T_{1/2} = 0.693 \qquad (2\text{-}11)$$

where 0.693 is the ln 2 (natural or Napierian logarithm of 2). Therefore,

$$T_{1/2} = \frac{0.693}{\lambda} = \frac{\ln 2}{\lambda}$$

and

$$\lambda = \frac{0.693}{T_{1/2}} = \frac{\ln 2}{T_{1/2}}$$

The mean or average life is the average expected lifetime for atoms of a radioactive nuclide. The mean life τ is related to the decay constant λ by

$$\tau = \frac{1}{\lambda} \qquad (2\text{-}12)$$

Since $T_{1/2} = (\ln 2)/\lambda$, the mean life may be calculated from the expression

$$\tau = 1.44 \, T_{1/2}$$

Illustrated in Figure 2-10 is the percent of the original activity of a radioactive sample, described as a function of time expressed in units of physical half-life. By replotting these data semilogarithmically (activity

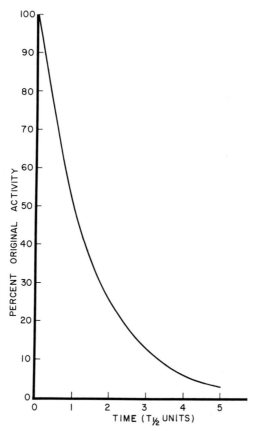

Fig 2-10. — Percent of the original activity of a radioactive sample, expressed as a function of time in units of half-life.

on a logarithmic axis, time on a linear axis), a straight line can be obtained, as shown in Figure 2-11.

Example 2-2

The physical half-life is 1.7 hr for ^{113m}In.

a. A sample of ^{113m}In has a mass of 2 μg. How many ^{113m}In atoms are present in the sample?

$$\text{Number of atoms } N_0 = \frac{(\text{No. of grams})(\text{No. of atoms/gm-atomic mass})}{\text{No. of grams/gm-atomic mass}}$$

$$= \frac{(2 \times 10^{-6} \text{ gm})(6.02 \times 10^{25} \text{ atoms/gm-atomic mass})}{113 \text{ gm/gm-atomic mass}}$$

$$= 1.07 \times 10^{16} \text{ atoms}$$

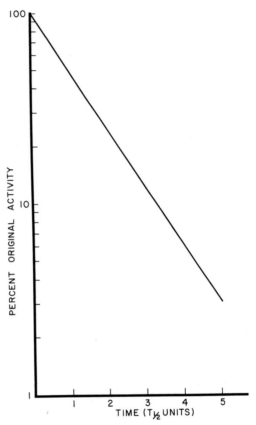

Fig 2-11. — A semilogarithmic graph of the data in Figure 2-10.

b. How many ^{113m}In atoms remain after 4 hr have elapsed?

$$\text{Number of atoms remaining} = N = N_0 e^{-\lambda t}$$

Since $\lambda = 0.693/T_{1/2}$:

$$N = N_0 e^{-(0.693/T_{1/2})t}$$
$$= (1.07 \times 10^{16} \text{ atoms})e^{-(0.693)4.0 \text{ hr}/1.7 \text{ hr}}$$

From the table in the Appendix for the exponential quantity e raised to selected powers

$$N = (1.07 \times 10^{16} \text{ atoms})(0.196)$$
$$= 2.10 \times 10^{15} \text{ atoms remaining}$$

c. What is the activity of the sample when $t = 4.0$ hr?

$$A = \lambda N = \frac{0.693}{T_{1/2}} N$$
$$= \frac{0.693 \ (2.1 \times 10^{15} \ \text{atoms})}{1.7 \ \text{hr} \ (3,600 \ \text{sec/hr})}$$
$$= 2.4 \times 10^{11} \ \text{dps}$$

In units of activity

$$A = \frac{2.4 \times 10^{11} \ \text{dps}}{3.7 \times 10^{10} \ \text{dps/Ci}} = 6.4 \ \text{Ci}$$

Because of the short physical half-life of ^{113m}In, a very small mass of this nuclide possesses high activity.

d. Specific activity is defined as the activity per unit mass of a radioactive sample. What is the specific activity of the ^{113m}In sample after 4 hr?

$$\text{Specific activity} = \frac{6.4 \ \text{Ci}}{2 \ \mu g} = 3.2 \ \frac{\text{Ci}}{\mu g}$$

e. Enough ^{113m}In must be obtained at 4 P.M. Thursday to provide 10 μCi at 1 P.M. Friday. How much ^{113m}In should be obtained?

$$A = A_0 e^{-\lambda t}$$
$$A_0 = A \ e^{\lambda t} = A \ e^{0.693t/T_{1/2}}$$
$$= (10 \ \mu\text{Ci}) \ e^{(0.693)(21 \ \text{hr})/1.7 \ \text{hr}}$$

From the table of exponential quantities in the Appendix, $A_0 = 51.5$ mCi = activity that should be obtained at 4 P.M. Thursday.

Example 2-3

The half-life of ^{99m}Tc is 6.0 hr. How much time t must elapse before a 10 mCi sample of ^{113m}In and a 2 mCi sample of ^{99m}Tc possess equal activities?

$$A_{99mTc} = A_{113mIn} \text{ at time } t$$
$$A_{0(99mTc)} \ e^{-(0.693)t/(T_{1/2})99mTc} = A_{0(113mIn)} \ e^{-(0.693)t/(T_{1/2})113mIn}$$
$$(2 \ \text{mCi}) \ e^{-(0.693)t/6.0 \ \text{hr}} = (10 \ \text{mCi}) \ e^{-(0.693)t/1.7 \ \text{hr}}$$
$$\frac{10 \ \text{mCi}}{2 \ \text{mCi}} = e^{(0.408 \ - \ 0.115)t}$$
$$5 = e^{0.293t}$$
$$t = 5.5 \ \text{hr before activities are equal}$$

This problem may be solved graphically by plotting the activity of each sample as a function of time. The time when activities are equal is indicated by the intersection of the curves for the nuclides.

Transient Equilibrium

Daughter nuclides produced during radioactive decay sometimes also are radioactive. For example, ^{222}Rn decays by alpha emission to ^{218}Po, an unstable nuclide which decays with a half-life of about 3 minutes. If the half-life of the parent is not much longer than the half-life of the daughter, then a condition of *transient equilibrium* may be established. After the time required to attain transient equilibrium has elapsed, the activity of the daughter decreases with an *apparent half-life* equal to the half-life of the parent. The apparent half-life reflects the simultaneous production and decay of the daughter nuclide. If no daughter atoms are present initially when $t = 0$, the number N_2 of daughter atoms present at any later time t may be computed with equation (2-13).

$$N_2 = \frac{\lambda_1}{\lambda_2 - \lambda_1} N_0(e^{-\lambda_1 t} - e^{-\lambda_2 t}) \qquad (2\text{-}13)$$

In equation (2-13), N_0 = number of parent atoms present when $t = 0$, λ_1 = decay constant of parent and λ_2 = decay constant of daughter. If $(N_2)_0$ daughter atoms are present when $t = 0$, then equation (2-13) may be rewritten as:

$$N_2 = (N_2)_0 \, e^{-\lambda_2 t} + \frac{\lambda_1}{\lambda_2 - \lambda_1} N_0(e^{-\lambda_1 t} - e^{-\lambda_2 t})$$

Transient equilibrium for the transition

$$^{132}\text{Te} \; (T_{1/2} = 78 \text{ hr}) \longrightarrow \; ^{132}\text{I} \; (T_{1/2} = 2.3 \text{ hr})$$

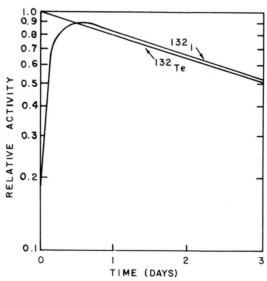

Fig 2-12. — Activities of parent ^{132}Te and daughter ^{132}I as a function of time, illustrating the condition of transient equilibrium that may be achieved when the half-life of the parent is not much greater than the half-life of the daughter.

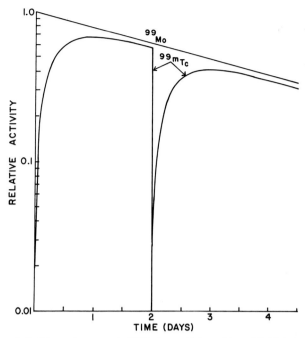

Fig 2-13.—Activities of parent (⁹⁹Mo) and daughter (⁹⁹ᵐTc) activities in a nuclide generator. About 14% of the parent nuclei decay without formation of ⁹⁹ᵐTc.

is illustrated in Figure 2-12. The activity of ^{132}I is greatest when parent (^{132}Te) and daughter (^{132}I) activities are equal. At all later times, the daughter activity exceeds the activity of the parent, and both nuclides decay with the half-life of the parent. After the moment of transient equilibrium, the ratio of the activities of parent (A_1) and daughter (A_2) can be shown to equal:

$$\frac{A_1}{A_2} = \frac{\lambda_2 - \lambda_1}{\lambda_2}$$

The principle of transient equilibrium underlies the production of short-lived isotopes (e.g., ⁹⁹ᵐTc and ¹¹³ᵐIn) in generators for radioactive nuclides used in nuclear medicine. For example, the activities of ⁹⁹ᵐTc ($T_{1/2}$ = 6.0 hr) and ⁹⁹Mo ($T_{1/2}$ = 66 hr) are plotted in Figure 2-13 as a function of time. The ⁹⁹ᵐTc activity remains less than that for ⁹⁹Mo because about 14% of the ⁹⁹Mo nuclei decay promptly to ⁹⁹Tc without passing through the isomeric state of ⁹⁹ᵐTc. The abrupt decrease in activity at 48 hr reflects the removal of ⁹⁹ᵐTc from the generator.

Secular Equilibrium

Secular equilibrium is established when the half-life of the parent nuclide is much greater than the half-life of the daughter. Since $\lambda_1 \ll \lambda_2$ if $T_{1/2\text{parent}} \gg T_{1/2\text{daughter}}$, equation (2-13) may be simplified by assuming that $\lambda_2 - \lambda_1 \simeq \lambda_2$ and that $e^{-\lambda_1 t} = 1$.

$$N_2 = \frac{\lambda_1}{\lambda_2 - \lambda_1} N_0(e^{-\lambda_1 t} - e^{-\lambda_2 t}) \simeq \frac{\lambda_1}{\lambda_2} N_0(1 - e^{-\lambda_2 t})$$

After several half-lives of the daughter have elapsed, $e^{-\lambda_2 t} \simeq 0$ and

$$N_2 = N_0 \left(\frac{\lambda_1}{\lambda_2}\right)$$

$$\lambda_2 N_2 = \lambda_1 N_0$$

$$\frac{0.693}{(T_{1/2})_2} N_2 = \frac{0.693}{(T_{1/2})_1} N_0 \tag{2-14}$$

$$\frac{N_2}{(T_{1/2})_2} = \frac{N_0}{(T_{1/2})_1} \tag{2-15}$$

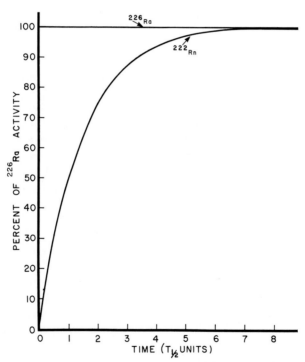

Fig 2-14.—Growth of activity and secular equilibrium of ^{222}Rn produced by decay of ^{226}Ra.

The terms $\lambda_1 N_0$ and $\lambda_2 N_2$ in equation (2-14) represent the activities of parent and daughter. These activities are equal after secular equilibrium has been achieved. Illustrated in Figure 2-14 are the growth of activity and the activity at equilibrium for ^{222}Rn produced in a closed environment by the decay of ^{226}Ra. Units for the abscissa (x-axis) in Figure 2-14 are multiples of the physical half-life of ^{222}Rn. The growth curve for ^{222}Rn approaches the decay curve for ^{226}Ra asymptotically. Seven half-lives of ^{222}Rn must elapse before the activity of the daughter equals 99% of the activity of the parent.

If the parent half-life is less than that for the daughter ($T_{1/2\text{parent}} < T_{1/2\text{daughter}}$, or $\lambda_1 > \lambda_2$), then a constant relationship is not achieved between the activities of parent and daughter. Instead, the activity of the daughter increases initially, reaches a maximum, and then decreases with a half-life intermediate between the parent and daughter half-lives.

Radioactive nuclides in secular equilibrium are used often in radiology. For example, energetic beta particles from ^{90}Y in secular equilibrium with ^{90}Sr are used to treat intraocular lesions. The ^{90}Sr- ^{90}Y ophthalmic irradiator decays with the physical half-life of ^{90}Sr (28 yr), whereas a source of ^{90}Y alone decays with the half-life of ^{90}Y (64 hr). Radium needles and capsules used in radiation therapy contain many decay products in secular equilibrium with long-lived ^{226}Ra.

NATURAL RADIOACTIVITY AND DECAY SERIES

Almost every radioactive nuclide found in nature may be classified as a member of one of three radioactive decay series. Each series consists of sequential transformations which begin with a long-lived parent and end with a stable nuclide. In a closed environment, products of intermediate transformations within each series are in secular equilibrium with the long-lived parent. These products decay with an apparent half-life equal to the half-life of the parent. All radioactive nuclides found in nature decay by emitting either alpha particles or negatrons. Consequently, each transformation in a radioactive decay series changes the mass number of the nucleus either by 4 (alpha decay) or by 0 (negatron decay).

The uranium series begins with ^{238}U ($T_{1/2} = 4.5 \times 10^9$ yr) and ends with stable ^{206}Pb. The mass number 238 of the parent nuclide is divisible by 4 with a remainder of 2. All members of the uranium series, including stable ^{206}Pb, also possess mass numbers divisible by 4 with a remainder of 2. Consequently, the uranium decay series sometimes is referred to as the "$4n + 2$ series," where n represents an integer between 51 and 59 (Fig 2-15). The nuclide ^{226}Ra and its decay products are members of the uranium decay series. A sample of ^{226}Ra decays with a half-life of 1,600 yr. However, 4.5×10^9 yr are required for the earth's supply of ^{226}Ra to de-

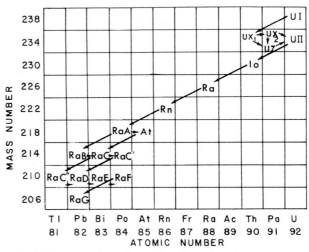

Fig 2-15. — Uranium (4*n* + 2) radioactive decay series.

crease to one-half, because ^{226}Ra in nature is in secular equilibrium with the parent nuclide ^{238}U.

Other radioactive series are the actinium or "4*n* × 3 series" (^{235}U → → ^{207}Pb) and the thorium or "4*n* series" (^{232}Th → → ^{208}Pb). Members of the hypothetical neptunium or "4*n* + 1 series" (^{241}Am → → ^{209}Bi) are not found in nature, because there is no long-lived parent for this series.

Nine naturally occurring radioactive nuclides are not members of a decay series. The nine nuclides, all with long half-lives, are ^{40}K, ^{50}V, ^{87}Rb, ^{115}In, ^{138}La, ^{144}Nd, ^{147}Sm, ^{176}Lu and ^{187}Re.

ARTIFICIAL RADIOACTIVITY

Many nuclides not found in nature may be produced by nuclear transmutation. Nuclear transmutation was observed by Rutherford in 1919[11] during his studies of alpha particles traversing an air-filled chamber. The transmutation occurring within the chamber was

$$\ce{_2^4He + _7^{14}N \rightarrow _8^{17}O + _1^1H}$$

where $_1^1$H represents protons detected during the experiment. The transmutation may be written more concisely as

$$_7^{14}N\ (\alpha,\ p)\ _8^{17}O$$

where $_7^{14}$N represents the bombarded nucleus, $_8^{17}$O the product nucleus, and (α, p) the incident and ejected particles, respectively.

In 1934, Curie and Joliot[8] detected radiation from aluminum bombarded by alpha particles. To explain their observations, Curie and Joliot suggested that the following transmutation occurred with a half-life of 2½ minutes:

$$_2^4\text{He} + {}_{13}^{27}\text{Al} \rightarrow {}_{15}^{30}\text{P} + {}_0^1\text{n}$$
$$_{15}^{30}\text{P} \rightarrow {}_{14}^{30}\text{Si} + {}_{+1}^{0}\beta + \nu$$

A large number of artificially radioactive nuclides have been produced since Curie and Joliot's discovery. Artificially radioactive nuclides may be produced in nuclear reactors, either as by-products of nuclear fission (e.g., ^{131}I, ^{137}Cs, ^{90}Sr) or by neutron bombardment of various materials (e.g., ^{14}C, ^{3}H, ^{32}P, ^{35}S, ^{60}Co, ^{198}Au). Other nuclides (e.g., ^{11}C, ^{22}Na, ^{28}Mg, ^{54}Mn) are produced in high-energy accelerators by bombarding materials with charged particles such as protons or deuterons.

Mathematics of Nuclide Production by Neutron Bombardment

The production of artificially radioactive nuclides by neutron bombardment within the core of a nuclear reactor may be described mathe-

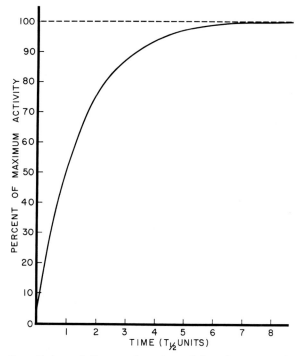

Fig 2-16. — Growth in activity as a function of time for a sample of ^{59}Co bombarded by slow neutrons in a nuclear reactor.

matically. The activity A of a sample bombarded for a time t, assuming no radioactivity when $t = 0$, may be written as:

$$A = \frac{\phi N \sigma}{3.7 \times 10^{10}} (1 - e^{-(0.963)t/T_{1/2}}) \tag{2-16}$$

where ϕ = Neutron flux in neutrons/sq cm-sec.

N = Number of target nuclei in the sample.

σ = Absorption cross section of target nuclei in sq cm (cross-sectional area presented to a neutron by a target nucleus is usually described in units of barns, with 1 barn = 10^{-24} sq cm).

$T_{1/2}$ = Half-life of the product nuclide.

A = Activity of the sample in curies.

When the bombardment time t is much greater than $T_{1/2}$, equation (2-16) reduces to

$$A_{max} = \frac{\phi N \sigma}{3.7 \times 10^{10}} \tag{2-17}$$

where A_{max} represents the maximum activity in curies. The curve in Figure 2-16 illustrates the growth of radioactivity in a sample of ^{59}Co bombarded by slow neutrons. This transmutation is written $^{59}_{27}$Co (n, γ) $^{60}_{27}$Co. The half-life of ^{60}Co is 5.3 yr.

Example 2-4

A 20-gm sample of ^{59}Co is positioned in the core of a reactor with an average neutron flux of 10^{14} neutrons/sq cm-sec. The absorption cross section for ^{59}Co is 36 barns.

a. What is the activity of the sample after 6.0 yr?

$$N = \frac{20 \text{ gm}(6.02 \times 10^{23}\text{atom/gm-atomic mass})}{59 \text{ gm/gm-atomic mass}} = 2.04 \times 10^{23} \text{ atoms}$$

$$A = \frac{\phi N \sigma}{3.7 \times 10^{10}} (1 - e^{-(0.693)t/T_{1/2}}) \tag{2-16}$$

$$A = \frac{(10^{14} \text{ neutrons/sq cm} - \text{sec})(2.04 \times 10^{23}\text{atoms})(36 \times 10^{-24}\text{sq cm})}{3.7 \times 10^{10} \text{ atom/sec} - \text{Ci}} [1 - e^{-(0.693)6.0\text{yr}/5.3\text{yr}}]$$

$$= 10,800 \text{ Ci}$$

b. What is the maximum activity for the sample?

$$A_{max} = \frac{\phi N \sigma}{3.7 \times 10^{10}}$$

$$= \frac{(10^{14} \text{ neutrons/sq cm} - \text{sec})(2.04 \times 10^{23}\text{atoms})(36 \times 10^{-24}\text{sq cm})}{3.7 \times 10^{10} \text{ atom/sec} - \text{Ci}} \tag{2-17}$$

$$= 19,800 \text{ Ci}$$

c. When does the sample activity reach 90% of its maximum activity?

$$(19,800 \text{ Ci})(0.9) = 17,800 \text{ Ci}$$

$$17,800 \text{ Ci} = 19,800 \text{ Ci}[1 - e^{-(0.693)t/5.3\text{yr}}]$$

$$17,800 \text{ Ci} = 19,800 - 19,800 \ e^{-0.131t}$$
$$19,800 \ e^{-0.131t} = 2,000$$
$$e^{-0.131t} = 0.10$$
$$0.131t = 2.30$$
$$t = 17.6 \text{ yr to reach } 90\% \ A_{max}$$

INFORMATION ABOUT RADIOACTIVE NUCLIDES

Decay schemes for many radioactive nuclei are listed in *Radiological Health Handbook,*[12] *Table of Isotopes,*[13] *Trilinear Chart of Nuclides,*[14] MIRD Pamphlets published by the Society of Nuclear Medicine,[15] *Radioatoms in Nuclear Medicine*[16] and *Nuclear Data Sheets.*[17]

Charts of the nuclides, obtainable from the General Electric Company, Schenectady, N.Y., and from Mallinckrodt Chemical Works, St. Louis, Mo., contain useful data concerning the decay of radioactive nuclides. A section of the chart from the General Electric Company is included in Figure 2-17. In this chart, isobars are positioned along 45-degree diagonals, isotones along vertical lines and isotopes along horizontal lines. Nuclei occupying shaded squares are stable and those in white squares are artificially radioactive. The energy of radiations emitted by various nuclei is expressed in units of MeV.

PROBLEMS

°1. The half-life of ^{132}I is 2.3 hr. What interval of time is required for 100 mCi of ^{132}I to decay to 25 mCi? What interval of time is required for decay of $^7/_8$ of the ^{132}I atoms? What interval of time is required for 100 mCi of ^{132}I to decay to 25 mCi, if the ^{132}I is in transient equilibrium with ^{132}Te ($T_{1/2} = 78$ hr)?

°2. What is the mass in grams of 100 mCi of pure ^{32}P? How many ^{32}P atoms constitute 100 mCi? What is the mass in grams of 100 mCi of Na$_3$^{32}PO$_4$ if all the phosphorus in the compound is radioactive?

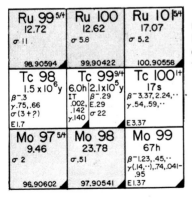

Fig 2-17.—Section from a chart of the nuclides. (Courtesy of Knolls Atomic Power Laboratory, Schenectady, N.Y., operated by the General Electric Company for the U.S. Department of Energy.)

°For those problems marked with an asterisk, answers are provided on the pages following the appendixes (see pp. 487–488).

3. Some ^{210}Bi nuclei decay by alpha emission and others by negatron emission. Write the equation for each mode of decay and identify the daughter nuclide.

°4. If a radioactive nuclide decays for an interval of time equal to its average life, what fraction of the original activity remains?

5. From the decay scheme for ^{131}I, determine the branching ratio for the mode of negatron emission that results in the release of gamma rays of 364 keV. From the decay scheme for ^{126}I, determine the branching ratios for the emission of negatrons and positrons with different maximum energies. Determine the branching ratios of ^{126}I for positron emission and electron capture.

°6. What are the frequency and wavelength of a 100-keV photon?

7. ^{126}I nuclei may decay be negatron emission, positron emission or electron capture. Write the equation for each mode of decay and identify the daughter nuclide.

°8. How much time is required before a 10-mCi sample of ^{99m}Tc ($T_{1/2} = 6.0$ hr) and a 25 mCi sample of ^{113m}In ($T_{1/2} = 1.7$ hr) possess equal activities?

9. From a chart of the nuclides determine:
   a. Whether ^{202}Hg is stable or unstable.
   b. Whether ^{193}Hg decays by negatron or positron emission.
   c. The nuclide that decays to ^{198}Hg by positron emission.
   d. The nuclide that decays to ^{198}Hg by negatron emission.
   e. The half-life of ^{203}Hg.
   f. The percent abundance of ^{198}Hg in naturally occurring mercury.
   g. The atomic mass of ^{204}Hg.

°10. How many atoms and grams of ^{90}Y are in secular equilibrium with 50 mCi of ^{90}Sr?

°11. How many millicuries of ^{24}Na should be ordered so that the sample activity will be 10 mCi when it arrives 24 hr later?

°12. Fifty grams of gold (^{197}Au) are subjected to a neutron flux of 10^{13} neutrons/sq cm-sec in the core of a nuclear reactor. How much time is required for the activity to reach 1,000 Ci? What is the maximum activity for the sample? What is the sample activity after 20 minutes? The cross section of ^{197}Au is 99 barns.

°13. The only stable isotope of arsenic is ^{75}As. What modes of radioactive decay would be expected for ^{74}As and ^{76}As?

14. For a nuclide X with the decay scheme

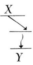

how many gamma rays are emitted per 100 disintegrations of X, if the coefficient for internal conversion is 0.25?

REFERENCES

1. Rutherford, E.: Uranium radiation and the electrical conduction produced by it, Phil. Mag. 47:109, 1899.
2. Boltwood, B., and Rutherford, E.: Production of helium by radium, Phil. Mag. 22:586, 1911.

3. Becquerel, H.: Sur les radiations émises par phosphorescence, Compt. Rend. 122:420, 1896.
4. Pauli, W.: In *Rapports du septieme conseil de physique Solvay, Bruxelles, 1933* (Paris: Gouthier-Villars & Cie, 1934).
5. Reines, F., and Cowan, C., Jr.: Detection of the free neutrino, Phys. Rev. 92: 830, 1953.
6. Villard, P.: Sur la réflexion et la réfraction des rayons cathodiques et des rayons déviables du radium, Compt. Rend. 130:1010, 1900.
7. Franck, P.: *Philosophy of Science* (Englewood Cliffs, N.J.: Prentice-Hall, Inc., 1957).
8. Curie, I., and Joliot, F.: Physique nucléaire: Un nouveau type de radioactivité, Compt. Rend. 198:254, 1934.
9. Anderson, C.: Cosmic-ray positive and negative electrons, Phys. Rev. 44: 406, 1933.
10. Liden, K.: The new special names of SI units in the field of ionizing radiations, Health Phys. 30:417, 1976.
11. Rutherford, E.: Collision of α particles with light atoms: I. Hydrogen, Phil. Mag. 37:537, 1919.
12. *Radiological Health Handbook* (rev. ed.; Washington, D.C.: U. S. Department of Health, Education and Welfare, Office of Technical Services, 1970).
13. Lederer, C., Hollander, J., and Perlman, I.: *Table of Isotopes* (New York: John Wiley & Sons, Inc., 1967).
14. Sullivan, W.: *Trilinear Chart of Nuclides* (2d ed.; Washington, D.C.: Government Printing Office, 1957).
15. Pamphlets of the Medical Internal Radiation Dose Committee of the Society of Nuclear Medicine, 475 Park Avenue South, New York, NY 10016.
16. Blichert-Toft, P.: *Radioatoms in Nuclear Medicine* (Sweden: Gothenburg, 1968).
17. *Nuclear Data Sheets* (New York: Academic Press).

3 / Interactions of Particulate Radiation

AN INTERACTION is *elastic* if the sum of the kinetic energies of the interacting entities is unchanged by the interaction. If the sum of the kinetic energies is changed, then the interaction is *inelastic*. Heavy, charged particles such as protons ($^1_1$H nuclei), deuterons ($^2_1$H nuclei) and alpha particles ($^4_2$He nuclei) usually interact inelastically with electrons of an absorbing medium. Electrons and other light particles with positive or negative charge interact with both electrons and nuclei of an absorber. Neutrons lose energy by colliding elastically and inelastically with nuclei of an absorber.

INTERACTIONS OF HEAVY, CHARGED PARTICLES

Protons, deuterons, alpha particles and other heavy, charged particles lose kinetic energy rapidly as they penetrate matter. Most of the energy is lost as the particles interact inelastically with electrons of the absorbing medium. The transfer of energy is accomplished by interacting electric fields, and physical contact is not required between the incident particles and the absorber electrons. Part of the energy lost by incident particles is used to raise electrons in the absorber to energy levels farther from the nucleus. This process is termed *excitation*. Sometimes, electrons are ejected from their atoms, a process known as *ionization*. Electrons ejected from atoms by impinging radiation are referred to as *primary electrons*. Some primary electrons have enough kinetic energy to produce additional ionization as they migrate from their site of liberation. Electrons ejected during interactions of primary electrons are termed *secondary electrons*. Delta (δ) rays are tracks of primary and secondary electrons in photographic emulsions and cloud chambers exposed to ionizing radiation.

Energy transferred to an electron in excess of its binding energy appears as kinetic energy of the ejected electron. An ejected electron and the residual positive ion constitute an *ion pair*, abbreviated IP. An average energy of 33.7 eV, termed the *W-quantity* or *W*, is expended by charged particles per ion pair produced in air.[1] The average energy required to remove an electron from nitrogen or oxygen is much less than 33.7 eV. The W-quantity includes the average kinetic energy of ejected electrons, together with the average energy lost as incident particles excite atoms, interact with nuclei and increase the rate of vibration of nearby molecules. On the average, 2.2 atoms are excited per ion pair produced in air.

The *specific ionization (SI)* is the number of primary and secondary ion pairs produced per unit length of path of the incident radiation. The specific ionization of alpha particles in air varies from about 30,000 to 70,000 IP/cm. The specific ionization of protons and deuterons is slightly less than that for alpha particles. The *linear energy transfer (LET)* is the average loss in energy per unit length of path of the incident radiation. The *LET* is the product of the specific ionization and the W-quantity.

$$LET = (SI)(W) \tag{3-1}$$

Example 3-1
Assuming that the average specific ionization is 40,000 IP/cm, calculate the average *LET* of alpha particles in air.

$$
\begin{aligned}
LET &= (SI)(W) \\
&= \left(40,000\ \frac{IP}{cm}\right)\left(33.7\ \frac{eV}{IP}\right) \\
&= 1,350\ \frac{keV}{cm}
\end{aligned}
$$

The range of ionizing particles in a particular medium is the straight-line distance traversed by the particles before they are stopped completely. For heavy particles with energy E, the range in a particular medium may be estimated from the average *LET*:

$$\text{Range} = \frac{E}{LET} \tag{3-2}$$

Example 3-2
Calculate the range in air for 4-MeV alpha particles with an average *LET* equal to the *LET* computed in Example 3-1.

$$
\begin{aligned}
\text{Range} &= \frac{E}{LET} \\
&= \frac{4\ MeV\ (10^6\ eV/MeV)}{1,350\ keV/cm\ (10^3\ eV/keV)} \\
&= \text{approximately 3 cm air}
\end{aligned}
$$

From Examples 3-1 and 3-2, it is apparent that alpha particles produce dense ionization but have limited range. Deuterons, protons and other heavy, charged particles also exhibit high specific ionization and a relatively short range. The density of soft tissue (1 gm/cc) is much greater

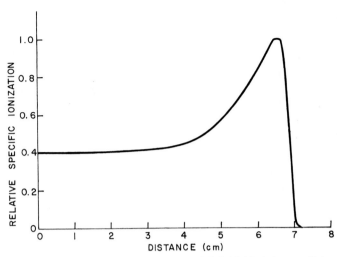

Fig 3-1.—The relative specific ionization of 7.7-MeV alpha particles from the decay of [214]Po, plotted as a function of the distance traversed in air.

than the density of air (1.29×10^{-3} gm/cc). Hence, alpha particles of a few MeV or less from radioactive nuclei penetrate soft tissue to depths of only a few microns ($1 \mu = 10^{-4}$ cm). For example, alpha particles from a radioactive source near or on the body penetrate only the most superficial layers of skin.

The specific ionization *(SI)* and *LET* are not constant along the entire path of monoenergetic charged particles traversing a homogeneous medium. The *SI* of 7.7-MeV alphas from [214]Po is plotted in Figure 3-1 as a function of the distance traversed in air. The increase in *SI* near the end of the path of the particles reflects the decreased velocity of the alphas. As the particles slow down, the *SI* increases because nearby atoms are influenced for a longer period. The region of increased *SI* is termed the *Bragg peak*. The rapid decrease in *SI* beyond the peak is due primarily to the capture of electrons by slowly moving alphas. Captured electrons reduce the charge of the alphas and decrease their ability to produce ionization.

A few attempts have been made to utilize beams of energetic, heavy particles in radiation therapy.[2, 3] If the Bragg peak of the particles is centered within the tumor, then maximum energy is delivered to the tumor with reduced energy deposited in surrounding normal tissue. Increased effectiveness of high-*LET* radiation for the destruction of tumor cells, and reduced scattering of radiation outside the primary beam, are other potential advantages of heavy-particle beams for radiation therapy.[3] One

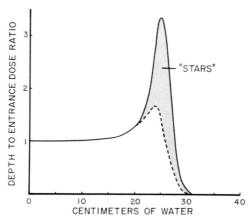

Fig 3-2.—Ratio of the specific ionization (or "dose") at depth to that on the surface for a "pure" beam of negative pions with an energy of 96 MeV at the surface. The shaded area depicts the contribution of nuclear fragments produced near the end of the path of the particles. (From Curtis, S., and Raju, M.: A calculation of the physical characteristics of negative pion beams—energy-loss distribution and Bragg curves, Radiat. Res. 34:239, 1968.)

disadvantage of heavy-particle beams is the complex, expensive equipment required for their production.

Recently, considerable interest has focused on the use of negative π mesons (negative pions) for radiation therapy.[3, 4] These particles have a mass 273 times the mass of the electron and are produced by bombarding targets with particles (e.g., protons or deuterons) accelerated to very high energies. Superimposed upon the Bragg peak for the pions is the energy released as slowly moving pions interact with nuclei of the absorbing medium, causing these nuclei to undergo spallation and produce "stars" (Fig 3-2). Currently, radiation therapy with negative pions is being contemplated or implemented at a few high-energy accelerators around the world.[3-5]

INTERACTIONS OF ELECTRONS

Interactions of negative and positive electrons may be divided into three categories:

1. Interactions with electrons.
2. Elastic interactions with nuclei.
3. Inelastic interactions with nuclei.

Scattering by Electrons

Negative and positive electrons traversing an absorbing medium transfer energy to electrons of the medium. Impinging electrons lose energy and are deflected at some angle with respect to their original direction. An electron receiving energy may be raised to an electron shell farther from the nucleus or may be ejected from the atom. The kinetic energy E_k of an ejected electron equals the energy E received minus the binding energy E_B of the electron:

$$E_k = E - E_B \qquad (3\text{-}3)$$

If the binding energy is negligible compared to the energy received, then the interaction may be considered as an elastic collision between "free" particles. The interaction is inelastic if the binding energy must be considered.

Incident negatrons and positrons are scattered by electrons with a probability that increases with the atomic number of the absorber. The probability for scattering by electrons decreases rapidly with increasing kinetic energy of the incident particles. That is, low-energy negatrons and positrons interact frequently with electrons of an absorber; the frequency of interaction diminishes rapidly as the kinetic energy of the incident particles increases.[6]

Ion pairs are produced by negatrons and positrons during both elastic and inelastic interactions. The specific ionization (IP/cm) in air at STP (standard temperature = 0 C, standard pressure = 760 mm Hg) may be estimated with equation (3-4) for negatrons and positrons with kinetic energy between 0 and 10 MeV.

$$SI = \frac{45}{(v/c)^2} \qquad (3\text{-}4)$$

In equation (3-4), v represents the velocity of an incident negatron or positron and c represents the speed of light *in vacuo* (3×10^8 m/sec).

Example 3-3

Calculate the SI and LET of 0.1-MeV electrons in air ($v/c = 0.548$). The LET may be computed from the specific ionization with equation (3-1), using an average W-quantity for electrons of 33.7 eV/IP.[7]

$$
\begin{aligned}
SI &= \frac{45}{(v/c)^2} \\
&= \frac{45}{(0.548)^2} \\
&= 150 \text{ IP/cm} \\
LET &= (SI)(W) \\
&= (150 \text{ IP/cm})(33.7 \text{ eV/IP}) \\
&= 5.06 \text{ keV/cm}
\end{aligned}
$$

After expending its kinetic energy, a positron combines with an electron in the absorbing medium. The particles annihilate each other and their mass appears as electromagnetic radiation, usually two 0.51-MeV photons moving in opposite directions. This interaction is termed *pair annihilation.*

Elastic Scattering by Nuclei

Electrons are deflected with reduced energy during elastic interactions with nuclei of an absorbing medium. The probability of elastic interactions with nuclei varies with Z^2 of the absorber and approximately with $(1/E_k^2)$, where E_k represents the kinetic energy of the incident electrons. The probability for elastic scattering by nuclei is slightly less for positrons than for negatrons with the same kinetic energy. Backscattering of negatrons and positrons in radioactive samples is due primarily to elastic scattering by nuclei.

Probabilities for elastic scattering of electrons by electrons and nuclei of an absorbing medium are about equal if the medium is hydrogen ($Z = 1$). In absorbers with higher atomic number, elastic scattering by nuclei occurs more frequently than electron scattering, because the nuclear scattering cross section varies with Z^2 and the cross section for scattering by electrons varies with Z.

Inelastic Scattering by Nuclei

A negative or positive electron passing near a nucleus may be deflected with reduced velocity. The interaction is inelastic if energy is released as electromagnetic radiation during the encounter. The radiated energy is known as *bremsstrahlung* (braking radiation). A bremsstrahlung photon may possess any energy up to the entire kinetic energy of the incident particle. For low-energy electrons, bremsstrahlung photons are radiated predominantly at right angles to the motion of the particles. The angle narrows as the kinetic energy of the electrons increases (Fig 3-

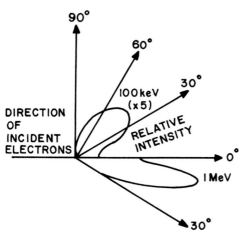

Fig 3-3. — Relative intensity of bremsstrahlung radiated at various angles, for electrons with kinetic energies of 100 keV and 1 MeV.[8, 9]

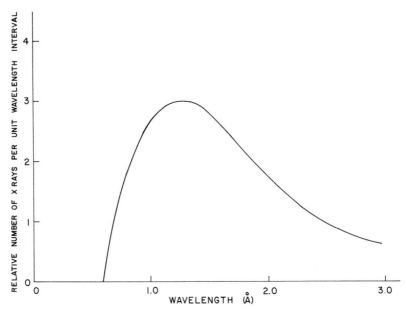

Fig 3-4. — Bremsstrahlung spectrum for a molybdenum target bombarded by electrons accelerated through 20 kV.[10]

3). The probability of bremsstrahlung production varies with Z^2 of the absorbing medium. A typical bremsstrahlung spectrum is illustrated in Figure 3-4. The shape of the spectrum is independent of the atomic number of the absorber.

The ratio of radiation energy loss (the result of inelastic interactions with nuclei) to the energy lost by excitation and ionization (the result of interactions with electrons) is approximately

$$\frac{\text{Radiation energy loss}}{\text{Ionization energy loss}} = \frac{E_k Z}{820} \tag{3-5}$$

where E_k represents the kinetic energy of the incident electrons in MeV, and Z is the atomic number of the absorbing medium. For example,

TABLE 3-1. — CLASSIFICATION OF
NEUTRONS ACCORDING TO
KINETIC ENERGY

TYPE	ENERGY RANGE
Slow	0–0.1 keV
Intermediate	0.1–20 keV
Fast	20 keV–10 MeV
High-energy	>10 MeV

excitation-ionization and bremsstrahlung contribute about equally to the energy lost by 10-MeV electrons traversing lead (Z = 82). The ratio of energy lost by the production of bremsstrahlung to that lost by ionization and excitation of atoms is important to the design of x-ray tubes.

Visible light is radiated by charged particles moving through a medium at a velocity exceeding the velocity of light in the medium. The visible light is named *Cerenkov radiation*.[11] Only a small fraction of the kinetic energy of high-energy electrons is lost by production of Cerenkov radiation.

INTERACTIONS OF NEUTRONS

Slow, intermediate and fast neutrons (Table 3-1) are present within the core of a nuclear reactor. Neutrons with various kinetic energies are emitted by ^{252}Cf, a nuclide that fissions spontaneously. This nuclide has been encapsulated into needles and used for implant therapy.[12, 13] Neutron beams are available from neutron generators (Fig 3-5) and cyclotrons, in which low-Z nuclei (e.g., ^{3}H or ^{9}Be) are bombarded by positively charged particles (e.g., nuclei of ^{1}H, ^{2}H or ^{4}He) moving at high velocities. For example, 14.1-MeV neutrons may be produced in a neutron generator by bombarding a tritium target with deuterons (^{2}H^{+}) accelerated through a potential difference of 150 kV. The energy distribution of neutrons from neutron generators and cyclotrons depends on the target material and on the type and energy of the bombarding particle. A few spectra for fast neutrons are shown in Figure 3-6.

Neutrons are uncharged particles that interact primarily by "billiard-

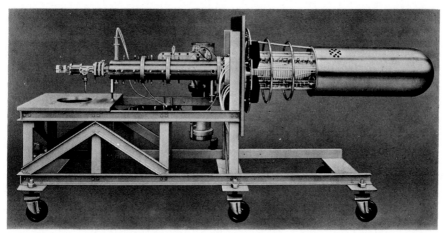

Fig 3-5. — A conventional neutron generator, in which a ^{3}H target is bombarded by fast-moving deuterons. (Courtesy of Texas Nuclear Corp., subsidiary of Nuclear-Chicago Corp.)

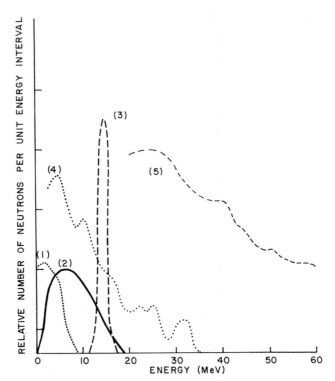

Fig 3-6.—Relative number of neutrons per unit energy interval, plotted as a function of the neutron energy in MeV. These spectra are only approximately correct, but illustrate the energy distribution of neutrons produced during selected nuclear reactions: *(1)* spectrum for neutrons released during nuclear fission; *(2)* spectrum for neutrons released when 16.1-MeV deuterons bombard a beryllium target;[14] *(3)* spectrum for neutrons resulting from bombardment of a tritium target by deuterons accelerated through 150 kV; *(4)* spectrum for neutrons released when a beryllium target is bombarded by 20-MeV ^{3}He ions; *(5)* neutron spectrum predicted for a beryllium target bombarded by helium ions or deuterons accelerated to very high energy. Spectra *(4)* and *(5)* are highly speculative. (Courtesy of J. Brennan, A. Raventos and M. Mendelsohn, University of Pennsylvania.)

ball" or "knock-on" collisions with absorber nuclei. A collision between neutron and nucleus is elastic if the total kinetic energy of the neutron and the nucleus is unchanged by the collision. A collision is inelastic if part of the kinetic energy is used to excite the nucleus. During an elastic knock-on collision, the energy transferred from neutron to nucleus is maximum if the mass of the nucleus equals the neutron mass. If the absorbing medium is tissue, then the energy transferred per collision is greatest for collisions of neutrons with nuclei of hydrogen, because the mass of a hydrogen nucleus (i.e., a proton) is close to the mass of a neutron. Most nuclei in tissue are hydrogen, and the cross section for elastic collision is greater for hydrogen than for other constituents of tissue. For these reasons, elastic collisions with hydrogen nuclei account for most of the energy deposited in tissue by neutrons with kinetic energies less than 20 MeV.

For neutrons with kinetic energy greater than 10 MeV, inelastic scattering also contributes to the energy lost in tissue. For example, inelastic interactions account for 30% of the energy deposited in tissue by 14.1-MeV neutrons.[15] Most inelastic interactions occur with nuclei other than hydrogen. Energetic charged particles (e.g., protons or alpha particles) often are ejected from nuclei excited by inelastic interactions with neutrons.

Certain materials (e.g., lithium, boron, cadmium and uranium) exhibit high cross sections for the capture of slow neutrons. Energetic, positively charged particles may be ejected by certain nuclei (e.g., ^{6}Li and ^{10}B) that capture neutrons. Other nuclei (e.g., ^{235}U and ^{239}Pu) fission spontaneously after absorbing a neutron. Some tumors concentrate compounds that contain atoms with high cross section for the capture of slow neutrons. Densely ionizing radiation is released if a tumor that has absorbed one of these compounds is exposed to slow neutrons. This radiation may deposit large amounts of energy within the tumor. For example, brain tumors have been irradiated with slow neutrons after the tumors have incorporated borax enriched with ^{10}B.[3, 18] The reaction within a tumor is

$$^{10}_{5}B(n, \alpha)^{7}_{3}Li$$

Both the alpha particles and the ^{7}Li nuclei are densely ionizing, short-range particles which deposit large amounts of energy within the tumor.

PROBLEMS

*1. Electrons with kinetic energy of 1.0 MeV have a specific ionization in air of about 60 IP/cm. What is the *LET* of these electrons in air?

*2. Alpha particles with 2.0 MeV have an *LET* in air of 0.175 keV/μ. What is the specific ionization of these particles in air?

*3. What is the ratio of bremsstrahlung to ionization and excitation energy loss for 200-keV electrons traversing a tungsten absorber (Z = 74)?

REFERENCES

1. Chappell, S., and Sparrow, J.: The average energy required to produce an ion pair in argon, nitrogen and air for 1- to 5-MeV alpha particles, Radiat. Res. 32:383, 1967.

*For those problems marked with an asterisk, answers are provided on the pages following the appendixes (see pp. 487–488).

2. Tobias, C., and Todd, P.: Heavy Charged Particles in Cancer Therapy, in del Regato, J. (ed.): *Proceedings of Conference on Radiobiology and Radiotherapy* (Washington, D.C.: Government Printing Office, 1967), p. 1.
3. Hendee, W., and Kirsch, W.: Effects of Ionizing Radiation upon Normal and Neoplastic Neural Tissue, in *The Experimental Biology of Brain Tumors* (Springfield, Ill.: Charles C Thomas, Publisher, 1972).
4. Rosen, L.: Possibilities and advantages of using negative pions in radiotherapy, Nucl. Appl. 5:379, 1968.
5. Kligerman, M., et al.: Current status of clinical pion radiotherapy, Radiology 125:489, 1977.
6. Bichsel, H.: Charged-Particle Interactions, in Attix, F., and Roesch, W. (eds.): *Radiation Dosimetry* (New York: Academic Press, 1968), vol. 1, p. 157.
7. Cole, A.: Absorption of 20-eV to 50,000 eV electron beams in air and plastic, Radiat. Res. 38:7, 1969.
8. Scherzer, O.: Über die Ausstrahlung bei der Bremsung von Protonen und schnellen Elektronen, Ann. Phys. 13:137, 1932.
9. Andrews, H.: *Radiation Biophysics* (Englewood Cliffs, N.J.: Prentice-Hall, 1961).
10. Wehr, M., and Richards, J.: *Physics of the Atom* (Reading, Mass.: Addison-Wesley Publishing Co., Inc., 1960), p. 159.
11. Jelley, J.: *Cerenkov Radiation and Its Applications* (New York: Pergamon Press, Inc., 1958).
12. Wright, C., et al.: Implantable californium-252 neutron sources for radiotherapy, Radiology 89:337, 1967.
13. Boulogne, A., and Evans, A.: Californium-252 neutron sources for medical applications, Int. J. Appl. Radiat. Isot. 20:453, 1969.
14. Bewley, D.: Physical aspects of the fast neutron beam, Br. J. Radiol. 36:81, 1963.
15. Randolph, M.: Energy deposition in tissue and similar materials by 14.1 MeV neutrons, Radiat. Res. 7:45, 1957.

4 / Production of X Rays

X RAYS WERE DISCOVERED by Röntgen[1] in 1895 during his investigations of "cathode rays" in gaseous discharge tubes. A number of studies of this historic discovery have been published.[2-5] Reproduced in Figure 4-1 is a radiograph Röntgen took of his wife's hand on December 22, 1895.

CONVENTIONAL X-RAY TUBES

Requirements for the efficient production of x rays include: (1) a source of electrons, (2) a large potential difference through which the electrons are accelerated, (3) an evacuated path for the accelerated electrons, (4) a target that absorbs the accelerated electrons and (5) an envelope to contain the vacuum. To attenuate undesired radiation, a ray-proof housing should be provided for the glass envelope. Elementary features of a conventional x-ray tube are illustrated in Figure 4-2, and modern x-ray tubes are shown in Figures 4-3 and 4-4.

Electron Source

Early x-ray tubes were not evacuated completely. Residual atoms of gas were ionized by an electric current, furnishing positive ions that were attracted to a negative electrode, termed the *cathode*. As the positive ions struck the cathode, electrons were released and accelerated toward a positively charged target called the *anode*. X rays were produced as the electrons were absorbed in the target. Gaseous x-ray tubes were unreliable and furnished only a small number of x rays. In 1913, Coolidge[6] improved the x-ray tube by using a wire filament heated with an electric current. Electrons were liberated or "boiled" from the surface of the heated filament. The release of electrons from a heated surface is termed *thermionic emission* or the *Edison effect*. Electrons liberated from the filament of the Coolidge tube were repelled by the negative charge of the filament and accelerated toward a positively charged target. X rays were produced as the electrons struck the target. The Coolidge tube was the prototype for x-ray tubes used today.

A metal with a high melting point is required for the filament of an x-ray tube. Tungsten filaments (melting point of tungsten = 3,370 C) are used in most modern tubes. A current of a few amperes raises the temperature of the filament, liberating electrons at a rate that increases with the filament current. The filament is mounted within a negatively

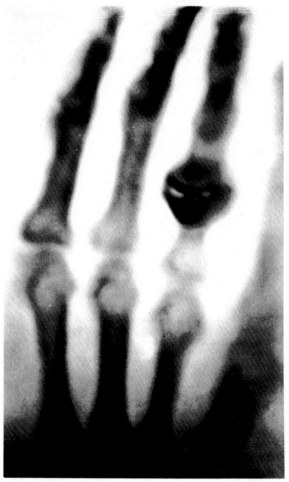

Fig 4-1.—A radiograph of the hand, taken by Röntgen with his wife as the subject. (Courtesy of Deutsches Röntgen-Museum, Remscheid-Lennep, West Germany.)

charged focusing cup. Collectively, these elements are termed the *cathode assembly.*

The focal spot is the volume of target within which electrons are absorbed and x rays are generated. For radiographs of the highest quality, electrons should be absorbed within a very small focal spot. To achieve a small focal spot, a small or "fine" filament is required. Radiographic quality sometimes is reduced by voluntary or involuntary motion of the

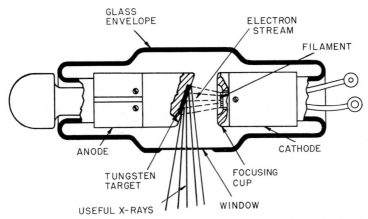

Fig 4-2.—A simplified x-ray tube with a stationary anode and a heated filament. (From Bloom, W., Hollenbach, J., and Morgan, J.: *Medical Radiographic Technic* [3d ed.; Springfield, Ill.: Charles C Thomas, Publisher, 1965].)

patient. The loss of image quality caused by motion of the patient may be reduced by using x-ray exposures of high intensity and short duration. However, the rate of emission of electrons from the filament required for these high-intensity exposures may exceed the capability of a small filament. Consequently, many x-ray tubes have two filaments. These tubes are termed *dual-focus tubes*. The smaller, fine filament is used when radiographs with high detail are desired and short, high-intensity exposures are not necessary. If high-intensity exposures of short duration are needed to limit the blurring effect of motion, the larger, coarse filament is used. The cathode assembly of a dual-focus x-ray tube is illustrated in Figure 4-5.

Tube Voltage

The potential difference between the filament and target of an x-ray tube influences the intensity and spectral distribution of x rays emerging

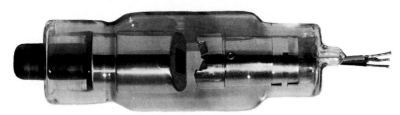

Fig 4-3.—A dual-focus x-ray tube with a stationary anode. (Courtesy of Machlett Laboratories, Inc.)

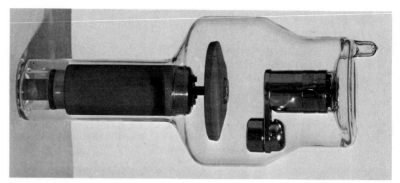

Fig 4-4. — A dual-focus x-ray tube with a rotating anode. (Courtesy of Machlett Laboratories, Inc.)

from the tube. At low tube voltages, electrons are released from the filament more rapidly than they are accelerated toward the target. A cloud of electrons, termed the *space charge,* accumulates around the filament and opposes the release of additional electrons from the filament. At low tube voltages, the electron flow across the x-ray tube is said to be *space-charge limited.* Curves in Figure 4-6 illustrate the influence of tube voltage and filament current upon the flow of electrons from filament to tar-

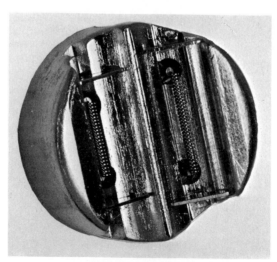

Fig 4-5. — Cathode assembly of a dual-focus tube. The small filament provides a smaller focal spot and a radiograph with greater detail, provided the patient does not move. The larger filament is used for high-intensity exposures of short duration. (Courtesy of Machlett Laboratories, Inc.)

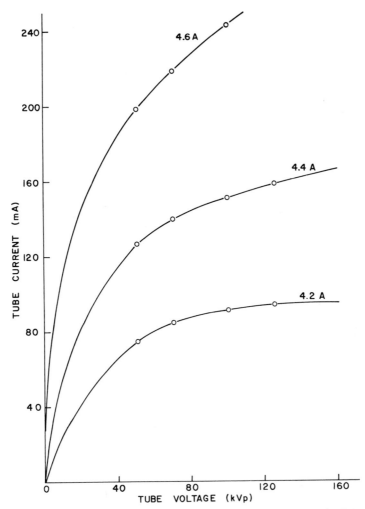

Fig 4-6.—Influence of tube voltage and filament current upon electron flow in a Machlett Dynamax x-ray tube with a rotating anode, 1 mm apparent focal spot and full-wave rectified voltage.

get. At low filament currents, a saturation voltage may be achieved, above which the current through the x-ray tube does not change. With a voltage at or above saturation, the tube current may be varied significantly only by changing the current through the filament. Hence, the tube current is said to be *temperature limited* or *filament-emission limited.* To obtain high tube currents and x rays with energy useful for diagnostic

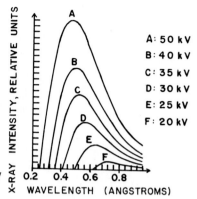

A: 50 kV
B: 40 kV
C: 35 kV
D: 30 kV
E: 25 kV
F: 20 kV

Fig 4-7.—X-ray spectra generated at different tube voltages, with a constant current through the x-ray tube. The x-ray tube contained a tungsten target.[7]

radiology, high filament currents and voltages between 40 and 140 kV must be used. With these filament currents and at lower tube voltages, the current through the x-ray tube is space-charge limited. Under these conditions, the influence of tube voltage upon tube current may be reduced with a *space-charge compensating circuit*. This circuit is discussed in Chapter 5.

Illustrated in Figure 4-7 is the influence of tube voltage upon the intensity and spectral distribution of bremsstrahlung x rays emerging from an x-ray tube containing a tungsten target. The efficiency of bremsstrahlung production increases with the energy of electrons striking the tar-

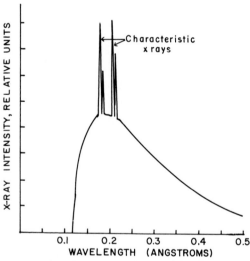

Fig 4-8.—X-ray spectrum illustrating the contribution of characteristic x rays produced as electrons fill holes in the K shell of tungsten.

get. Consequently, the number of bremsstrahlung photons emerging from an x-ray tube increases rapidly as the voltage is increased across the x-ray tube. At tube voltages of 70 kilovolts peak (kVp) and higher, a characteristic peak on the x-ray spectrum reflects the emission of characteristic x rays produced as electrons fill vacancies in the K shell of tungsten atoms (Fig 4-8).

During the interaction of an electron with a target nucleus, a bremsstrahlung photon may emerge with energy equal to the total kinetic energy of the electron. The maximum energy of the photons depicted in Figure 4-8 reflects the peak voltage applied across the x-ray tube, described in units of kilovolts peak. Photons of maximum energy in an x-ray beam also possess the shortest or minimum wavelength. The minimum wavelength λ_{min} for an x-ray beam may be computed if the peak voltage across the x-ray tube is known, because the peak voltage is equal numerically to the maximum energy $h\upsilon_{max}$ of photons in the x-ray beam:

$$h\upsilon_{max} = \frac{hc}{\lambda_{min}}$$

$$h\upsilon_{max} \ (\text{keV}) = \frac{(6.62 \times 10^{-34} \ \text{J-sec})(3 \times 10^{8} \ \text{m/sec})(10^{10} \ \text{Å/m})}{\lambda_{min} \ (1.6 \times 10^{-16} \ \text{J/keV})}$$

The minimum wavelength λ_{min} is expressed in units of angstroms.

$$\lambda_{min} = \frac{12.4}{h\upsilon_{max}}$$

$$= \frac{12.4}{\text{kVp}} \tag{4-1}$$

In equation (4-1) the maximum voltage is expressed in units of kilovolts and the minimum wavelength in units of angstroms.

Example 4-1

Calculate the maximum energy and minimum wavelength for an x-ray beam generated at 100 kVp.

Maximum energy (keV) = Maximum tube voltage (kVp)

Since the maximum tube voltage is 100 kVp, the maximum energy of the photons is 100 keV:

$$\lambda_{min} = \frac{12.4}{100 \ \text{kVp}}$$

$$= 0.124 \ \text{Å}$$

Tube Vacuum

To prevent collisions between molecules of air and electrons accelerated between the filament and target, x-ray tubes are evacuated to pressures less than 10^{-5} mm Hg. Removal of air also reduces the deterioration of the hot filament by oxidation. The method of evacuation includes "outgassing" procedures to remove the gas occluded in components of the x-ray tube. Nevertheless, tubes occasionally become "gassy," either after prolonged use or because the vacuum seal is not perfect. Filaments are destroyed rapidly in gassy tubes.

Envelope and Housing

A vacuum-tight glass envelope surrounds other components required for the efficient production of x rays. The x-ray tube is mounted inside a metal case or housing which is grounded electrically and usually contains oil. The oil insulates the housing from the high voltage applied to the tube, and also absorbs heat radiated from the anode. Shockproof cables that deliver high voltage to the x-ray tube enter the housing through insulated openings. A bellows in the housing permits heated oil to expand when the tube is used. Often, the bellows is connected to a switch that interrupts the operation of the x-ray tube if the oil reaches a temperature incompatible with the heat-storage capacity of the tube housing. A lead sheath inside the metal housing attenuates radiation emerging from the x-ray tube in undesired directions. A cross section of an x-ray tube and its housing is shown in Figure 4-9.

Target and Anode

The efficiency of x-ray production is the ratio of energy emerging as x radiation from the x-ray tube target divided by the energy deposited by

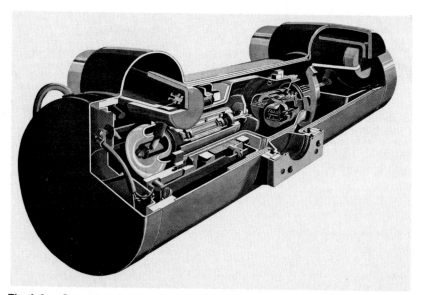

Fig 4-9.—Cutaway of a rotating-anode x-ray tube positioned in its housing. (Courtesy of Machlett Laboratories, Inc.)

electrons impinging on the target. The rate P [in watts (W)] at which electrons deposit energy in a target is given by:

$$P = VI$$

where V = tube voltage in volts, and I = tube current in amperes. The rate P' at which energy is released as x radiation is:[8]

$$P' = 0.9 \times 10^{-9} ZV^2I \tag{4-2}$$

where Z = atomic number of target. Hence, the efficiency of x-ray production is

$$\text{Efficiency} = \frac{P'}{P} = \frac{0.9 \times 10^{-9} ZV^2I}{VI}$$
$$= 0.9 \times 10^{-9} ZV \tag{4-3}$$

From equation (4-3), it is apparent that the efficiency of x-ray production increases with the atomic number of the target and the voltage across the x-ray tube. However, x-ray production is very inefficient, even in targets with high atomic number. For example, the efficiency of x-ray production is only about 0.6% for a tungsten target receiving electrons accelerated through 100 kV.

Example 4-2
In 1 second, 6.25×10^{17} electrons (100 mA) are accelerated through a constant potential difference of 100 kV. At what rate is energy deposited in the target?

$$P = (10^5V)(0.1 \text{ A})$$
$$= 10^4 \text{ W}$$

For x-ray tubes operated at conventional voltages, less than 1% of the energy deposited in the target appears as x radiation. Almost all of the energy delivered by impinging electrons is degraded to heat within the target. Four requirements which a target must satisfy are: (1) high atomic number, (2) high melting point, (3) high conductivity of heat and (4) reasonable cost. Tungsten satisfies these four requirements reasonably well, and is the target of most x-ray tubes used in diagnostic radiology.

The high rate of energy deposition in the small target of an x-ray tube heats the target to a very high temperature. Hence, a target with a high melting point is required. Furthermore, the target must have high thermal conductivity to transfer heat rapidly from the target to its surroundings. Stationary targets usually consist of a block of tungsten about 0.1 in. thick embedded in a large copper anode. The anode absorbs most of the heat produced in the target. Heat is removed from the stationary anode in various ways. In some stationary anode tubes, cooling oil is circulated through a hollow copper anode. In others, cool water is circulated

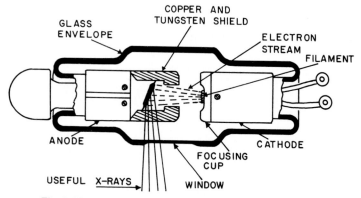

Fig 4-10. — Therapy x-ray tube with a hooded anode.

through coils surrounding an extension of the copper anode. Sometimes, air is blown across cooling fins on one end of the anode.

Rotating anodes are used in almost all diagnostic x-ray tubes. A rotating anode increases the volume of tungsten absorbing energy from impinging electrons, thereby reducing the temperature attained by any portion of the anode. Rotating anodes are composed of either pure tungsten or a mixture of tungsten and rhenium, and may be laminated with a backing of metal such as molybdenum. The anode is attached to the rotor of a small induction motor by a stem which usually is composed of molybdenum. Anodes rotate at speeds up to 10,000 rpm. The induction motor is energized for about 1 second before high voltage is applied to the x-ray tube. The delay ensures that electrons do not strike the target before the anode reaches its maximum speed of rotation. Energy deposited in the rotating anode is radiated to the oil bath surrounding the glass envelope of the x-ray tube.

Secondary electrons may be ejected from a target bombarded by high-speed electrons. X rays may be produced as these electrons are absorbed by the glass envelope or by metallic components of the x-ray tube. X rays produced away from the target are referred to as *off-focus x rays*. Also, electrons accumulated by the glass envelope may perturb the motion of electrons traveling from filament to target, increasing the size of the focal spot. Hence, secondary electrons should be removed before they reach the glass envelope or other components of the x-ray tube. Some stationary anode x-ray tubes possess a hooded anode similar to that illustrated in Figure 4-10. Secondary electrons ejected from the target are absorbed in the copper sleeve. Off-focus x rays produced in the copper are absorbed by the tungsten shield surrounding the copper sleeve.

The quality of a radiologic image is reduced by off-focus x rays emerg-

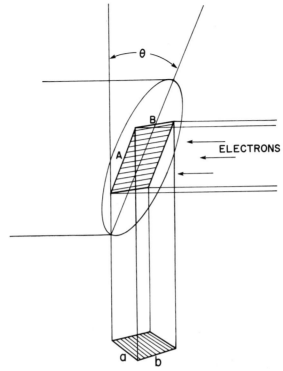

Fig 4-11.—Illustration of the line-focus principle which reduces the apparent size of the focal spot.

ing from a diagnostic x-ray tube. The production of off-focus x radiation is greater in x-ray tubes with large surfaces of high-Z elements such as tungsten. Hence, the production of off-focus radiation is greater in an x-ray tube with a rotating anode than in a tube equipped with a stationary anode. For example, off-focus radiation contributes as much as 25% of the total amount of radiation emerging from some x-ray tubes with rotating anodes.[9] Off-focus x radiation may be reduced by collimating the x-ray beam as close as possible to the target.

For radiologic images of highest quality, the volume of the target from which x rays emerge should be as small as possible. To reduce the "apparent size" of the focal spot, the target of an x-ray tube is mounted at a very steep angle with respect to the motion of the incident electrons (Fig 4-11). With the target at this angle, x rays appear to originate within a focal spot much smaller than the volume of the target absorbing energy from the impinging electrons. This reduction in the apparent size of the focal spot is termed the *line-focus principle*. Most diagnostic x-ray tubes

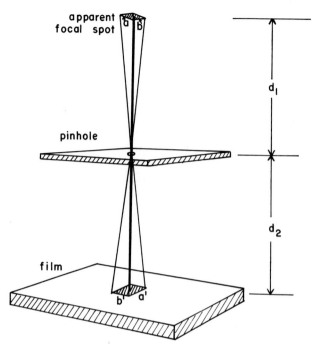

Fig 4-12. — Pinhole method for determining the size *ab* of the apparent focal spot.

use a target angle between 6 and 17 degrees. In Figure 4-11, side *a* of the projected or apparent focal spot may be calculated by

$$a = A \sin \theta \tag{4-4}$$

where *A* is the corresponding dimension of the true focal spot and θ is the target angle.

Example 4-3

Using Figure 4-11 and equation (4-4), calculate *a* if $A = 7$ mm and $\theta = 17$ degrees.

$$
\begin{aligned}
a &= A \sin \theta \\
&= (7 \text{ mm})(\sin 17 \text{ degrees}) \\
&= (7 \text{ mm})(0.29) \\
&= 2 \text{ mm}
\end{aligned}
$$

Side *b* of the apparent focal spot equals side *B* of the true focal spot because side *B* is perpendicular to the electron beam. However, side *B* is less than side *A* of the true focal spot, because the width of a filament always is less than its length. The apparent focal spot usually is square.

The line-focus principle is used in x-ray tubes with stationary and rotating anodes. Dual-focus diagnostic x-ray tubes furnish two apparent focal spots, one for fine-focus (e.g., 0.6 mm) and another for coarse-focus (e.g., 1.5 mm) radiography. Which apparent focal spot is used is determined by the tube current desired. The small filament is used when a low (e.g., 100 mA) tube current is satisfactory. The coarse filament is used when a larger tube current (e.g., 200 mA or greater) is required to reduce exposure time. Apparent focal spots of very small dimensions (e.g., 0.1 mm) are available with certain x-ray tubes.

The apparent size of the focal spot of an x-ray tube may be measured with a pinhole x-ray camera.[10, 11] A hole with a diameter of a few hundredths of a millimeter is drilled in a plate opaque to x rays. The plate is positioned between the x-ray tube and an x-ray film. The size of the image of the hole is measured on the exposed film. From the dimensions of the image and the position of the pinhole, the size of the apparent focal spot may be computed. For example, the dimension a of the apparent focal spot in Figure 4-12 may be computed from the corresponding dimension a' in the image by

$$a = a' \left(\frac{d_1}{d_2}\right) \qquad (4\text{-}5)$$

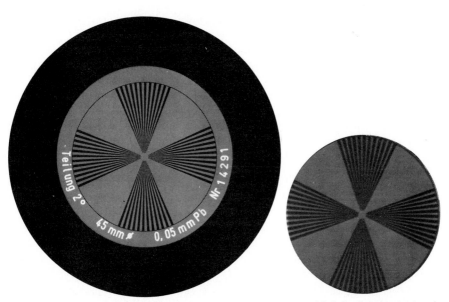

Fig 4-13.—Contact radiograph *(left)* and x-ray image *(right)* of a star test pattern. From the diameter of the blur zone in the x-ray image, the effective size of the focal spot may be computed. (From Hendee, W., Chaney, E., and Rossi, R.: *Radiologic Physics, Equipment and Quality Control* [Chicago: Year Book Medical Publishers, Inc., 1977].)

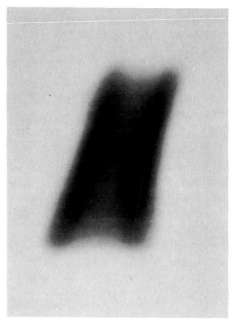

Fig 4-14. — Pinhole image of a "double banana" x-ray focal spot. (From Hendee, W., Chaney, E., and Rossi, R.: *Radiologic Physics, Equipment and Quality Control* [Chicago: Year Book Medical Publishers, Inc., 1977].)

where d_1 is the distance from target to pinhole and d_2 is the distance from pinhole to film.

Focal spot size also can be measured with a resolution test object such as the star pattern shown in Figure 4-13. The x-ray image of the pattern on the right of Figure 4-13 reveals a blur zone where the spokes of the test pattern are indistinct. From the diameter of the blur zone, the effective size of the focal spot can be computed in any dimension. This effective focal spot size may differ from pinhole camera measurements of the focal spot along the same dimension, because the diameter of the blur zone is influenced not only by the actual focal spot dimensions, but also by the distribution of x-ray intensity across the focal spot.[12] In most diagnostic x-ray tubes, this distribution is not uniform. Instead, the intensity tends to be concentrated at the edges of the focal spot in a direction perpendicular to the electron beam. The concentration of x-ray intensity at the edges of the focal spot is shown in the pinhole image in Figure 4-14. A focal spot with this configuration is called a *double banana* focal spot.

For most x-ray tubes, the size of the focal spot is not constant. Instead, it varies with both the tube current and the voltage applied to the x-ray tube.[13] This influence is shown in Figure 4-15 for the dimension of the focal spot parallel to the motion of impinging electrons. On the left of Figure 4-15, the growth or "blooming" of the focal spot with tube current is illustrated. The gradual reduction of the same focal spot dimension

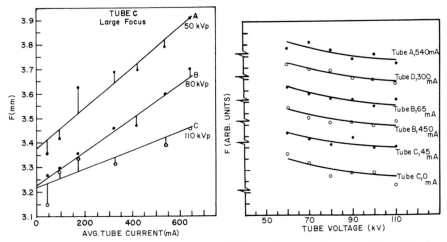

Fig 4-15.—Influence of tube current *(left)* and tube voltage *(right)* on the focal-spot size in a direction parallel to the motion of impinging electrons. (From Chaney, E., and Hendee, W.: Effects of x-ray tube current and voltage on effective focal-spot size, Med. Phys. 1:141, 1974.)

with increasing levels of peak kilovoltage is shown on the right of Figure 4-15.

Low-energy x rays generated in a tungsten target are attenuated severely during their escape from the target. For targets mounted at a small angle, the attenuation is greater for x rays emerging along the anode side

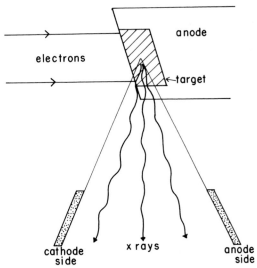

Fig 4-16.—The heel effect is produced by increased attenuation of x rays in the sloping target near the anode side of the x-ray beam.

of the x-ray beam than for those emerging along the side of the beam nearest the cathode (Fig 4-16). Consequently, the x-ray intensity decreases from the cathode to the anode side of the beam. This variation in intensity across an x-ray beam is termed the *heel effect*. The heel effect is noticeable particularly for x-ray beams used in diagnostic radiology, because the x-ray energy is relatively low and the target angles are steep. To compensate for the heel effect, a filter may be installed in the tube housing near the exit portal for the x-ray beam. The thickness of the filter increases from the anode to the cathode side of the x-ray beam. Positioning thicker portions of a patient near the cathode side of the x-ray beam also helps to compensate for the heel effect.

The heel effect increases with the steepness of the target angle and limits the maximum useful field size obtainable with any particular target angle. For example, a target angle no steeper than 12 degrees is recommended for x-ray examinations using 14 by 17 in. film at a 40-in. distance from the x-ray tube, whereas targets as steep as 7 degrees may be used if field sizes no larger than 10 by 10 in. are required at a 40-in. distance.

Targets with an angle of about 30 degrees are used in most therapy x-ray tubes. These targets furnish an apparent focal spot with dimensions between 5 and 7 mm. The larger focal spots reduce the nonuniformity in intensity across the x-ray beam, providing an x-ray beam that is reasonably uniform over a wide area. In therapy tubes operated at conventional voltages (140–400 kVp), x-rays are generated predominantly in a slightly forward direction with respect to the motion of impinging electrons. X rays generated in the forward direction pass through a thickness of target greater than that traversed by x rays released at angles nearer 90 degrees. Hence, the increased intensity of x rays in the forward direction is compensated by the increased attenuation of these photons, and a relatively uniform x-ray beam is obtained when the target angle is about 30 degrees. The target in an x-ray tube designed for operation at conventional voltages (<400 kVp) is termed a *reflectance target*, because the x-ray beam emerges at a right angle to the motion of electrons in the x-ray tube. With tube voltages of 1 million volts or more, x rays are produced predominantly in the direction of motion of the electrons impinging upon the target. *Transmission targets* are used in x-ray tubes designed for operation at these voltages. Usually, these targets consist of a thin layer of gold plated upon a water-cooled copper anode. X rays emerge from the target parallel to the path of electrons in the x-ray tube.

SPECIAL PURPOSE X-RAY TUBES

Many x-ray tubes have been designed for special applications. A few of these special purpose tubes are discussed in this chapter.

Grid-Controlled X-Ray Tubes

In a grid-controlled x-ray tube, the focusing cup within the cathode assembly is maintained a few hundred volts negative with respect to the filament over most of the voltage cycle applied to the x-ray tube. During this period, the negative potential of the focusing cup prevents the flow of electrons from the filament to the target across the tube. Only when the negative potential is removed can electrons flow across the x-ray tube. That is, applying and removing the potential difference between the focusing cup and the filament provides an off–on switch for the production of x rays. Grid-controlled x-ray tubes are used for very short exposures such as those required during angiographic radiography and cinefluorography.

X-Ray Tubes for Contact Therapy

X-ray tubes with thin, hollow anodes have been designed for the treatment of conditions of the skin. Contact therapy (Chaoul) x-ray tubes are operated at a voltage between 30 and 50 kVp. With the anode of a contact therapy x-ray tube positioned 1–5 cm above the skin surface, a large quantity of low-energy x rays may be delivered to the skin in a short time. The x-ray intensity decreases rapidly over the first few millimeters below the skin surface, primarily because of the rapid decrease in intensity with increasing distance from a radiation source only 1–5 cm away. The high attenuation of low-energy x rays in tissue also contributes to the rapid falloff in x-ray intensity below the surface.

Grenz-Ray X-Ray Tubes

Dermatologic conditions sometimes are treated with x rays generated at a voltage between 5 and 15 kVp. X rays produced at these voltages are termed *grenz rays* (grenz = border or boundary). To reduce the attenuation of x rays emerging from grenz-ray and contact therapy x-ray tubes, thin windows of beryllium are mounted in the glass envelope at the exit portal for the x-ray beam. Very high intensities of low-energy ("soft") x rays are emitted by grenz-ray tubes.

Stereographic X-Ray Tubes

Stereographic x-ray tubes (Fig 4-17) are similar to conventional rotating-anode x-ray tubes, except that the rotating anode is bombarded by two beams of electrons furnished by independent cathode assemblies. Stereographic x-ray tubes are used for stereoradiographic and stereofluoroscopic x-ray examinations.

Field-Emission X-Ray Tubes

In a field-emission x-ray tube, the cathode is a metal needle with a tip about 1 μ in diameter. Electrons are extracted from the cathode by an intense electric field rather than by thermionic emission. At diagnostic

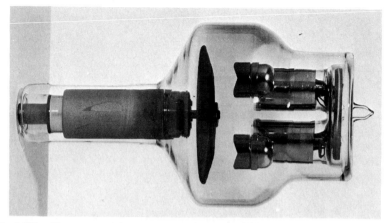

Fig 4-17.—Stereographic x-ray tube with two cathode assemblies and a rotating anode. (Courtesy of Machlett Laboratories, Inc.)

tube voltages, the rate of electron extraction is too low to provide tube currents adequate for most examinations, and field-emission x-ray tubes have been limited to pediatric radiography where lower tube currents can be tolerated. Field-emission tubes also have been used for high-voltage chest radiography because the higher tube voltage (300 kVp) enhances the extraction of electrons from the cathode.

Molybdenum Target X-Ray Tubes

For low-voltage studies of soft-tissue structures (e.g., mammography), x-ray tubes with molybdenum targets sometimes are preferred over tubes with tungsten targets. In the voltage range of 25–45 kVp, K-characteristic x rays can be produced in molybdenum but not in tungsten. These characteristic molybdenum x rays yield a concentration of x rays on the low-energy side of the x-ray spectrum (Fig 4-18), which enhances the visualization of soft-tissue structures.

RATINGS FOR X-RAY TUBES

Maximum Tube Voltage

The maximum voltage to be applied between cathode and anode is specified for every x-ray tube. This "voltage rating" depends upon the characteristics of the applied voltage (e.g., single phase or three phase) and upon the properties of the x-ray tube (e.g., distance between cathode and anode, shape of cathode and anode, and shape of the glass envelope). For example, the voltage rating for a Dunlee Duratron 300-13 rotating-anode x-ray tube is:

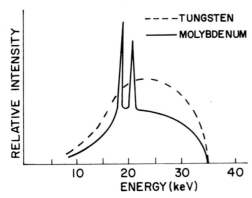

Fig 4-18. — X-ray spectrum from molybdenum *(solid line)* and tungsten *(dashed line)* target x-ray tubes. (From Hendee, W., Chaney, E., and Rossi, R.: *Radiologic Physics, Equipment and Quality Control* [Chicago: Year Book Medical Publishers, Inc., 1977].)

Maximum voltage: 150 kVp, fully rectified, with transformer center-grounded, voltage balanced to ground.

Occasional transient surges in voltage may be tolerated by an x-ray tube, provided the voltage surges exceed the voltage rating by only a few percent.

Maximum Filament Current and Voltage

Limitations are placed on the current and voltage delivered to coarse and fine filaments of an x-ray tube. For example, current and voltage ratings for the coarse (apparent focal spot of 2 mm) and fine (apparent focal spot of 1 mm) filaments of the Dunlee Duratron 300-13 tube are:

Small focal spot (1 mm): 3.0–8.5 V, 3.0–5.5 A. Large focal spot (2 mm): 4.0–14.0 V, 3.0–5.5 A. Operation of the filament at maximum current results in a reduction in filament life and should be done only intermittently.

The current rating for the filament should be reduced for continuous operation of the x-ray tube, because the temperature of the filament rises steadily as current flows through the filament.

Maximum Energy

Maximum-energy ratings are provided for the target, anode and housing of an x-ray tube.[14] These ratings are expressed in *heat units*, where for single-phase electric power

$$\text{Number of heat units (hu)} = (\text{Tube voltage})(\text{Tube current})(\text{Time})$$
$$= (\text{kVp})(\text{mA})(\text{sec})$$

If the tube voltage and current are constant, then 1 hu = 1 J of energy. For three-phase power, the number of heat units is computed as

$$\text{Number of heat units (hu)} = (\text{Tube voltage})(\text{Tube current})(\text{Time})(1.35)$$
$$= (\text{kVp})(\text{mA})(\text{sec})(1.35)$$

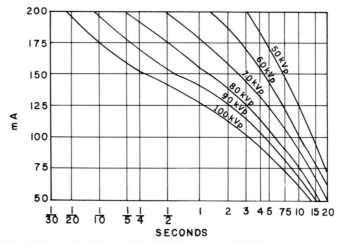

Fig 4-19. — Rating chart for a Machlett Dynamax "25" x-ray tube with a 1 mm focal spot and single-phase, fully rectified voltage. (Courtesy of Machlett Laboratories, Inc.)

Energy ratings for the anode and the tube housing are expressed in terms of heat-storage capacities, which indicate the number of heat units that may be absorbed without damage to these components. For example, maximum-energy ratings for the anode of a Dunlee Duratron 300-13 rotating-anode tube are:

Anode heat-storage capacity: 300,000 hu.

The heat-storage capacity of the x-ray tube housing also is important because heat is transferred from the anode to the tube housing. As an example, the housing heat-storage capacity is 1,500,000 hu for the housing usually used with a Machlett Dynamax "69" x-ray tube.

To determine whether the target of an x-ray tube might be damaged by a particular combination of tube voltage, tube current and exposure time, rating charts furnished with the x-ray tube should be consulted. For example, the rating chart reproduced in Figure 4-19 should be consulted before energizing the small filament of a Machlett Dynamax "25" x-ray tube supplied with single-phase, fully rectified voltage. To use this chart, a horizontal line is drawn between the desired tube current on the ordinate and the curve for the desired tube voltage. From the intersection of the horizontal line and the voltage curve, a vertical line crosses the abscissa at the maximum exposure time recommended for the x-ray tube. The area under each voltage curve encompasses combinations of tube current and exposure time that do not exceed the target-loading capacity when the x-ray tube is operated at that voltage. The area

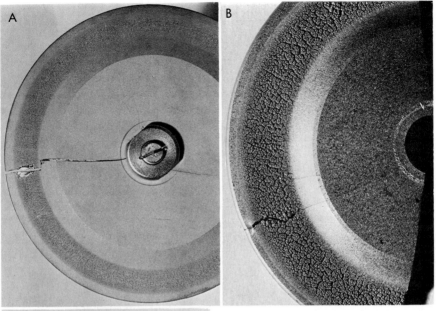

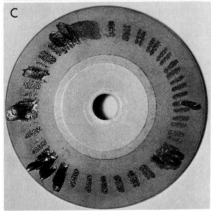

Fig 4-20. — Rotating targets damaged by excessive loading or improper rotation of the target. **A,** target cracked by lack of rotation. **B,** target damaged by slow rotation and excessive loading. **C,** target damaged by slow rotation. (From Bavor, G.: Motor controls and starting requirements for rotating anode x-ray tubes, Cathode Press 19:3, 1962.)

above each curve reflects combinations of tube current and exposure time that overload the x-ray tube and might damage the target. Often, switches are incorporated into an x-ray circuit to prevent the operator from exceeding the energy rating for the x-ray tube. Shown in Figure 4-20 are a few targets damaged by excess loading or improper rotation of the target.

An anode thermal-characteristics chart describes the rate at which energy may be delivered to an anode without exceeding its capacity for storing heat (Fig 4-21). Included in the chart is consideration of the rate

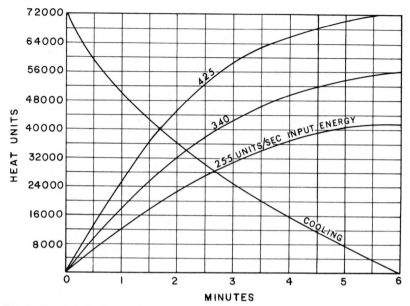

Fig 4-21.—Anode thermal-characteristics chart for a Machlett Dynamax "25" rotating anode x-ray tube. The anode heat-storage capacity is 72,000 heat units. (Courtesy of Machlett Laboratories, Inc.)

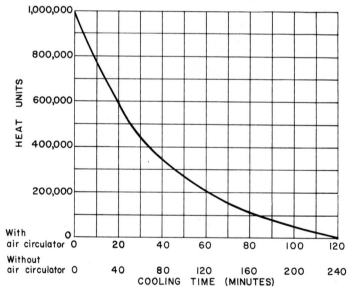

Fig 4-22.—Housing-cooling chart for a Machlett Dynamax "25" x-ray tube. (Courtesy of Machlett Laboratories, Inc.)

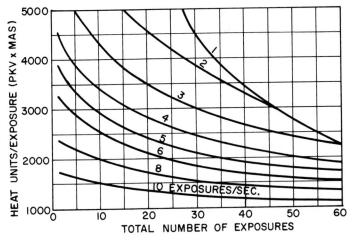

Fig 4-23. — Angiographic rating chart for a Machlett Super Dynamax x-ray tube, 1.0 mm focal spot, full-wave rectification, single phase.

at which heat is radiated from the anode to the insulating oil and housing. For example, the delivery of 425 hu/sec to the anode of a Machlett Dynamax "25" x-ray tube exceeds the anode heat-storage capacity after 5.5 min. The delivery of 340 hu/sec could be continued indefinitely. The cooling curve in Figure 4-21 shows the rate at which the anode cools after storing a certain amount of heat.

The housing-cooling chart in Figure 4-22 depicts the rate at which the tube housing cools after storing a certain amount of heat. Data describe the rate of cooling with and without forced circulation of air. Charts similar to those in Figures 4-21 and 4-22 are used to insure that multiple exposures in rapid succession do not damage an x-ray tube or its housing.

When a number of exposures are made over a short interval of time, a target-heating problem is created which is not covered adequately in any of the charts described above. This target-heating problem is caused by heat deposition in the focal track of the rotating anode at a more rapid rate than heat dissipation. To prevent this buildup of heat from damaging the target, an additional tube-rating chart should be consulted. This chart, termed an angiographic-rating chart because the problem of rapid successive exposures occurs frequently in angiographic radiography, is illustrated in Figure 4-23 for a Machlett Super Dynamax x-ray tube. Use of this chart is depicted in Example 4-8.

For x-ray tubes supplied with single-phase (1ϕ), fully rectified voltage, the peak current through the x-ray tube is about 1.4 times the average current. The average current nearly equals the peak current in x-ray generators supplied with three-phase (3ϕ) voltage. For this reason, the number of heat units for an exposure from a 3ϕ generator is computed as $1.35 \times$ (kVp)(mA)(time). For long exposures or a series of exposures with an x-ray tube supplied with 3ϕ voltage, more energy is delivered to the target, and the number of exposures in a given interval of time must be reduced.[15] Separate rating charts usually are provided for 1ϕ or 3ϕ operation of an x-ray tube.

Example 4-4

From the tube-rating chart in Figure 4-19, is a radiographic technique of 150 mA, 1 second at 100 kVp permissible?

The maximum exposure time is slightly longer than 0.25 second for 150 mA at 100 kVp. Therefore, the proposed technique is unacceptable.

Is 100 mA at 100 kVp for 1.5 seconds permissible?

The maximum exposure time is 3 seconds for 100 mA at 100 kVp. Therefore, the proposed technique is acceptable.

Example 4-5

Five minutes of fluoroscopy at 4 mA and 100 kVp are to be combined with eight 0.5-second spot films at 100 kVp and 100 mA. Is the technique permissible according to Figures 4-19 and 4-21?

The technique is acceptable according to the tube-rating chart in Figure 4-19. The rate of delivery of energy to the anode during fluoroscopy is (100 kVp)(4 mA) = 400 hu/sec. From Figure 4-21, after 5 minutes approximately 60,000 hu have been accumulated by the anode. The eight spot films contribute an additional 40,000 hu [(100 kVp)(100 mA)(0.5 sec) 8 = 40,000 hu]. After all exposures have been made, the total amount of heat stored in the anode is 40,000 + 60,000 = 100,000 hu. This amount of heat exceeds the anode heat-storage capacity of 72,000 hu. Consequently, the proposed technique is unacceptable.

Example 4-6

Three minutes of fluoroscopy at 3 mA and 85 kVp are combined with four 0.25-second spot films at 85 kVp and 150 mA. From Figure 4-20, what time must elapse before the procedure may be repeated?

The rate of delivery of energy to the anode is (85 kVp)(3 mA) = 255 hu/sec, resulting in a heat load of 31,000 hu after 3 minutes. To this head load is added (85 kVp)(150 mA)(0.25 sec)(4) = 12,750 hu for the four spot films, yielding a total heat load of 43,750 hu. From the position on the vertical axis corresponding to this heat load, a horizontal line is extended to intersect the anode-cooling curve at 1.4 minutes. From this intersection, the anode must cool until its residual heat load is (72,000 − 43,750) = 28,250 hu, so that when the 43,750 hu from the next procedure is added to the residual heat load, the total heat load does not exceed the 72,000 hu anode heat-storage capacity. The time corresponding to a residual heat load of 28,250 hu is 2.6 minutes. Hence, the cooling time required between procedures is (2.6 − 1.4) = 1.2 minutes.

Example 4-7

From Figures 4-19 and 4-21, it is apparent that three exposures per minute are acceptable, if each exposure is taken at 0.5 second, 125 mA and 100 kVp. Could this procedure be repeated each minute for 1 hour?

Rate of transfer of energy to the housing

$$= (100 \text{ kVp})(125 \text{ mA})(0.5 \text{ sec})(3 \text{ exposures/min})$$
$$= 18,750 \text{ hu/min}$$

At the end of 1 hr, (18,750 hu/min)(60 min/hr) = 1,125,000 hu will have been delivered to the housing. The heat-storage capacity of the housing is only 1 million hu. Without forced circulation of air, the maximum rate of energy dissipation from the housing is estimated to be approximately 12,500 hu/min (Fig 4-22). With air circulation, the rate of energy dissipation is 25,000 hu/min. Therefore, the procedure is unacceptable if the housing is not air-cooled and acceptable if the housing is cooled by forced circulation of air.

Example 4-8

From Figure 4-23, how many consecutive exposures can be made at a rate of 6 exposures per second, if each exposure is taken at 85 kVp, 500 mA and 0.05 second?

Each exposure produces (85 kVp)(500 mA)(0.05 sec) = 2,125 hu. A horizontal line from this position on the y-axis intersects the 6 exposures per second curve at a position corresponding to 20 exposures. Hence, no more than 20 exposures should be made at a rate of 6 exposures per second.

PROBLEMS

1. Explain why tube current is more likely to be limited by space charge in an x-ray tube operated at low voltage and high tube current than in a tube operated at high voltage and low current. Would you expect the tube current to be space-charge limited or filament-emission limited in an x-ray tube used for mammography? What would you expect for an x-ray tube used for chest radiography at 120 kVp and 100 mA?

*2. How many electrons flow from cathode to anode each second in an x-ray tube with a tube current of 50 mA? (1 A = 1 coulomb/sec). If the tube voltage is constant and equals 100 kV, at what rate (J/sec) is energy delivered to the anode?

3. Explain why off-focus radiation is reduced greatly by shutters placed near the target of the x-ray tube.

*4. An apparent focal spot of 1 mm is projected from an x-ray tube. The true focal spot is 5 mm. What is the target angle? Why is the heel effect greater in an x-ray beam from a target with a small target angle?

*5. From Figure 4-19, is a radiographic technique of 125 mA for 3 seconds at 90 kVp permissible? Is a 4-second exposure at 90 kVp, 100 mA permissible?

°For those problems marked with an asterisk, answers are provided on the pages following the appendixes (see pp. 487–488).

Why does the number of milliampere-seconds permitted for a particular voltage increase as the exposure time is increased?

*6. From Figures 4-19 and 4-21, is it permissible to combine four 0.5-second spot films/min at 90 kVp and 100 mA with 4 minutes of fluoroscopy at 90 kVp and 4 mA? If the technique is not permitted, then how many spot films should be eliminated to reduce the total heat delivered to the anode to a permissible level?

*7. From Figure 4-22, how many exposures are permitted each minute over a period of 1 hour, if each exposure is made for 1 second at 100 mA and 90 kVp? The tube is operated with forced circulation of air.

*8. What kinetic energy do electrons possess when they reach the target of an x-ray tube operated at 250 kVp? What is the approximate ratio of bremsstrahlung to characteristic radiation produced by these electrons? Calculate the minimum wavelength of x-ray photons generated at 250 kVp.

*9. A lead plate is positioned 20 in. from the target of a diagnostic x-ray tube. The plate is 50 in. from a film cassette. The plate has a hole 0.1 mm in diameter. The image of the hole is 5 mm. What is the size of the apparent focal spot?

*10. The target slopes at an angle of 12 degrees in a diagnostic x-ray tube. Electrons are focused along a strip of the target 2 mm wide. How long is the strip if the apparent focal spot is 2 mm × 2 mm?

REFERENCES

1. Röntgen, W.: Über eine neue Art von Strahlen (vorläufige Mitteilung), Sitzungs-Berichte der Physikalisch-medicinischen Gesellschaft zu Würzburg 9:132, 1895.

2. Klickstein, H.: William Conrad Röntgen: On a new kind of rays—a bibliographical study, in *Mallinckrodt Classics of Radiology* (St. Louis: Mallinckrodt Chemical Works, 1966), vol. 1.

3. Etter, L. (ed.): *The Science of Ionizing Radiation* (Springfield, Ill.: Charles C Thomas, Publisher, 1965).

4. Glasser, O.: *Dr. W. C. Röntgen* (2d ed.; Springfield, Ill.: Charles C Thomas, Publisher, 1958).

5. Donizetti, P.: *Shadow and Substance: The Story of Medical Radiography* (Oxford: Pergamon Press, Inc., 1967).

6. Coolidge, W.: A powerful röntgen ray tube with a pure electron discharge, Phys. Rev. 2:409, 1913.

7. Ulrey, C.: An experimental investigation of the energy in the continuous x-ray spectra of certain elements, Phys. Rev. 11:401, 1918.

8. Botden, P.: Modern Trends in Diagnostic Radiologic Instrumentation, in Moseley, R., and Rust, J. (eds.): *The Reduction of Patient Dose by Diagnostic Radiologic Instrumentation* (Springfield, Ill.: Charles C Thomas, Publisher, 1964), p. 15.

9. Ter-Pogossian, M.: *The Physical Aspects of Diagnostic Radiology* (New York: Harper & Row, 1967), p. 107.

10. International Commission on Radiological Units and Measurements: *Methods of Evaluating Radiological Equipment and Materials.* Recommendations of the ICRU. National Bureau of Standards Handbook 89, 1962.

11. Parrish, W.: Improved method of measuring x-ray tube focus, Rev. Sci. Instrum. 38:1779, 1967.

12. Hendee, W., and Chaney, E.: X-ray focal spots: practical considerations, Appl. Radiol. 3:25, 1974.
13. Chaney, E., and Hendee, W.: Effects of x-ray tube current and voltage on effective focal-spot size, Med. Phys. 1:141, 1974.
14. Hallock, A.: A review of methods used to calculate heat loading of x-ray tubes extending the life of rotating anode x-ray tubes, Cathode Press 15:1, 1958.
15. Hallock, A.: Introduction to three phase rating of rotating anode tubes, Cathode Press 23:30, 1966.

5 / X-Ray Circuits

ELECTRIC CIRCUITS in modern x-ray generators are complex and vary from one type of generator to another. Fortunately, x-ray generators may be understood conceptually by studying a few simple circuits. A simple x-ray generator is depicted in the circuit diagram in Figure 5-1. This diagram may be divided into: (1) a primary circuit, (2) a filament circuit and (3) a high-voltage circuit. Each of these parts may be discussed independently of the other two.

THE PRIMARY CIRCUIT

The rudimentary primary circuit in Figure 5-1 contains an autotransformer A with switches S_1 and S_2, a primary winding P of a high-voltage transformer, a voltmeter V, a timer, and a switch S, which is operated by the remote exposure switch S_w.

Autotransformer

An *autotransformer* consists of a length of wire coiled around a laminated iron core. Alternating voltage (usually 110, 220 or 440 V) from the "line" or "mains" is applied across a small number of windings referred to as the autotransformer primary. Alternating voltage is induced across the remaining windings of the transformer. By connecting the kilovolt-major switch S_1 and the kilovolt-minor switch S_2 to different "taps" on the autotransformer, the alternating voltage applied to the primary P of the high-voltage transformer may be varied. For example, when the kilovolt-minor switch is fixed and a voltage of 100 V is supplied to a particular autotransformer, the data in Table 5-1 depict the variation in voltage across the high-voltage primary as the position of the kilovolt-major switch is changed.

TABLE 5-1.—VOLTAGE ACROSS PRIMARY OF HIGH-VOLTAGE TRANSFORMER FOR DIFFERENT POSITIONS OF KILOVOLT-MAJOR SWITCH (SECONDARY OF HIGH-VOLTAGE TRANSFORMER IS OPEN)

KILOVOLT-MAJOR POSITION	VOLTAGE ACROSS PRIMARY
1	120
3	140
5	160
7	180
9	200

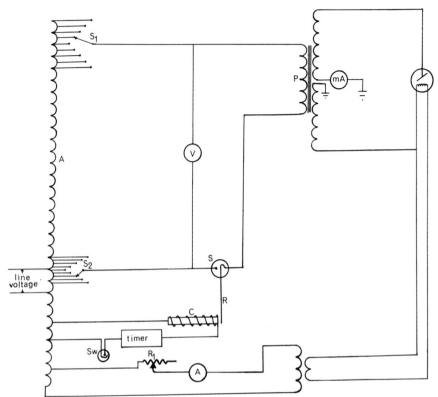

Fig 5-1. — Circuit diagram for an elementary x-ray generator.

Small changes in the voltage applied to the high-voltage primary P are accomplished with the kilovolt-minor switch S_2. Usually, a change of ten steps in the kilovolt-minor switch or push-button array furnishes the same change in voltage across P as that provided by a change of one step in the kilovolt-major switch. This difference in sensitivity of voltage regulation is related to the greater number of turns of the autotransformer included between taps for switch S_1 compared to the number included between taps for switch S_2. Kilovolt-major and kilovolt-minor switches should not be adjusted during exposure, because contacts between the switches and taps on the autotransformer may be damaged by electric arcing.

Sometimes a variable resistance (rheostat) is substituted for the closely spaced taps and selector switch or push-button array S_1 of the kilovolt-minor control. In principle, a large rheostat could replace the entire autotransformer. However, this substitution is not desirable, because it would lower the efficiency of the voltage divider and reduce the stability of the voltage supplied to the primary of the high-voltage transformer.

Primary Voltmeter

The voltage across the primary of the high-voltage transformer may be measured by a "load-on" or a "preread" voltmeter V. When switch S is open, the load-on voltmeter indicates the "open circuit" voltage across the primary of the high-voltage transformer. The voltmeter reading is reduced when switch S is closed, because voltage is applied across components of the primary circuit other than the primary of the high-voltage transformer. As the current increases in the primary circuit, the difference between the voltage indicated before and during exposure increases. To compensate for this reduction in voltage during exposure, the voltage indicated by a load-on voltmeter before exposure must be higher than the voltage desired for the exposure. With a load-on voltmeter, the pre-exposure voltage required for a certain voltage during exposure is determined by consulting a chart furnished with the x-ray generator.

A preread voltmeter consists of a variable resistance in series with a voltmeter. The resistance is varied until the voltmeter reading before exposure reflects the voltage across the transformer primary during exposure. For an x-ray generator with a preread voltmeter, the kilovolt-major and kilovolt-minor controls are adjusted until the voltmeter indicates the voltage desired across the x-ray tube during exposure. No attention is paid to the decreased reading of the preread voltmeter during exposure.

The voltage applied to the x-ray tube depends upon the voltage induced across the secondary of the high-voltage transformer. When no load is placed across the secondary (i.e., when no current flows in the high-voltage circuit), the voltage V_s across the transformer secondary is

$$V_s = V_p \frac{N_s}{N_p} \tag{5-1}$$

In equation (5-1), V_p is the primary voltage and N_s/N_p is the ratio of secondary to primary turns in the transformer. When current flows in the high-voltage circuit, the voltage across the transformer secondary decreases from that predicted by equation (5-1). Listed in Table 5-2 are voltages across the primary and secondary of a high-voltage transformer with different currents flowing in the high-voltage circuit. For a given primary voltage, the voltage decreases across the transformer secondary (and across the x-ray tube) as the current increases in the high-voltage circuit. Charts may be compiled that relate the voltage across an x-ray tube to the voltage delivered to the transformer primary and to the current in the high-voltage circuit. These charts are consulted when a primary voltage is selected for a particular exposure. Often, the scale of a load-on voltmeter provides a direct indication of tube voltage. If only a

TABLE 5-2. — VOLTAGES ACROSS PRIMARY AND
SECONDARY OF HIGH-VOLTAGE TRANSFORMER
FOR DIFFERENT CURRENTS FLOWING IN
HIGH-VOLTAGE CIRCUIT

PRIMARY VOLTAGE (V)	SECONDARY VOLTAGE (kV)		
	NO LOAD	100 mA	500 mA
100	58	50	34
120	71	62	48
140	84	76	60
160	96	88	74
180	110	101	86
200	122	114	100

few different currents flow through the high-voltage circuit and the x-ray
tube, then a separate scale for each current may be provided on the voltmeter (Fig 5-2).

A kilovoltmeter compensation circuit eliminates the need for more
than one voltage scale on the voltmeter. This circuit consists of a variable
resistance and a few windings of the autotransformer connected in parallel with the voltmeter. As different tube currents are selected, the resistance in the compensation circuit changes to provide a "bucking voltage," which causes the voltmeter to indicate the voltage across the x-ray
tube during exposure. Sometimes the bucking voltage is varied by
changing the number of turns of the autotransformer included in the kilovoltmeter compensation circuit.

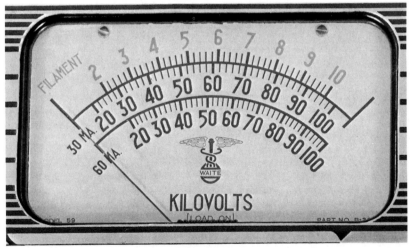

Fig 5-2. — A load-on voltmeter that indicates tube voltage for two different
tube currents. (Courtesy of Picker X-Ray Corp.)

Line-Voltage Compensation

In some x-ray generators, a line-voltage compensation voltmeter is connected across a few windings of the autotransformer. Usually, this meter replaces the voltmeter connected across the primary of the high-voltage transformer. A line-voltage compensation circuit is used often in x-ray generators with kilovolt-major and kilovolt-minor switches or push-button arrays which designate the voltage across the x-ray tube for each setting of the switches or push-buttons. A switch that selects the voltage supplied to the autotransformer is adjusted until the voltage indicated by the compensation voltmeter reaches a desired value. Often, the desired value is indicated by a mark on the face of the compensation voltmeter. With a line-voltage compensation voltmeter, the voltage supplied to the autotransformer and, consequently, to all components of the x-ray circuit, is relatively constant from one use of the x-ray generator to the next. To compensate for changes in the voltage across the x-ray tube as current is varied in the high-voltage circuit, a variable resistance may be placed in series with the compensation voltmeter. This resistance increases with current through the x-ray tube, causing the voltage indicated by the compensation voltmeter to decrease. The indicated voltage is returned to the desired value by adjusting the selector switch for line voltage. Therefore, with increasing current through the x-ray tube, the voltage is increased across the primary of the high-voltage transformer. This increase in voltage across the transformer primary compensates for the reduction in tube voltage caused by the higher current in the high-voltage circuit. With a variable resistance in series with the line-voltage compensation voltmeter, the tube voltage designated by the kilovolt-major and kilovolt-minor controls is accurate for all currents through the x-ray tube.

Exposure Switch

The switch S closes the primary circuit and permits current to flow through the primary of the high-voltage transformer. With many x-ray generators, the exposure switch is operated by hand or foot and may be positioned at some distance from the generator console. A remote switch (S_w) is included in Figure 5-1. When the switch is closed, current flows through coil C and magnetizes the soft-iron core within the coil. The insulated rod R is attracted to the magnetized core, closing the switch S in the primary circuit. This type of switch, termed a *contactor*, is inadequate for exposures shorter than about $1/60$ second. Gas-filled tubes (thyratrons) and solid-state devices (silicon-controlled rectifiers) are used when an exposure switch with a rapid response is required.

Usually incorporated within the circuit for the exposure switch is a timer which terminates the exposure after a selected interval of time has elapsed. A mechanical (spring-driven), synchronous or impulse timer is used for therapy x-ray generators and for some diagnostic x-ray generators. Exposures shorter than about $1/120$ second require an electronic timer.[1]

Timers used with diagnostic x-ray generators may be checked and adjusted accurately with the aid of a radiation detector and an oscilloscope. The accuracy of a timer may be estimated by exposing a small disk that is rotating upon an x-ray film. The disk is relatively opaque to x rays and contains a small hole along its edge. For a 1ϕ x-ray generator, the number of images of the hole recorded by the radiograph should correspond to the number of x-ray pulses that occurred during the interval used for the exposure. For example, a full-wave rectified, single-phase x-ray generator produces 2 pulses per voltage cycle or 12 pulses during an exposure interval of 0.1 second. If the timer is accurate, 12 images of the hole should be present on a radiograph obtained by an exposure of 0.1 second to a full-wave rectified, single-phase x-ray beam.

To estimate timer accuracy for a 3ϕ x-ray unit, the same method may be applied provided that the disk is rotated at a known frequency, usually by coupling the disk to a small synchronous motor. During exposure, the hole in the disk sweeps out an arc of exposed film, and the length of the arc is an indication of exposure time. For example, a disk rotating at 60 revolutions/second will yield a 180-degree arc of exposed film for an exposure time of $1/120$ second (8 msec).

Phototiming

After a desired amount of radiation has reached an x-ray film, an exposure may be terminated by a phototimer. A simplified phototiming circuit is shown in Figure 5-3. X rays transmitted through the patient and grid produce light as they strike a small (e.g., 4 by 4 in.) fluorescent screen. The light is directed onto the photocathode of a photomultiplier tube.* As the light is absorbed, electrons are liberated from the photocathode and accelerated toward the anode of the photomultiplier tube. The number of electrons increases as the electrons strike electrodes (dynodes) on their way to the anode. The resulting electric signal from the photomultiplier tube charges the capacitor C†. After the capacitor

*Photomultiplier tubes are discussed further in Chapter 11.

†A capacitor (or condenser) is composed of two conducting plates separated by an insulator. A potential difference exists between the plates when one plate stores a charge opposite in sign to that stored on the other plate.

$$V = \frac{Q}{C}$$

where V is the potential difference between the plates in volts, Q is the charge on either plate in coulombs and C is the "capacitance" of the capacitor in farads.

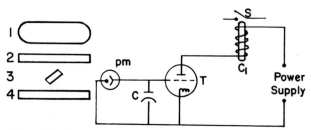

Fig 5-3. — A simplified phototiming circuit: *(1)* patient, *(2)* grid, *(3)* fluorescent screen, *(4)* film cassette.

reaches a certain voltage, the gas-filled thyratron tube T discharges through coil C_1. When current flows through coil C_1, the exposure switch opens in the primary circuit. In summary, the exposure switch opens after a selected number of x rays have passed through the patient and impinged on the film cassette. The density control of the phototimer determines the number of photons that are transmitted before the exposure is terminated. By adjusting the density control, radiographs of greater or lesser density may be achieved, according to the preference of the operator. With a phototimer, radiographs of acceptable density are obtained irrespective of variations in patient thickness and radiographic technique.[2]

THE FILAMENT CIRCUIT

Filament Transformer

Alternating voltage for the filament circuit in Figure 5-1 is supplied by the autotransformer. Part of the voltage from the autotransformer is applied across the primary of the filament transformer. The voltage V_s induced across the secondary is proportional to N_s/N_p, the ratio of secondary to primary turns on the filament transformer. The ratio N_s/N_p is less than 1 for a filament transformer, providing a voltage of 5–15 V across the secondary of the transformer. A transformer used to reduce voltage (e.g., a filament transformer) is a "step-down transformer"; a transformer that increases voltage (e.g., a high-voltage transformer) is a "step-up transformer."

Usually, the cathode assembly of the x-ray tube is connected to the secondary of the high-voltage transformer. The filament transformer isolates the high voltage of the cathode assembly from ground potential. The primary and secondary of most filament transformers are coiled around a soft-iron core and insulated from each other and from the core by oil.

Selection of Filament Current

In Figure 5-1, the voltage across the primary of the filament transformer is changed with the variable resistance R_1 connected in series with the transformer primary. The voltage across the transformer primary determines the voltage induced across the transformer secondary and, consequently, the voltage applied across the filament of the x-ray tube. The current through the filament and, therefore, the filament temperature vary with the filament voltage. The current through the x-ray tube varies with the temperature of the filament. Hence, the variable resistance R_1 may be used to regulate the current through the x-ray tube.

The tube current may be varied continuously if a variable resistance such as R_1 (Fig 5-1) is placed in the filament circuit. For variation of the tube current in discrete steps, a set of fixed resistances and a selector switch or push-button array may be substituted for the variable resistance. A coil sometimes is substituted for the variable resistance or set of fixed resistances and selector switch. The self-inductance* of the coil

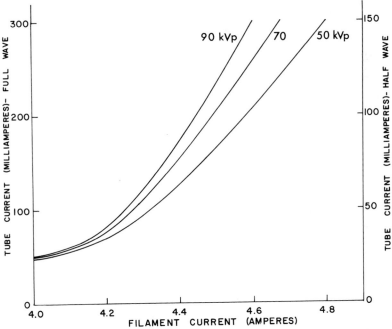

Fig 5-4. — Typical filament-increment chart used to select the filament current necessary for a desired tube current at a specific tube voltage. (Courtesy of Picker X-Ray Corp.)

*The self-inductance of a coil describes the voltage induced across the coil in opposition to a changing current in the coil.

and, therefore, its impedance to the flow of current may be varied continuously or in discrete steps.

If the current through an x-ray tube is space-charge limited, then the current varies with the voltage across the x-ray tube as well as with the filament current. To obtain a desired tube current at a particular tube voltage, a filament current may be selected from a filament-increment chart (Fig 5-4).

Space-Charge Compensation

A filament-increment chart is not provided with newer x-ray generators. Instead, a space-charge transformer is positioned in the filament circuit in parallel with a small section of the autotransformer. The voltage induced across the secondary of this transformer is applied across the primary of the filament transformer in opposition to the voltage supplied directly by the autotransformer. With the space-charge transformer connected to the kilovolt-major switch, the opposing voltage supplied to the filament transformer increases with the voltage across the x-ray tube. Consequently, the filament current and temperature decrease with increasing voltage across the x-ray tube, and the current through the x-ray tube remains constant. In this manner, the space-charge compensating circuit eliminates the dependence of tube current upon the voltage applied across the x-ray tube.

Stabilization of Filament Voltage

A current of less than 6 A usually flows through the filament of an x-ray tube. The current flowing from filament to target in the x-ray tube usually does not exceed 1,200 mA. Small fluctuations in filament current cause large changes in the temperature of the filament and in the current through the x-ray tube. To reduce the fluctuation in tube current, most manufacturers include a voltage stabilizer (constant-voltage transformer) in the filament circuit. The voltage supplied by the voltage stabilizer varies by less than $\pm 0.1\%$ for fluctuations in line voltage as large as $\pm 10\%$.

Tube-Current Stabilization

The current in an x-ray tube is affected by factors other than fluctuations in the voltage supplied to the filament. For example, a series of exposures may raise the temperature of the x-ray tube, increasing the filament temperature and tube current for a particular setting of the tube-current control. Over a long period, evaporation of tungsten from the heated filament and anode may cause the deposition of a layer of tungsten upon the glass envelope of the x-ray tube. The deposited tungsten attenuates x-ray photons and reduces the intensity of the x-ray beam produced by a certain current through the x-ray tube. Also, the diameter of the filament is reduced by evaporation. As the diameter decreases, the resistance of the filament increases and a selected filament current heats the filament to a higher temperature.

A circuit for improving the stability of the current through an x-ray tube may be added to the high-voltage circuit. This circuit changes the current through the filament of the x-ray tube in response to variations in current through the x-ray tube. If a circuit to stabilize the tube current is included in the high-voltage circuit, then a voltage stabilizer and space-charge compensating circuit may not be needed in the filament circuit.

HIGH-VOLTAGE CIRCUIT

Self-Rectification

The voltage induced across the secondary of the high-voltage transformer may be applied directly to the x-ray tube. Under normal circumstances, electrons flow through the x-ray tube only when the cathode is negative and the target is positive. Consequently, a pulsating direct current flows in the x-ray tube and high-voltage circuit. Since the x-ray tube permits current to flow in one direction only, the x-ray tube acts as a rectifier and the mode of rectification is termed *self-rectification.*

The *inverse half-cycle* is the portion of the alternating-voltage cycle during which no current flows in the high-voltage circuit and x-ray tube. When the current in the high-voltage circuit is zero, no voltage is dropped across components of the circuit other than the x-ray tube. Hence, the voltage across the x-ray tube during the inverse half-cycle exceeds that applied across the x-ray tube during the conducting portion of the voltage cycle. The x-ray tube and high-voltage cables must be constructed to withstand this higher voltage. Also, electrons may be released from a target heated during prolonged bombardment by electrons. These electrons may be accelerated from target to cathode during the inverse half-cycle and may damage the filament or cathode assembly of the x-ray tube.

Suppression of Inverse Voltage

A circuit that suppresses the voltage across the x-ray tube during the inverse half-cycle may be included in the primary circuit of a self-rectified x-ray generator. An inverse-voltage suppression circuit is diagramed in Figure 5-5 and is used often for x-ray tubes with currents less than 30 mA. The rectifier R_e allows current to flow in one direction only. During the inverse half-cycle, the current flows through the shunt resistance R. The large voltage drop across R reduces the voltage applied to the primary of the high-voltage transformer. Hence, the voltage across the x-ray tube is reduced during the inverse half-cycle.

A current in the high-voltage circuit and x-ray tube requires a much larger current in the primary circuit. Since the current through a rectifier

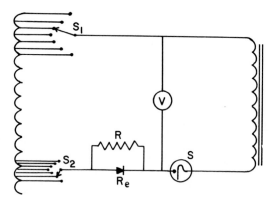

Fig 5-5. — Circuit for suppressing the voltage across an x-ray tube during the inverse half-cycle.

must not exceed a certain maximum, many rectifiers would be required to suppress the inverse voltage across an x-ray tube with a high tube current. For an x-ray tube with a high tube current, methods are used to remove the voltage completely from the tube during the inverse cycle.

Rectifiers

Current flows through a rectifier in one direction only. The rectifier symbol > designates the direction of current flow. By convention, the direction of current flow in a circuit is opposite to the motion of electrons in the circuit.

$> |$

Current $\rightarrow$

$\leftarrow$ Electrons

Rectifier tubes (sometimes called *diodes, kenotrons* or *valves*) were used in x-ray circuits for many years (Fig 5-6). In these devices, electrons are released from a large, heated tungsten filament, which may be impregnated with thorium to increase the emission of electrons. The electrons are attracted to a cylinder surrounding the filament when the cylinder is positive and the filament is negative. The voltage drop across the rectifier tube is relatively low (4–6 kVp), because electrons are emitted in excess by the filament and because the cylindrical anode is easily accessible. Although low-energy x rays are produced as the electrons strike the anode, most of these x rays are absorbed by the glass envelope of the rectifier tube. To attenuate x rays further and to reduce the hazard of exposure of personnel to high voltage, rectifiers usually are placed in the insulated tank for the high-voltage transformer.

Solid-state, barrier-layer rectifiers have replaced rectifier tubes in new-

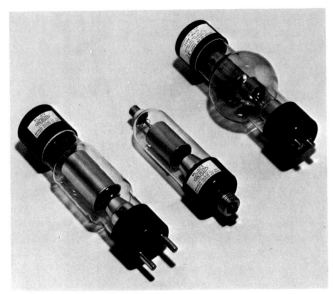

Fig 5-6.—Typical rectifier tubes used in x-ray circuits. (Courtesy of Machlett Laboratories, Inc.)

er x-ray generators. Certain semiconducting elements (e.g., selenium, germanium, copper oxide and silicon) conduct electrons in one direction only. A rectifier element or cell is constructed by plating a conductor with a thin "barrier layer" of one of these semiconducting elements. A cell resembles a dime in thickness and size. A rectifier stack is a group of cells assembled upon an insulated rod passing through holes in the center of the cells. Rectifier stacks composed of selenium or silicon cells are used in modern x-ray generators. The drop in voltage in the conducting direction across a silicon rectifier is lower and more constant than that across a selenium rectifier. However, selenium rectifiers are less expen-

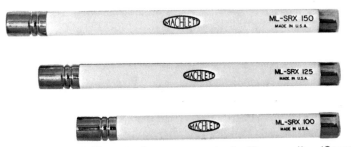

Fig 5-7.—Typical rectifier stacks composed of silicon cells. (Courtesy of Machlett Laboratories, Inc.)

sive than silicon rectifiers. Advantages of solid-state rectifiers over valve tubes include: (1) longer life (no filament burnout or deactivation), (2) no radiation hazard, (3) greater current stability, (4) lower voltage drop in the conducting direction, (5) smaller size and (6) elimination of voltage supplies for tube filaments.[3] Rectifier stacks of silicon cells are shown in Figure 5-7.

Half-Wave Rectification

If two rectifiers are added to the high-voltage circuit, then voltage is not applied across the x-ray tube during the inverse half-cycle. Some of the problems encountered with self-rectification (e.g., increased insulation and the possibility of electron flow from target to cathode) are eliminated by this mode of rectification, termed *half-wave rectification*. Illustrated in Figure 5-8 are a circuit for half-wave rectification and the tube voltage and current produced when this circuit is used. Half-wave rectification is almost never used in modern x-ray generators.

Full-Wave Rectification

Full-wave rectification is achieved by placing four rectifiers in the high-voltage circuit. In Figure 5-9, electrons follow the path *ABFEDCGH* when end *A* of the secondary of the high-voltage transformer is negative. When the voltage across the secondary reverses polarity, the

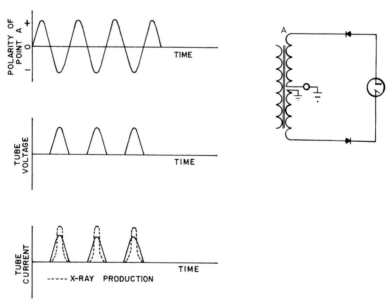

Fig 5-8.—A circuit for half-wave rectification **(right),** with resulting tube voltage, tube current and efficiency for production of x rays. Rectifiers indicate the direction of current flow.

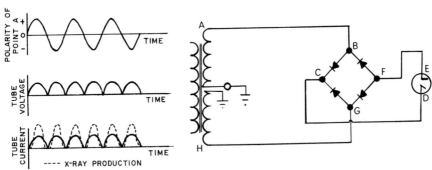

Fig 5-9.—A circuit for full-wave rectification **(right),** with resulting tube voltage, tube current and efficiency for production of x rays.

electron path is *HGFEDCBA*. With full-wave rectification, the x-ray tube filament is negative and the x-ray tube target is positive during both half-cycles of the voltage across the high-voltage transformer. Hence, full-wave rectification doubles the number of voltage pulses of desired polarity applied across the x-ray tube in a given interval of time. Also, the effective tube current is higher with full-wave rectification, because the current is not averaged over half-cycles of tube voltage during which the current is zero. Almost always, full-wave rectification is used in x-ray generators with tube currents greater than 100 mA.

The voltage across an x-ray tube may be kept nearly constant by placing a circuit with high capacitance in parallel with the x-ray tube. Constant-voltage circuits are used frequently in x-ray generators for radiation therapy.

Center-Tapped High-Voltage Secondary

The center of the secondary of the high-voltage transformer almost always is grounded electrically (Figs 5-8 and 5-9). A center tap that is grounded electrically decreases the potential difference between each end of the high-voltage secondary and ground and reduces the insulation required for the high-voltage cables and transformer. For example, if a voltage of 100 kVp is induced across a transformer secondary with a grounded center tap, then one end of the secondary is 50 kVp positive with respect to ground, and the other end is 50 kVp negative with respect to ground. A milliammeter for measuring the current through the x-ray tube may be inserted between the center tap and ground. The meter is at ground potential and may be installed on the console of the x-ray generator without danger to the operator.

Villard Voltage-Doubling Circuit

Circuits have been designed to increase the tube voltage above that furnished by the secondary of the high-voltage transformer. An example

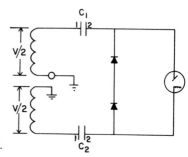

Fig 5-10. — Villard voltage-doubling circuit.

is the Villard voltage-doubling circuit illustrated in Figure 5-10. Suppose a maximum voltage V is induced across the transformer secondary. During the inverse half-cycle, a voltage $V/2$ is developed across each of the capacitors C_1 and C_2. When the polarity reverses, Plate 1 of C_2 is $V/2$ volts negative with respect to ground and Plate 2 of C_2 is $V/2$ volts negative with respect to Plate 1. Therefore, the filament of the x-ray tube is $(V/2 + V/2)$ or V volts negative with respect to ground. Similarly, Plate 1 of C_1 is $V/2$ volts positive with respect to ground during the conducting half-cycle, and Plate 2 of C_1 is $V/2$ volts positive with respect to Plate 1. Consequently, the target is V volts positive with respect to ground. With a voltage V induced across the transformer secondary, a potential difference of $2V$ exists between filament and target of the x-ray tube. Even greater amplification of voltage is possible with Villard circuits connected in cascade.

THREE-PHASE CIRCUITS

Many newer diagnostic x-ray generators are designed to use three-phase power. Single-phase (1ϕ) and three-phase (3ϕ) voltages are compared in Figure 5-11. Both voltages are full-wave rectified. The solid envelope in the diagram for 3ϕ voltage describes the voltage across an x-ray tube when full-wave rectified, 3ϕ voltage is used. Dotted lines in this diagram indicate how the envelope is produced. With 3ϕ voltage and six rectifiers in the high-voltage circuit, the fluctuation in tube voltage (percent ripple) is about 13%. During each cycle, six voltage pulses are applied across the x-ray tube and six x-ray pulses are produced. Hence, a 3ϕ circuit with six rectifiers is termed a *six-pulse circuit*. With six more rectifiers added to the high-voltage circuit, the percent ripple may be reduced to 3 or 4%. With 12 rectifiers in the high-voltage circuit, either 6 or 12 x-ray pulses may be produced during each cycle. An x-ray generator that releases 12 x-ray pulses per cycle is termed a 3ϕ, 12-pulse unit.

With 1ϕ, full-wave rectified voltage across an x-ray tube, the average

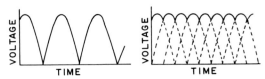

Fig 5-11.—Single-phase **(left)** and three-phase **(right)** voltages across an x-ray tube. Both voltages are full-wave rectified. The three-phase voltage is furnished by a six-pulse circuit.

current (more correctly, *effective current**) through the tube is about 71% of the peak current. With 3φ voltage and a six-pulse circuit, the average tube current is about 95% of the peak current. Target-loading capacities are based upon the peak current through the x-ray tube. Without exceeding the target-loading capacity of an x-ray tube, the average tube current often may be higher in a 3φ circuit than in a 1φ circuit. The higher average current permits a reduction in the time required for a particular diagnostic exposure. As an example of this reduction, spot-film radiographic techniques with 1φ and 3φ voltage are compared in Table 5-3. Part of the reduction in milliampere-seconds indicated in the table results from an increase in the average tube current permissible with 3φ tube voltage. The rest of the milliampere-second reduction with 3φ voltage reflects an increase in the efficiency of x-ray production resulting from a higher average voltage across the x-ray tube. For high-intensity exposures of short duration, 3φ generators are preferred over 1φ x-ray generators.[4] Other advantages of 3φ generators include an increase in the average energy of x radiation produced at a specific tube voltage and a reduction in the loading of the power supply for the x-ray generator. The principal disadvantage of a 3φ x-ray generator is its higher cost. Problems associated with starting, timing and stopping exposures from 3φ generators have been solved satisfactorily.[5, 6]

TABLE 5-3.—COMPARISON OF SPOT-FILM RADIOGRAPHIC TECHNIQUES WITH 1φ AND 3φ GENERATORS

QUANTITY	1φ	3φ
kVp	90–100	90–100
mA	200	250
sec	0.20	0.10
Focal spot	1.5 mm	1.5 mm
mAs	40	25

*The effective or root mean square (rms) value of an alternating voltage or current oscillating with a sinusoidal waveform is $1/\sqrt{2}$ or 0.71 times the maximum or peak value.

RESONANT-TRANSFORMER X-RAY GENERATORS

The resonant frequency ν_r of an alternating-current circuit is

$$\nu_r = \frac{1}{2\pi \sqrt{LC}}$$

where L represents the total inductance and C the total capacitance of the circuit. Alternating current encounters minimum impedance in a circuit if the current oscillates at the resonant frequency. In a resonant-transformer x-ray generator, current supplied to the primary of the high-voltage transformer oscillates at the resonant frequency (often 180 hertz†) of the high-voltage circuit. Since the current induced in the transformer secondary oscillates at the same frequency as that in the primary, the current in the high-voltage circuit encounters minimum impedance. Consequently, a resonant-transformer x-ray generator provides maximum tube current for a particular voltage across the secondary of the high-voltage transformer. Resonant-transformer x-ray generators are used frequently in radiation therapy.

PROBLEMS

*1. A peak voltage of 200 V is applied to the primary of a high-voltage transformer with a turn ratio of 500:1. What peak voltage is induced across the secondary under a no-load condition?

*2. A 1:10 filament transformer provides a peak voltage of 12 V to the filament of an x-ray tube. What peak voltage should be applied to the transformer primary if the voltage across the filament is 90% of the voltage across the transformer secondary under a no-load condition?

3. A technologist notices that when an exposure is made, the reading decreases on the voltmeter on the console of the x-ray generator. The technologist compensates for the voltage depression by selecting a higher tube voltage before exposure. Is this technique correct?

*4. A spinning disk is used to check the timer of a 1φ, full-wave rectified x-ray generator. An exposure of 0.05 second is made. How many images of the hole in the disk should be present in the radiograph?

5. Can a spinning disk be used to check the timer of a 3φ, 12-pulse x-ray generator?

*6. An impedance loss of 20 kVp occurs in the high-voltage circuit of a radiographic generator operated at 500 mA. The generator is line-voltage compensated. The high-voltage transformer has a turn ratio of 500:1. What voltage should be tapped from the autotransformer to provide a tube voltage of 90 kVp?

*7. What effect does the rotational speed of a spinning disk have upon the accuracy of a timer test?

†A hertz (Hz) is a unit of frequency equal to 1 cycle per second.
*For those problems marked with an asterisk, answers are provided on the pages following the appendixes (see pp. 487–488).

8. In Figure 5-1, why should the voltmeter be on the left of the exposure switch rather than on the right?

REFERENCES

1. Jaundrell-Thompson, F., and Ashworth, W.: *X-Ray Physics and Equipment* (2d ed.; Oxford: Blackwell Scientific Publications, 1970).
2. Chaney, E., Hendee, W., and Hare, D.: Performance evaluation of photo-timers, Radiology 118:715, 1976.
3. Rogers, T.: Solid state rectification in x-ray transformers, Cathode Press 22:36, 1965.
4. Morgan, J.: The development and application of multi-phase x rays in medical radiography: Jerman Memorial Lecture, Radiol. Technol. 40:57, 1968.
5. *Three Phase Generation of X Rays*, Publication 5-122, Picker X-Ray Corp., White Plains, N.Y.
6. Kanamori, H.: Advantages of three-phase roentgen units, Acta Radiol. [Diagn.] 6:91, 1967.

6 / Interactions of X and Gamma Rays

GAMMA- AND x-ray photons are attenuated (absorbed or scattered) in many ways as they traverse a medium. Of the various attenuating processes, photoelectric and Compton interactions are the most important to radiology. Interactions of less importance include coherent scattering, pair production and photodisintegration.

ATTENUATION OF A BEAM OF X OR γ RAYS

The number of photons that are attenuated in a medium depends on the number of photons traversing the medium. This relationship may be expressed as

$$P = \mu I$$

where P is the rate of removal of photons from a beam by absorption and scattering, I is the number of photons traversing the attenuating medium and μ is the attenuation coefficient of the medium for the photons of interest. If all the photons possess the same energy (i.e., the beam is monoenergetic) and if the photons are attenuated under conditions of good geometry (i.e., the beam is narrow and contains no scattered photons), then the number I of photons penetrating a thin slab of matter of thickness x is

$$I = I_0 e^{-\mu x} \tag{6-1}$$

In equation (6-1), I_0 represents the number of photons in the beam before the thin slab of matter is in position. The number I_d of photons absorbed or scattered from the beam is

$$
\begin{aligned}
I_d &= I_0 - I \\
&= I_0 - I_0 e^{-\mu x} \\
&= I_0 (1 - e^{-\mu x}) \tag{6-2}
\end{aligned}
$$

The exponent of e must possess no units. Therefore, the units for μ are 1/cm if the thickness x is expressed in centimeters, 1/in. if x is expressed in inches, etc. An attenuation coefficient with units of 1/length is called a *linear attenuation coefficient*.

The *mean path length* is the average distance traveled by x- or γ-ray photons before interaction in a particular medium. The mean path length sometimes is termed the *mean free path* or *relaxation length*, and may be shown to equal $1/\mu$, where μ is the total linear attenuation coefficient. Occasionally, the thickness of an attenuating medium may be expressed as a multiple of the mean free path of photons of a particular energy in the medium.

The probability is $e^{-\mu x}$ that a photon traverses a slab of thickness x without interacting. This probability is the product of probabilities that the photon does not interact by any of the five processes mentioned earlier:

$$e^{-\mu x} = (e^{-\omega x})(e^{-\tau x})(e^{-\sigma x})(e^{-\kappa x})(e^{-\pi x}) = e^{-(\omega + \tau + \sigma + \kappa + \pi)x}$$

The coefficients ω, τ, σ, κ and π represent attenuation by coherent scattering (ω), photoelectric absorption (τ), Compton scattering (σ), pair production (κ) and photodisintegration (π). The *total linear attenuation coefficient* may be written:

$$\mu = \omega + \tau + \sigma + \kappa + \pi \tag{6-3}$$

Often, coherent scattering, photodisintegration and pair production are negligible, and μ is written:

$$\mu = \tau + \sigma \tag{6-4}$$

In general, attenuation coefficients vary with the energy of the x- or γ-ray photons and with the atomic number of the absorber. Linear attenuation coefficients depend also upon the density of the absorber. Mass attenuation coefficients, denoted by the subscript m and computed by dividing linear attenuation coefficients by the density ρ of the attenuating medium, do not vary with the density of the medium.

$$\mu_m = \frac{\mu}{\rho} \qquad \omega_m = \frac{\omega}{\rho} \qquad \tau_m = \frac{\tau}{\rho} \qquad \sigma_m = \frac{\sigma}{\rho} \qquad \kappa_m = \frac{\kappa}{\rho} \qquad \pi_m = \frac{\pi}{\rho}$$

Mass attenuation coefficients usually have units of sq cm/gm or sq cm/mg. Total mass attenuation coefficients for air, water, sodium iodide and lead are plotted in Figure 6-1 as a function of the energy of incident photons.

When mass attenuation coefficients are used, thicknesses x_m are expressed in units such as gm/sq cm or mg/sq cm. The thickness of an attenuating medium may be expressed also as the number of atoms or electrons per unit area. Symbols x_a and x_e denote thicknesses in units of atoms per sq cm and electrons per sq cm. These thicknesses may be computed from the linear thickness x by

$$x_a\left(\frac{\text{atoms}}{\text{sq cm}}\right) = \frac{x(\text{cm})\rho(\text{gm/cc})N_0(\text{atoms/gm-atomic mass})}{M(\text{gm/gm-atomic mass})}$$

$$= \frac{x\rho N_0}{M} \tag{6-5}$$

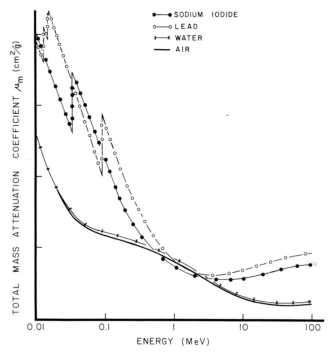

Fig 6-1. — Total mass attenuation coefficients μ_m for selected materials as a function of the energy of incident photons in MeV.

$$x_e\left(\frac{\text{electrons}}{\text{sq cm}}\right) = x_a\left(\frac{\text{atoms}}{\text{sq cm}}\right)Z\left(\frac{\text{electrons}}{\text{atom}}\right)$$
$$= x_a Z \qquad (6\text{-}6)$$

In these equations, M is the gram-atomic mass of the attenuating medium, Z is the atomic number of the medium and N_0 is Avogadro's number (6.02×10^{23}) or the number of atoms per gram-atomic mass. Total atomic and electronic attenuation coefficients μ_a and μ_e, to be used with thicknesses x_a and x_e, may be computed from the linear attenuation coefficient μ by

$$\mu_a\left(\frac{\text{sq cm}}{\text{atom}}\right) = \frac{\mu(\text{cm}^{-1})M(\text{gm/gm-atomic mass})}{\rho(\text{gm/cc})N_0(\text{atoms/gm-atomic mass})}$$
$$= \frac{\mu M}{\rho N_0} \qquad (6\text{-}7)$$

$$\mu_e\left(\frac{\text{sq cm}}{\text{electron}}\right) = \frac{\mu_a(\text{sq cm/atom})}{Z(\text{electrons/atom})}$$
$$= \frac{\mu_a}{Z} \qquad (6\text{-}8)$$

The number I of photons penetrating a thin slab of matter may be computed with any of the following expressions:

$$I = I_0 e^{-\mu x} \qquad\qquad I = I_0 e^{-\mu_a x_a}$$
$$I = I_0 e^{-\mu_m x_m} \qquad\qquad I = I_0 e^{-\mu_e x_e}$$

Example 6-1

A narrow beam containing 2,000 monoenergetic photons is reduced to 1,000 photons by a slab of copper 1 cm thick. What is the total linear attenuation coefficient of the copper slab for these photons?

$$I = I_0 e^{-\mu x} \qquad\qquad (6\text{-}1)$$

$$\frac{I_0}{I} = e^{\mu x}$$

$$\ln \frac{I_0}{I} = \mu x$$

$$\ln\left(\frac{2,000 \text{ photons}}{1,000 \text{ photons}}\right) = \mu(1 \text{ cm})$$

$$\ln 2 = \mu(1 \text{ cm})$$

$$\mu = \frac{\ln 2}{1 \text{ cm}}$$

$$\mu = \frac{0.693}{1 \text{ cm}}$$

$$\mu = 0.693 \text{ cm}^{-1}$$

The thickness of a slab of matter required to reduce the intensity (or exposure rate – see chap. 9) of an x- or γ-ray beam to one half is the *half-value layer* (HVL) or half-value thickness (HVT) for the beam. The half-value layer describes the "quality" or penetrating ability of the beam. The HVL in Example 6-1 is 1 cm of copper. The HVL of a monoenergetic beam of x- or γ-ray photons in any medium is

$$\text{HVL} = \frac{\ln 2}{\mu} \qquad\qquad (6\text{-}9)$$

where $\ln 2 = 0.693$ and μ is the total linear attenuation coefficient of the medium for photons in the beam. The measurement of half-value layers for monoenergetic and polyenergetic beams is discussed in Chapter 9.

Example 6-2

a. What are the total mass (μ_m), atomic (μ_a) and electronic (μ_e) attenuation coefficients of the copper slab described in Example 6-1? Copper has a density of 8.9 gm/cc, a gram-atomic mass of 63.6 and an atomic number of 29.

$$\mu_m = \mu/\rho$$
$$= \frac{0.693 \text{ cm}^{-1}}{8.9 \text{ gm/cc}}$$
$$= 0.078 \text{ sq cm/gm}$$

$$\mu_a = \frac{\mu M}{\rho N_0} \tag{6-7}$$

$$= \frac{(0.693 \text{ cm}^{-1})(63.6 \text{ gm/gm-atomic mass})}{(8.9 \text{ gm/cc})(6.02 \times 10^{23} \text{ atoms/gm-atomic mass})}$$

$$= 8.2 \times 10^{-24} \text{ sq cm/atom}$$

$$\mu_e = \frac{\mu_a}{Z} \tag{6-8}$$

$$= \frac{8.2 \times 10^{-24} \text{ sq cm/atom}}{29 \text{ electrons/atom}}$$

$$= 2.8 \times 10^{-25} \text{ sq cm/electron}$$

b. To the 1-cm copper slab, 2 cm of copper are added. How many photons remain in the beam emerging from the slab?

$$I = I_0 e^{-\mu x} \tag{6-1}$$

$$= (2,000 \text{ photons})e^{-(0.693 \text{ cm}-1)(3 \text{ cm})}$$

$$= (2,000 \text{ photons})e^{-2.079}$$

$$= (2,000 \text{ photons})(0.125)$$

$$= 250 \text{ photons}$$

One centimeter of copper reduces the number of photons to one-half. Since the beam is narrow and monoenergetic, 2 cm of copper reduce the number to one-fourth. Only one eighth of the original number of photons remains after the beam has traversed 3 cm of copper.

c. What is the thickness x_e in electrons per square centimeter for the 3-cm slab?

$$x_e = x_a Z$$

$$= \frac{x \rho N_0 Z}{M}$$

$$= \frac{(3 \text{ cm})(8.9 \text{ gm/cc})(6.02 \times 10^{23} \text{ atoms/gm-atomic mass})(29 \text{ electrons/atom})}{(63.6 \text{ gm/gm-atomic mass})}$$

$$= 7.3 \times 10^{24} \text{ electrons/sq cm}$$

d. Repeat the calculation in part b, using the electronic attenuation coefficient.

$$I = I_0 e^{-\mu_e x_e} \tag{6-1}$$

$$= (2,000 \text{ photons})e^{-\left(2.8 \times 10^{-25} \frac{\text{sq cm}}{\text{electron}}\right)\left(7.3 \times 10^{24} \frac{\text{electrons}}{\text{sq cm}}\right)}$$

$$= (2,000 \text{ photons})e^{-2.079}$$

$$= (2,000 \text{ photons})(0.125)$$

$$= 250 \text{ photons}$$

Under conditions of good geometry, a beam of monoenergetic photons is attenuated exponentially. Exponential attenuation is described by equation (6-1) and depicted in Figure 6-2. The relationship

$$\ln\left(\frac{I}{I_0}\right) = -\mu x$$

may be derived from equation (6-1). From this expression, it is apparent

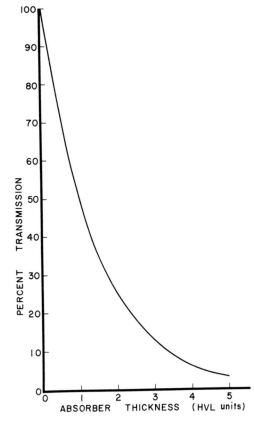

Fig 6-2. — Percent transmission of a narrow beam of monoenergetic photons as a function of the thickness of an attenuating slab in units of half-value layer (HVL). Absorption conditions satisfy requirements for "good geometry."

that the logarithm of the number I of photons varies linearly with the thickness of the attenuating slab. Hence, a straight line is obtained when the logarithm of the number of x- or γ-ray photons is plotted as a function of thickness (Fig 6-3). However, it should be emphasized that a semilogarithmic plot of the number of photons versus the thickness of the attenuating slab yields a straight line only if all photons possess the same energy and the conditions for attenuation fulfill requirements for good geometry.

In general, the total attenuation coefficient of a particular medium decreases as the energy of incident photons increases. Consequently, photons of low energy are attenuated more rapidly than photons of higher energy. A beam containing x- or γ-ray photons of different energies is "harder" (i.e., the penetrating ability of the beam is greater) after it has traversed a medium, because photons of lower energy are removed selectively from the beam. The transmission of a polyenergetic beam

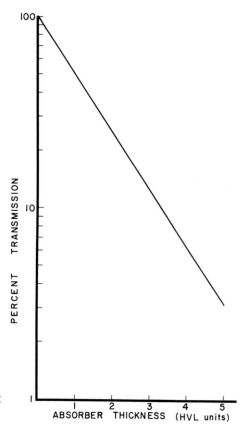

Fig 6-3. — Semilogarithmic plot
of data in Figure 6-2.

does not yield a straight line when plotted on a semilogarithmic graph as
a function of the thickness of an attenuating medium (Fig 6-4). To remove low-energy photons and increase the penetrating ability of an x-ray
beam from a diagnostic or therapy x-ray unit, filters of aluminum, copper, tin or lead may be placed in the beam. For most diagnostic x-ray
units, the added filters are usually 1–3 mm of aluminum.

Because the energy distribution changes as a polyenergetic x-ray
beam penetrates an attenuating medium, no single value for the attenuation coefficient may be used in equation (6-1) to compute the attenuation
of the x-ray beam. However, from the measured half-value layer an *effective attenuation coefficient* may be computed (see Example 6-1):

$$\mu_{eff} = \frac{\ln 2}{HVL}$$

The *average effective energy* of an x-ray beam is the energy of monoenergetic photons that have an attenuation coefficient in a particular medium

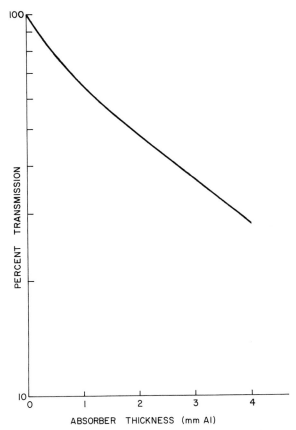

ABSORBER   THICKNESS   (mm Al)

Fig 6-4. — Semilogarithmic plot of the number of x rays in a polyenergetic beam as a function of the thickness of an attenuating medium. The penetrating ability (HVL) of the beam increases continuously with thickness, because lower-energy photons are removed selectively from the beam. The straight-line relationship illustrated in Figure 6-3 for a narrow beam of monoenergetic photons is not achieved for a polyenergetic x-ray beam.

equal to the effective attenuation coefficient for the x-ray beam in the same medium. The effective energy of an x-ray beam is discussed further in Chapter 9.

Example 6-3

An x-ray beam produced at 200 kVp has a HVL of 1.5 mm Cu.

a. What are the effective linear and mass attenuation coefficients?

$$\mu_{eff} = \frac{\ln 2}{1.5 \text{ mm Cu}}$$
$$= 0.46 \ (\text{mm Cu})^{-1}$$

$$(\mu_m)_{\text{eff}} = \frac{\mu_{\text{eff}}}{\rho}$$
$$= \frac{0.46(\text{mm Cu})^{-1}(10 \text{ mm/cm})}{8.9 \text{ gm/cc}}$$
$$= 0.52 \text{ sq cm/gm}$$

b. What is the average effective energy of the beam?

Monoenergetic photons of 96 keV possess a total mass attenuation coefficient of 0.52 sq cm/gm in copper. Consequently, the average effective energy of the x-ray beam is 96 keV.

COHERENT SCATTERING

Photons are deflected or scattered with negligible loss of energy by the process of coherent or Rayleigh scattering. Coherent scattering sometimes is referred to as *classical scattering*, because the interaction may be described completely by methods of classical physics. The classic description assumes that a photon interacts with electrons of an atom as a group rather than with a single electron within the atom. Usually, the photon is scattered in a direction near that of the incident photon. Although photons with energies up to 150–200 keV may scatter coherently in media with high atomic number, this interaction is important in tissue only for low-energy photons. The importance of coherent scattering is reduced further because little energy is deposited in the attenuating medium. However, coherent scatter sometimes reduces the resolution of scans obtained with low-energy, γ-emitting nuclides (e.g., ^{125}I) used in nuclear medicine.

PHOTOELECTRIC ABSORPTION

During a photoelectric interaction, the total energy of an x- or γ-ray photon is transferred to an inner electron of an atom (Fig 6-5). The electron is ejected from the atom with kinetic energy E_k, where E_k equals the photon energy $h\nu$ minus the binding energy E_B required to remove the electron from the atom:

$$E_k = h\nu - E_B \tag{6-10}$$

The ejected electron is called a *photoelectron*.

Example 6-4

What is the initial kinetic energy of a photoelectron ejected from the K shell of lead ($E_B = 88$ keV) by photoelectric absorption of a photon with 100 keV?

$$E_k = h\nu - E_B$$
$$= 100 \text{ keV} - 88 \text{ keV}$$
$$= 12 \text{ keV}$$

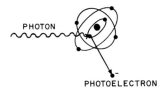

PHOTON

PHOTOELECTRON

Fig 6-5.—Photoelectric absorption of a photon with energy *hv*. The photon disappears and is replaced by an electron ejected from the atom with kinetic energy $E_k = hv - E_B$, where E_B is the binding energy of the electron. Characteristic radiation and Auger electrons are emitted as electrons cascade to replace the ejected photoelectron.

The average binding energy is only 0.5 keV for K electrons in soft tissue. Consequently, a photoelectron ejected from the K shell of an atom in tissue possesses a kinetic energy about 0.5 keV less than the energy of the incident photon.

Photoelectrons resulting from the interaction of low-energy photons are released approximately at a right angle to the motion of the incident photons. As the energy of the photons increases, the average angle decreases between incident photons and released photoelectrons (Fig 6-6).

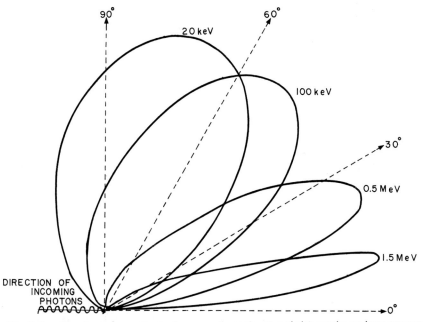

Fig 6-6.—Electrons are ejected approximately at a right angle as low-energy photons interact photoelectrically. As the energy of the photons increases, the angle decreases between incident photons and ejected electrons.

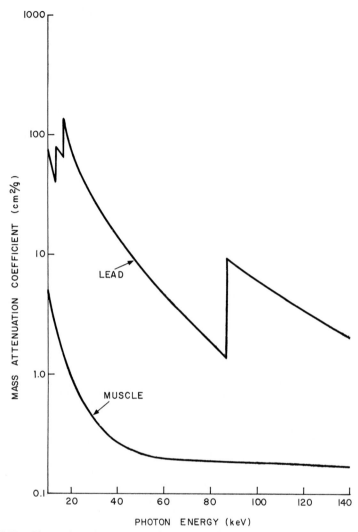

Fig 6-7.—Photoelectric mass attenuation coefficients of lead and soft tissue as a function of photon energy. K- and L-absorption edges are depicted for lead.

An electron ejected from an inner shell leaves a vacancy or hole which is filled immediately by an electron from an energy level farther from the nucleus. Only rarely is a hole filled by an electron from outside the atom. Instead, electrons usually cascade from higher to lower energy levels, producing a number of characteristic photons and Auger electrons with energies that, when added together, equal the binding energy of the ejected photoelectron. Characteristic photons and Auger electrons released during photoelectric interactions in tissue possess an energy usually less than 0.5 keV. These low-energy photons and electrons are absorbed rapidly in surrounding tissue.

The probability of photoelectric interaction decreases rapidly as the photon energy is increased. In general, the mass attenuation coefficient τ_m for photoelectric absorption varies roughly as $1/(h\nu)^3$, where $h\nu$ is the photon energy. In Figure 6-7, the photoelectric mass attenuation coefficients τ_m of tissue and lead are plotted as a function of the energy of incident photons. Discontinuities in the curve for lead are termed *absorption edges,* and occur at photon energies equal to the binding energies of electrons in inner electron shells. Photons with energy less than the binding energy of K-shell electrons interact photoelectrically only with electrons in the L shell and in shells even farther from the nucleus. Photons with energy equal to or greater than the binding energy of K electrons interact predominantly with these electrons. Similarly, photons with energy less than the binding energy of L-shell electrons interact only with electrons in M and more distant shells. That is, most photons interact photoelectrically with electrons that have a binding energy nearest to the energy of the photons. Hence, the photoelectric attenuation coefficient increases abruptly at photon energies equal to the binding energies of electrons in different shells. Absorption edges for photoelectric attenuation in soft tissue occur at photon energies that are very low and are not shown in Figure 6-7. Iodine and barium exhibit K-absorption edges at energies of 33 and 37 keV. Compounds containing these elements are used routinely as contrast agents in diagnostic radiology (chap. 10).

At all photon energies depicted in Figure 6-7, the photoelectric attenuation coefficient for lead ($Z = 82$) is greater than that for soft tissue ($\overline{Z} = 7.4$).* In general, the photoelectric mass attenuation coefficient varies with Z^3. For example, the number of 15-keV photons absorbed primarily by photoelectric interaction in bone ($\overline{Z} = 11.6$) is approximately four times greater than the number of 15-keV photons absorbed in an equal mass of soft tissue. Selective attenuation of photons in media with different atomic numbers and different physical densities is the principal reason for the usefulness of low-energy x rays for producing images in diagnostic radiology.

COMPTON (INCOHERENT) SCATTERING

Gamma- and x-ray photons with energy between 30 keV and 30 MeV interact in soft tissue predominantly by Compton scattering. During a Compton interaction, part of the energy of an incident photon is trans-

---

*$\overline{Z}$ represents the effective atomic number of a mixture of elements. The determination of $\overline{Z}$ is discussed in Chapter 7.

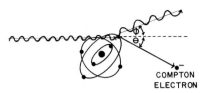

Fig 6-8. — Compton scattering of an x- or γ-ray photon by a loosely bound electron. Scattering angles θ and ϕ for the electron and photon are shown.

ferred to a loosely bound or "free" electron within the attenuating medium. The electron recoils at an angle θ with respect to the motion of the incident photon, and the photon is scattered at an angle ϕ (Fig 6-8). The kinetic energy of the recoil or Compton electron equals the energy lost by the photon, assuming that the binding energy of the electron is negligible. Although the photon may be scattered at any angle ϕ with respect to its original direction, the Compton electron is confined to an angle θ which is 90 degrees or less with respect to the motion of the incident photon. Both θ and ϕ decrease with increasing energy of the incident photons (Fig 6-9).

During a Compton interaction, the change in wavelength of the x- or γ-ray photon is

$$\Delta\lambda = 0.0243 \, (1 - \cos \phi) \tag{6-11}$$

where ϕ is the scattering angle of the photon and $\Delta\lambda$ is the change in wavelength in angstroms. The wavelength λ' of the scattered photon is

$$\lambda' = \lambda + \Delta\lambda \tag{6-12}$$

where λ is the wavelength of the incident photon. The energies $h\nu$ and $h\nu'$ of the incident and scattered photons are

$$
\begin{aligned}
h\nu \, (\text{keV}) &= \frac{hc}{\lambda} \\
&= \frac{(6.62 \times 10^{-34} \, \text{J-sec})(3 \times 10^8 \, \text{m/sec})}{\lambda(\text{Å})(10^{-10} \, \text{m/Å})(1.6 \times 10^{-19} \, \text{J/eV})(10^3 \, \text{eV/keV})} \\
&= \frac{12.4}{\lambda(\text{Å})}
\end{aligned} \tag{6-13}
$$

Also,

$$h\nu' \, (\text{keV}) = \frac{12.4}{\lambda'(\text{Å})} \tag{6-14}$$

Example 6-5

A 210-keV photon is scattered at an angle of 80 degrees during a Compton interaction. What are the energies of the scattered photon and the Compton electron?

The wavelength λ of the incident photon is

$$\lambda = \frac{12.4}{h\nu} \qquad \text{(6-13)}$$
$$= \frac{12.4}{210 \text{ keV}}$$
$$= 0.059 \text{ Å}$$

The change in wavelength $\Delta\lambda$ is

$$\Delta\lambda = 0.0243 \, (1 - \cos \phi) \qquad \text{(6-11)}$$
$$= 0.0243 \, (1 - \cos 80)$$
$$= 0.0243 \, (1 - 0.174)$$
$$= 0.020 \text{ Å}$$

The wavelength λ' of the scattered photon is

$$\lambda' = \lambda + \Delta\lambda \qquad \text{(6-12)}$$
$$= (0.059 + 0.020) \text{ Å}$$
$$= 0.079 \text{ Å}$$

The energy of the scattered photon is

$$h\nu' = \frac{12.4}{\lambda'} \qquad \text{(6-14)}$$
$$= \frac{12.4}{0.079 \text{ Å}}$$
$$= 160 \text{ keV}$$

The energy of the Compton electron is

$$E_k = h\nu - h\nu'$$
$$= (210 - 160) \text{ keV}$$
$$= 50 \text{ keV}$$

Example 6-6

A 20-keV photon is scattered by a Compton interaction. What is the maximum energy transferred to the recoil electron?

The energy transferred to the electron is greatest when the change in wavelength of the photon is maximum; $\Delta\lambda$ is maximum when $\phi = 180$ degrees.

$$(\Delta\lambda)_{\text{max}} = 0.0243[1 - \cos (180)]$$
$$= 0.0243[1 - (-1)]$$
$$= 0.0486 \text{ Å}$$
$$\approx 0.05 \text{ Å}$$

The wavelength λ of a 20-keV photon is

$$\lambda = \frac{12.4}{h\nu} \qquad \text{(6-13)}$$
$$= \frac{12.4}{20 \text{ keV}}$$
$$= 0.62 \text{ Å}$$

The wavelength λ' of the photon scattered at 180 degrees is

$$\begin{aligned}
\lambda' &= \lambda + \Delta\lambda \\
&= (0.62 + 0.05) \text{ Å} \\
&= 0.67 \text{ Å}
\end{aligned} \tag{6-12}$$

The energy $h\nu'$ of the scattered photon is

$$\begin{aligned}
h\nu' &= \frac{12.4}{\lambda'} \\
&= \frac{12.4}{0.67 \text{ Å}} \\
&= 18.6 \text{ keV}
\end{aligned} \tag{6-14}$$

The energy E_k of the Compton electron is

$$\begin{aligned}
E_k &= h\nu - h\nu' \\
&= (20.0 - 18.6) \text{ keV} \\
&= 1.4 \text{ keV}
\end{aligned}$$

When a low-energy photon undergoes a Compton interaction, most of the energy of the incident photon is retained by the scattered photon. Only a small fraction of the energy is transferred to the electron.

Example 6-7

A 2-MeV photon is scattered by a Compton interaction. What is the maximum energy transferred to the recoil electron?

The wavelength λ of a 2-MeV photon is

$$\begin{aligned}
\lambda &= \frac{12.4}{h\nu} \\
&= \frac{12.4}{2,000 \text{ keV}} \\
&= 0.0062 \text{ Å}
\end{aligned} \tag{6-13}$$

The change in wavelength of a photon scattered at 180 degrees is 0.0486 Å (see Example 6-6). Hence, the wavelength λ' of the photon scattered at 180 degrees is

$$\begin{aligned}
\lambda' &= \lambda + \Delta\lambda \\
&= (0.0062 + 0.0486) \text{ Å} \\
&= 0.0548 \text{ Å}
\end{aligned} \tag{6-12}$$

The energy $h\nu'$ of the scattered photon is

$$\begin{aligned}
h\nu' &= \frac{12.4}{\lambda'} \\
&= \frac{12.4}{0.0548 \text{ Å}} \\
&= 226 \text{ keV}
\end{aligned} \tag{6-14}$$

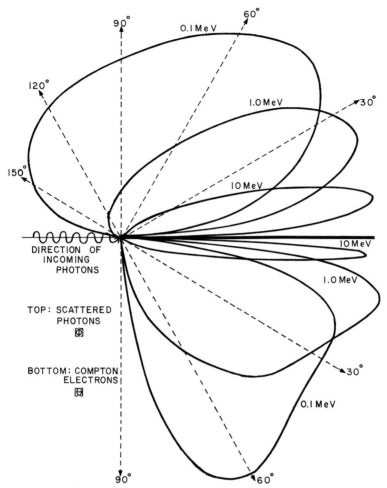

Fig 6-9. — Electron scattering angle θ and photon scattering angle ϕ as a function of the energy of incident photons. Both θ and ϕ decrease as the energy of incident photons increases.

The energy E_k of the Compton electron is

$$E_k = h\nu - h\nu'$$
$$= (2,000 - 226) \text{ keV}$$
$$= 1,774 \text{ keV}$$

When a high-energy photon is scattered by the Compton process, most of the energy is transferred to the Compton electron. Only a small fraction of the energy of the incident photon is retained by the scattered photon.

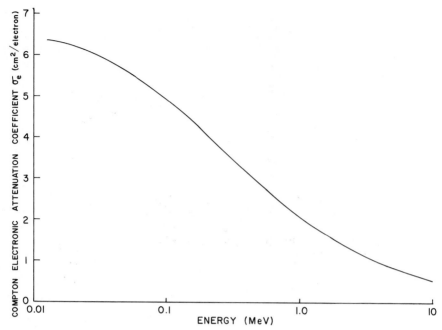

Fig 6-10. — Compton electronic attenuation coefficient as a function of photon energy.

Example 6-8

Show that, irrespective of the energy of the incident photon, the maximum energy is 255 keV for a photon scattered at 180 degrees and 511 keV for a photon scattered at 90 degrees.

The wavelength λ' of a scattered photon is

$$\lambda' = \lambda + \Delta\lambda \qquad (6\text{-}12)$$

For photons of very high energy, λ is very small and may be neglected relative to $\Delta\lambda$.

$$\lambda' \simeq \Delta\lambda$$

For photons scattered at 180 degrees,

$$
\begin{aligned}
\lambda' &\simeq 0.0243 \left[1 - \cos{(180)}\right] \\
&\simeq 0.0243 \left[1 - (-1)\right] \\
&\simeq 0.0486 \ \mathring{A} \\
h\nu' &= \frac{12.4}{\lambda'} \\
&\simeq \frac{12.4}{0.0486 \ \mathring{A}} \\
&\simeq 255 \ \text{keV}
\end{aligned}
\qquad (6\text{-}14)
$$

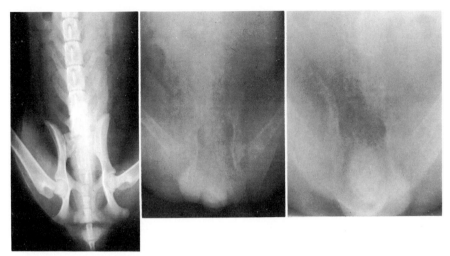

Fig 6-11.—Radiographs taken at 70 kVp, 250 kVp and 1.25 MeV (^{60}Co). These films illustrate the loss of radiographic contrast as the energy of the incident photons increases.

For photons scattered at 90 degrees,

$$\lambda' \simeq 0.0243\ [1 - \cos(90)]$$
$$\simeq 0.0243\ (1 - 0)$$
$$\simeq 0.0243\ \overset{\circ}{A}$$
$$h\nu' = \frac{12.4}{\lambda'} \tag{6-14}$$
$$\simeq \frac{12.4}{0.0243\ \overset{\circ}{A}}$$
$$\simeq 511\ keV$$

The Compton electronic attenuation coefficient σ_e is plotted in Figure 6-10 as a function of the energy of incident photons. The coefficient decreases gradually with increasing photon energy. The Compton mass attenuation coefficient varies directly with the electron density (electrons per gram) of the absorbing medium, because Compton interactions occur primarily with loosely bound electrons. A medium with more unbound electrons will attenuate more photons by Compton scattering than will a medium with fewer electrons. The Compton mass attenuation coefficient is nearly independent of the atomic number of the attenuating medium. For this reason, radiographs exhibit very poor contrast when exposed by high-energy photons. When most of the photons in a beam of x or γ rays interact by Compton scattering, little selective attenuation occurs in different materials with different atomic number. The image in a radiograph obtained by exposing a patient to high-energy photons is not the result of differences in atomic number between different regions of the patient. Instead, the image reflects differences in physical density (gm/cc) between the different regions (e.g., bone and soft tissue). The loss of radiographic contrast with increasing energy of incident photons is depicted in Figure 6-11 and discussed more completely in Chapter 10.

PAIR PRODUCTION

An x- or γ-ray photon may interact by pair production while near a nucleus in an attenuating medium. A pair of electrons, one negative and one positive, appears in place of the photon. Since the energy equivalent to the mass of an electron is 0.51 MeV, the creation of two electrons requires 1.02 MeV. Consequently, photons with energy less than 1.02 MeV do not interact by pair production. During pair production, energy in excess of 1.02 MeV is released as kinetic energy of the two electrons

$$h\nu \text{ (MeV)} = 1.02 + (E_k)_{e-} + (E_k)_{e+}$$

Although the nucleus recoils slightly during pair production, the small amount of energy transferred to the recoiling nucleus usually may be neglected. Pair production is depicted in Figure 6-12.

Occasionally, pair production occurs near an electron rather than near a nucleus. For 10-MeV photons in soft tissue, for example, about 10% of all pair-production interactions occur in the vicinity of an electron. An interaction near an electron is termed *triplet production*, because the electron receives energy from the photon and is ejected from the atom. Hence, three ionizing particles, two negative electrons and one positive electron, are released during triplet production. To conserve momentum, the threshold energy for triplet production must be 2.04 MeV. The ratio of triplet to pair production increases with the energy of incident photons and decreases as the atomic number of the medium is increased.

The mass attenuation coefficient κ_m for pair production varies almost

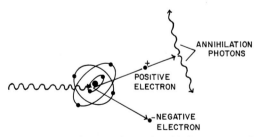

Fig 6-12.—Pair-production interaction of a high-energy photon near a nucleus. Annihilation photons are produced when the positron and an electron annihilate each other.

linearly with the atomic number of the attenuating medium. The coefficient increases slowly with energy of the incident photons. In soft tissue, pair production accounts for only a small fraction of the interactions of x and γ rays with energy between 1.02 and 10 MeV. Positive electrons released during pair production produce annihilation radiation identical to that produced by positrons released from radioactive nuclei.

Example 6-9

A 5.0-MeV photon near a nucleus interacts by pair production. Residual energy is shared equally between the negative and positive electron. What are the kinetic energies of these particles?

$$h\nu \text{ (MeV)} = 1.02 + (E_k)_{e-} + (E_k)_{e+}$$
$$(E_k)_{e-} = (E_k)_{e+} = \frac{(h\nu - 1.02) \text{ MeV}}{2}$$
$$= \frac{(5.00 - 1.02) \text{ MeV}}{2}$$
$$= (E_k)_{e+} = 1.99 \text{ MeV}$$

Described in Figure 6-13 are the relative importances of photoelectric, Compton and pair-production interactions in media of different atomic number, plotted as a function of the energy of incident photons. The curves in Figure 6-13 reflect atomic numbers and photon energies for which adjacent effects are equally probable. In muscle or water ($\overline{Z}$ = 7.45), the probabilities of photoelectric interaction and Compton scatter-

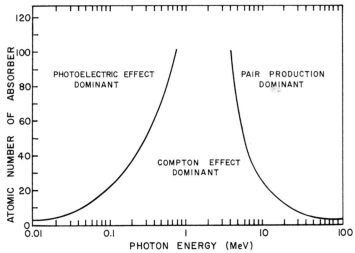

Fig 6-13. — Relative importance of the three principal interactions of x and γ rays.

TABLE 6-1.—VARIABLES THAT INFLUENCE THE
PRINCIPAL MODES OF INTERACTION OF X AND γ RAYS

MODE OF INTERACTION	DEPENDENCE OF LINEAR ATTENUATION COEFFICIENT ON			
	PHOTON ENERGY $h\nu$	ATOMIC NUMBER Z	ELECTRON DENSITY ρ_e	PHYSICAL DENSITY ρ
Photoelectric	$\dfrac{1}{(h\nu)^3}$	Z^3	—	ρ
Compton	$\dfrac{1}{h\nu}$	—	ρ_e	ρ
Pair production	$h\nu$ (above 1.02 MeV)	Z	—	ρ

ing are equal at a photon energy of 35 keV. However, equal energies are not deposited in tissue at 35 keV by each of these modes of interaction; all of the photon energy is deposited during a photoelectric interaction, whereas only part of the photon energy is deposited during a Compton interaction. Equal deposition of energy in tissue by photoelectric and Compton interactions occurs for 60-keV, rather than 35-keV, photons.

A summary of the variables that influence the linear attenuation coefficients for photoelectric, Compton and pair-production interactions is given in Table 6-1.

PHOTODISINTEGRATION

Except for pair production, interactions of x- and γ-ray photons with nuclei are important only if the photons have very high energy. One exception to this rule is the reaction

$$^9\text{Be } (h\nu, \text{ n}) \, ^8\text{Be}$$

which occurs with a threshold energy of 1.65 MeV. A beryllium foil emits neutrons after irradiation by photons with energy equal to or exceeding 1.65 MeV. A silver foil adjacent to the beryllium is activated by the neutrons and emits gamma rays. If no gamma radiation is emitted by adjacent beryllium and silver foils after exposure of the foils to a supervoltage x-ray beam, then x rays with energy equal to or exceeding 1.65 MeV are not present in the beam. If the tube voltage is increased until gamma rays are detected, then the most energetic x rays in the beam possess an energy of 1.65 MeV. At this voltage, the voltmeter on the console of the supervoltage generator should indicate 1.65 MV. Other combinations of foils may be used to determine the energy of x rays in beams of higher energy. Photodisintegration interactions are important also during computation of the shielding required for beams of high-energy photons.

PROBLEMS

1. The tenth-value layer is the thickness of a slab of matter necessary to attenuate a beam of x- or γ-ray photons to one-tenth the intensity with no attenuator present. Assuming good geometry and monoenergetic photons, show that the tenth-value layer equals $2.30/\mu$, where μ is the total linear attenuation coefficient.

°2. The mass attenuation coefficient of copper is 0.0589 sq cm/gm for 1.0-MeV photons. The number of 1.0-MeV photons in a narrow beam is reduced to what fraction by a slab of copper 1 cm thick? The density of copper is 8.9 gm/cc.

°3. Copper has a density of 8.9 gm/cc and a gram-atomic mass of 63.56. The total atomic attenuation coefficient of copper is 8.8×10^{-24} sq cm/atom for 500-keV photons. What thickness of copper in centimeters is required to attenuate 500-keV photons to one half of the original number?

4. Assume that the exponent μx in the equation $I = I_0 e^{-\mu x}$ is equal to or less than 0.1. Show that, with an error less than 1%, the number of photons transmitted is $I_0(1 - \mu x)$ and the number attenuated is $I_0\mu x$. (Hint: Expand the term $e^{-\mu x}$ into a series.)

°5. K- and L-shell binding energies for cesium are 28 keV and 5 keV, respectively. What are the kinetic energies of photoelectrons released from the K and L shells as 40-keV photons interact in cesium?

6. The binding energies of electrons in different shells of an element may be determined by measuring the transmission of a monoenergetic beam of photons through a thin foil of the element as the energy of the beam is varied. Explain why this method works.

°7. Compute the energy of a photon scattered at 45 degrees during a Compton interaction, if the energy of the incident photon is 150 keV. What is the kinetic energy of the Compton electron? Is the energy of the scattered photon increased or decreased if the photon scattering angle is increased to more than 45 degrees?

°8. A γ ray of 2.75 MeV from ^{24}Na undergoes pair production in a lead shield. The negative and positive electrons possess equal kinetic energy. What is this kinetic energy?

9. Prove that, regardless of the energy of the incident photon, a photon scattered at an angle greater than 60 degrees during a Compton interaction cannot undergo pair production.

°For those problems marked with an asterisk, answers are provided on the pages following the appendixes (see pp. 487–488).

7 / Radiation Intensity and Exposure

To describe a beam of ionizing radiation, the amount or "quantity" of radiation must be defined at one or more locations within the beam. In 1928, the roentgen was defined as a unit of radiation quantity for x-rays of medium energy. The definition of the roentgen has been revised many times since 1928, with each revision reflecting an increased understanding of the interactions of electromagnetic radiation and of the equipment used to detect these interactions. Over this same period, many other units of radiation quantity have been proposed. In 1958, the International Commission on Radiation Units and Measurements (ICRU) organized a continuing study of the units of radiation quantity. Results of this study are described in the ICRU Report 19.[1] Recommendations in this report concerning units for radiation intensity and exposure are discussed in this chapter. Recommendations concerning units for radiation dose are included in Chapter 8.

RADIATION INTENSITY

Consider a sphere with unit cross-sectional area exposed to x- or γ-ray photons. The rate at which photons pass through the sphere is termed the *photon intensity* or *photon flux density* ϕ, expressed in units of photons per area-time. If all the photons traverse the sphere in approximately the same direction, then the sphere may be replaced by a plane oriented at a right angle to the motion of the photons. The number Φ of photons passing through the sphere or plane in a finite interval of time t is the product

$$\Phi = \phi t \tag{7-1}$$

provided ϕ is constant over the interval of time. The symbol Φ represents the photon fluence, with units of photons per area (e.g., photons per square meter). If ϕ varies with time, then the number Φ of photons traversing the sphere or plane in time t is

$$\Phi = \int_{0}^{t} \phi(t)dt \tag{7-2}$$

where $\phi(t)$ implies that the photon flux density is expressed as a function of the time t.

If all the photons possess the same energy $h\nu$, then the energy flux density ψ may be computed by

$$\psi = \phi h\nu \tag{7-3}$$

where $h\nu$ is expressed in units of energy per photon (e.g., J/photon or MeV/photon) and ψ is described in units of energy per area-time. If the energy flux density is constant over the time interval t, then the energy fluence Ψ in units of energy per area (e.g., J/sq m or MeV/sq m) is

$$\Psi = \psi t \tag{7-4}$$

If the energy flux density varies with time, the energy fluence is

$$\Psi = \int_0^t \psi(t)dt \tag{7-5}$$

where $\psi(t)$ indicates that the energy flux density is expressed as a function of time t. The energy fluence of monoenergetic photons may be found also by

$$\Psi = \Phi h\nu \tag{7-6}$$

If the radiation beam consists of photons of m different energies, then the energy flux density may be expressed

$$\psi = \sum_{i=1}^m f_i \phi h\nu_i \tag{7-7}$$

where f_i represents the fraction of photons with energy $h\nu_i$ in the beam. The symbol

$$\sum_{i=1}^m$$

indicates that ψ is determined by adding the products $f_i \phi h\nu_i$ for each photon energy. If the distribution of photon energies is continuous, as in an x-ray beam, then the summation sign must be replaced by an integral. The expression becomes

$$\psi = \int_a^b \phi(h\nu)d(h\nu) \tag{7-8}$$

where a and b represent the minimum and maximum photon energies, and $\phi(h\nu)$ implies that the photon flux density must be described as a function of the photon energy $h\nu$. Expressions similar to equations (7-1) through (7-8) may be derived for beams of charged or uncharged particles.

Although photon and energy flux densities and fluences are important in many computations in radiologic physics, these quantities cannot be measured easily. Hence, units have been defined that are related more closely to common methods for measuring radiation quantity. One of these units is the roentgen.

RADIATION EXPOSURE

Primary ion pairs (electrons and positive ions) are produced as ionizing radiation interacts with atoms of an attenuating medium. Secondary ion pairs are produced as the primary ion pairs dissipate their energy by ionizing nearby atoms. The total number of ion pairs (IP) produced is proportional to the energy that the radiation deposits in the medium. The concept of *radiation exposure* is based upon the assumption that the absorbing medium is air. If Q is the total charge (negative *or* positive) liberated as x or γ rays interact in a small volume of air of mass m, then the radiation exposure X at the location of the small volume is

$$X = \frac{Q}{m} \tag{7-9}$$

The total charge reflects the production of both primary and secondary ion pairs, with the secondary ion pairs produced both inside and outside of the small volume of air. The unit of radiation exposure is the *roentgen* (R).

$$1 \text{ R} = 2.58 \times 10^{-4} \text{ coulomb/kg air}$$

This definition of the roentgen is equivalent numerically to an older definition:

$$1 \text{ R} = 1 \text{ esu}/0.001293 \text{ gm air}$$
$$= 1 \text{ esu/sq cm air at STP}^\circ$$

The roentgen is applicable only to x- and γ-radiation less than about 3 MeV. Consequently, this unit should not be used with charged-particle beams or with x- and γ-ray photons greater than about 3 MeV.

With the W-quantity equal to 33.7 eV/IP for x and γ rays in air, the energy absorbed in a unit mass of air during an exposure X in roentgens is

Energy absorbed in air
$$= \frac{[X(\text{R})](2.58 \times 10^{-4} \text{ coulomb/kg-R})(33.7 \text{ eV/IP})(1.6 \times 10^{-19} \text{ J/eV})}{(1.6 \times 10^{-19} \text{ coulomb/IP})}$$
$$= 86.9 \times 10^{-4} X \frac{\text{J}}{\text{kg}} \tag{7-10}$$

$^\circ$STP = Standard temperature (0 C) and pressure (1 atm or 760 mm Hg).

Energy and Photon Fluence per Roentgen

From equation (7-10), the energy absorbed in air is $86.9 \times 10^{-4} X$ (J/kg) during an exposure of X R. The absorbed energy also is

Energy absorbed in air = [Energy fluence][Total energy absorption coefficient]

$$= \Psi\left(\frac{J}{sq\ m}\right)(\mu_{en})_m\left(\frac{sq\ m}{kg}\right)$$

Energy absorbed in air $= \Psi(\mu_{en})_m\left(\frac{J}{kg}\right)$ (7-11)

where $(\mu_{en})_m$ is the total mass energy absorption coefficient for x- or γ-ray photons that contribute to the energy fluence. The coefficient $(\mu_{en})_m$ is defined as

$$(\mu_{en})_m = \mu_m\left(\frac{\overline{E}_a}{h\nu}\right)$$

where μ is the total mass attenuation coefficient of air for photons of

TABLE 7-1.—MASS ENERGY ABSORPTION
COEFFICIENTS FOR SELECTED
MATERIALS AND PHOTON ENERGIES°

PHOTON ENERGY (MeV)	MASS ENERGY ABSORPTION COEFFICIENT $(\mu_{en})_m$(sq m/kg)			
	AIR	WATER	COMPACT BONE	MUSCLE
0.01	0.466	0.489	1.90	0.496
0.02	0.0516	0.0523	0.251	0.0544
0.03	0.0147	0.0147	0.0743	0.0154
0.04	0.00640	0.00647	0.0305	0.00677
0.05	0.00384	0.00394	0.0158	0.00409
0.06	0.00292	0.00304	0.00979	0.00312
0.08	0.00236	0.00253	0.00520	0.00255
0.10	0.00231	0.00252	0.00386	0.00252
0.20	0.00268	0.00300	0.00302	0.00297
0.30	0.00288	0.00320	0.00311	0.00317
0.40	0.00296	0.00329	0.00316	0.00325
0.50	0.00297	0.00330	0.00316	0.00327
0.60	0.00296	0.00329	0.00315	0.00326
0.80	0.00289	0.00321	0.00306	0.00318
1.0	0.00280	0.00311	0.00297	0.00308
2.0	0.00234	0.00260	0.00248	0.00257
3.0	0.00205	0.00227	0.00219	0.00225
4.0	0.00186	0.00205	0.00199	0.00203
5.0	0.00173	0.00190	0.00186	0.00188
6.0	0.00163	0.00180	0.00178	0.00178
8.0	0.00150	0.00165	0.00165	0.00163
10.0	0.00144	0.00155	0.00159	0.00154

°From National Bureau of Standards Handbook 85.[3]

energy $h\nu$. The term $\overline{E}_a$ represents the average energy transformed into kinetic energy of electrons and positive ions per photon absorbed or scattered from the x- or γ-ray beam.[2] The average energy $\overline{E}_a$ is corrected for bremsstrahlung produced as electrons interact with nuclei within the attenuating medium. Mass energy absorption coefficients for a few media, including air, are listed in Table 7-1.

Combining equations (7-10) and 7-11),

$$\Psi \, (\mu_{en})_m = 86.9 \times 10^{-4} \, (X)$$

The energy fluence per roentgen (Ψ/X) is

$$\frac{\Psi}{X} = \frac{86.9 \times 10^{-4}}{(\mu_{en})_m} \qquad (7\text{-}12)$$

where $(\mu_{en})_m$ is expressed in units of sq m/kg, Ψ in J/sq m and X in roentgens.

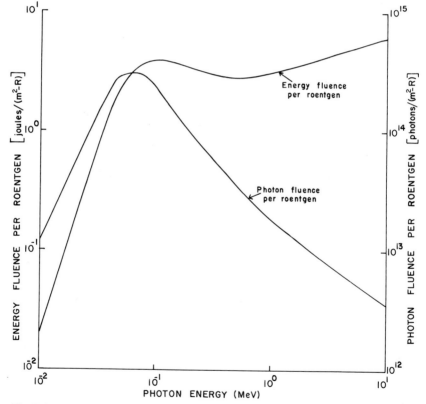

Fig 7-1.—Photon and energy fluence per roentgen, plotted as a function of the photon energy in MeV.

For monoenergetic photons, the photon fluence per roentgen, Φ/X, is the quotient of the energy fluence per roentgen divided by the energy per photon.

$$\frac{\Phi}{X} = \frac{\Psi}{X(h\nu)(1.6 \times 10^{-13} \text{ J/MeV})}$$

From equation (7-12),

$$\frac{\Phi}{X} = \frac{54.3 \times 10^9}{h\nu(\mu_{en})_m} \tag{7-13}$$

with $h\nu$ expressed in MeV and Φ in units of photons per square meter.

The photon and energy fluence per roentgen are plotted in Figure 7-1 as a function of photon energy. At lower photon energies, the large influence of photon energy upon the energy absorption coefficient of air is reflected in the rapid change in the energy and photon fluence per roentgen. Above 100 keV, the energy absorption coefficient is relatively constant, and the energy fluence per roentgen does not vary greatly.[4] However, the photon fluence per roentgen decreases steadily as the energy per photon increases.

Example 7-1

Compute the energy and photon fluence per roentgen for ^{60}Co γ rays. The average energy of the photons is 1.25 MeV and the total energy absorption coefficient is 2.67×10^{-3} sq m/kg (Table 7-1).

$$\frac{\Psi}{X} = \frac{86.9 \times 10^{-4}}{(\mu_{en})_m} \tag{7-12}$$

$$= \frac{86.9 \times 10^{-4} \text{ J/kg}}{2.67 \times 10^{-3} \text{ sq m/kg}}$$

$$= 3.25 \frac{\text{J}}{\text{sq m-R}}$$

$$\frac{\Phi}{X} = \frac{54.3 \times 10^9}{(h\nu)(\mu_{en})_m} \tag{7-13}$$

$$= \frac{54.3 \times 10^9 \text{ MeV/kg}}{(1.25 \text{ MeV/photon})(2.67 \times 10^{-3} \text{ sq m/kg})}$$

$$= 1.63 \times 10^{13} \frac{\text{photons}}{\text{sq m-R}}$$

Ionization Measurements

With designation of the energy absorbed per kilogram of air as E_a, equation (7-11) may be rewritten as:

$$\Psi = \frac{E_a}{(\mu_{en})_m}$$

In a unit volume of air, the energy absorbed per kilogram is

$$E_a = \frac{E}{\rho}$$

where E is the energy deposited in the unit volume by impinging x and γ radiation and ρ is the density of air (1.29 kg/cu m at STP). If J is the number of primary and secondary ion pairs produced as a result of this energy deposition, then

$$E = JW$$

where $W = 33.7$ eV/IP. The energy fluence Ψ is

$$\Psi = \frac{JW}{\rho(\mu_{en})_m} \tag{7-14}$$

Example 7-2

A 1 cu m volume of air at STP is exposed to a photon fluence of 10^{15} photons sq m. Each photon possesses 0.1 MeV. The total energy absorption coefficient of air is 2.31×10^{-3} sq m/kg for 0.1-MeV photons. How many ion pairs are produced inside and outside of the 1 cc volume? How much charge is measured if all the ion pairs are collected?

$$\Psi = \Phi h\nu \tag{7-6}$$

$$= \left(10^{15} \frac{\text{photons}}{\text{sq m}}\right)\left(0.1 \frac{\text{MeV}}{\text{photon}}\right)\left(1.6 \times 10^{-13} \frac{\text{J}}{\text{MeV}}\right)$$

$$= 1.6 \times 10^1 \frac{\text{J}}{\text{sq m}}$$

$$= \frac{JW}{\rho(\mu_{en})_m}$$

$$J = \frac{\Psi\rho(\mu_{en})_m}{W} \tag{7-14}$$

$$= \frac{(1.6 \times 10^1 \text{ J/sq m})(1.29 \text{ kg/cu m})(2.31 \times 10^{-3} \text{ sq m/kg})(10^{-6} \text{ cu m/cc})(1 \text{ cc})}{(33.7 \text{ eV/IP})(1.6 \times 10^{-19} \text{ J/eV})}$$

$$= 88 \times 10^8 \text{ ion pairs}$$

The charge Q collected is

$$Q = \left(88 \times 10^8 \text{ IP}\right)\left(1.6 \times 10^{-19} \frac{\text{coulomb}}{\text{IP}}\right)$$

$$= 1.41 \times 10^{-9} \text{ coulomb}$$

It is not possible to measure all of the ion pairs resulting from the deposition of energy in a small volume of air exposed to x or γ radiation. In particular, secondary ion pairs may escape measurement if they are produced outside the "collecting volume" of air. However, the small volume may be chosen so that energy lost outside the collecting volume by ion pairs created within equals energy lost inside the collecting volume by ion pairs that originate outside. When this condition of *electron equilibrium* is satisfied, the number of ion pairs collected inside the small volume of air equals the total ionization J. The principle of electron equilibrium is used in the free air ionization chamber.

Free Air Ionization Chamber

X- or γ-ray photons incident upon a free air ionization chamber are collimated by a tungsten or gold diaphragm into a beam with cross-sectional area A (Fig 7-2). Inside the chamber, the beam traverses an electric field between parallel electrodes A and B, with the potential of electrode B highly negative. Electrode A is grounded electrically and is divided into two guard electrodes and a central collecting electrode. The guard electrodes ensure that the electric field is uniform over the collecting volume of air between the electrodes. To measure the total ionization accurately, the range of electrons liberated by the incident radiation must be less than the distance between each electrode and the air volume exposed directly to the x- or γ-ray beam. Furthermore, for electron equilibrium to exist, the photon flux density must remain constant across the chamber, and the distance from the diaphragm to the border of the collecting volume must exceed the electron range. If all of these requirements are satisfied, then the number of ion pairs liberated by the incident photons per unit volume of air is

$$\frac{IP}{\text{Unit volume}} = \frac{N}{AL}$$

where N is the number of ion pairs collected, A is the cross-sectional area of the beam at the center of the collecting volume and L is the length of the collecting volume. The charge Q (positive or negative) collected by the chamber is

$$Q = N\left(1.6 \times 10^{-19} \frac{\text{coulomb}}{IP}\right)$$

Since 1 R equals 2.58×10^{-4} coulombs/kg air, the number of roentgens X corresponding to a charge Q in a free air ionization chamber is

$$X = \left(\frac{1}{2.58 \times 10^{-4} \text{ coulombs/kg-R}}\right) \frac{Q}{AL\rho} \tag{7-15}$$

where ρ is the density of air.

To prevent ion pairs from recombining, the potential difference between the electrodes of a free air ionization chamber must be great enough to attract all ion pairs to the electrodes. A voltage this great is referred to as a *saturation voltage*. Ionization currents in a free air chamber subjected to different exposure rates are plotted in Figure 7-3 as a function of the potential difference across the electrodes. For any partic-

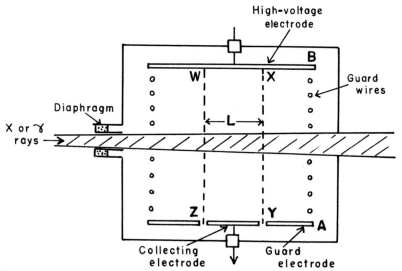

Fig 7-2.—A free air ionization chamber. The collecting volume of length *L* is enclosed within the region *WXYZ*. The air volume exposed directly to the x- or γ-ray beam is depicted by the hatched area.

ular voltage, there is an exposure rate above which significant recombination occurs. Unless the potential difference is increased, an exposure rate higher than this limiting value is measured incorrectly, because some of the ion pairs recombine and are not collected. Errors due to the recombination of ion pairs may be especially severe during the measurement of exposure rates from a pulsed beam of x rays.[5]

Free air ionization chambers are used primarily with x-ray beams generated at a tube voltage between 50 and 300 kVp. Electrodes in these chambers are separated by about 12 cm. This distance exceeds the range of photoelectrons liberated by x rays generated at tube voltages less than 100 kVp (Table 7-2). However, photons greater than about 100 keV produce very few photoelectrons, and the small error introduced by inadequate separation of electrodes at tube voltages greater than 100 kVp may be eliminated almost completely with a small correction factor. For x rays produced at tube voltages between 20 and 50 kVp, the electrodes are separated by less than 10 cm.[6] Free air chambers are used only infrequently for x rays generated at tube voltages less than 20 kVp.

The range of electrons liberated in air increases rapidly with the energy of incident x- or γ-ray photons (see Table 7-2). Electrodes would have to be separated by about 4 m in a chamber used to measure x rays generated at 1,000 kVp. Above 1,000 kVp free air ionization chambers would become very large, and uniform electric fields would be difficult to

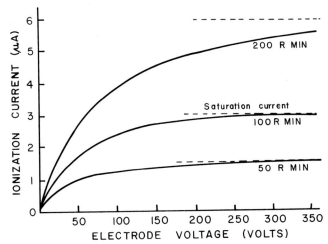

Fig 7-3.—Current in a free air ionization chamber as a function of the potential difference across the electrodes of the chamber. Saturation currents are shown for different exposure rates. Data were obtained with a chamber with electrodes 1 cm apart. (From Johns, H., and Cunningham, J.: *The Physics of Radiology* [3d ed.; Springfield, Ill.: Charles C Thomas, Publisher, 1969].)

achieve. Other problems, such as a reduction in the efficiency of ion-pair collection, are also encountered with chambers designed for high-energy x and γ rays. With some success, chambers containing air at a pressure of several atmospheres have been designed for high-energy photons. Problems associated with the design of free air ionization chambers for high-energy x and γ rays contribute to the decision to confine the roentgen to x and γ rays with energy less than about 3 MeV.

A few corrections usually are applied to measurements with a free air ionization chamber. These include:

TABLE 7-2.—RANGE AND PERCENT OF TOTAL IONIZATION PRODUCED BY PHOTOELECTRONS AND COMPTON ELECTRONS FOR X RAYS GENERATED AT 100, 200 AND 1,000 kVp°

X-RAY TUBE VOLTAGE (kVp)	PHOTOELECTRONS		COMPTON ELECTRONS		ELECTRODE SEPARATION IN FREE AIR IONIZATION CHAMBER
	RANGE IN AIR (cm)	% OF TOTAL IONIZATION	RANGE IN AIR (cm)	% OF TOTAL IONIZATION	
100	12	10	0.5	90 ⎫	12 cm
200	37	0.4	4.6	99.6 ⎬	
1,000	290	0	220	100	4 m

°From Meredith and Massey.[8]

1. Correction for attenuation of the x or γ rays by air between the diaphragm and the collecting volume.
2. Correction for the recombination of ion pairs within the chamber.
3. Correction for air density and humidity.
4. Correction for ionization produced by photons scattered from the primary beam.
5. Correction for the loss of ionization caused by inadequate separation of the chamber electrodes.

These and other corrections to measurements with free air ionization chambers have been discussed by Wyckoff and Attix.[7] With corrections applied, measurements of radiation exposure with a free air ionization chamber are accurate to within ± 0.5%. Free air ionization chambers are used to calibrate exposure rates for x- and γ-ray beams in standards laboratories such as the National Bureau of Standards in the United States and the National Physical Laboratory in Great Britain.

Thimble Chambers

Free air ionization chambers are too fragile and bulky for routine use. However, the amount of ionization collected in a small volume of air is independent of the medium surrounding the collecting volume, provided the medium has an atomic number equal to the effective atomic number of air. Consequently, large distances required for electron equilibrium in the free air chamber may be replaced by lesser thicknesses of a more dense material, provided the atomic number is not changed.

The effective atomic number $\overline{Z}$ of a material is the atomic number of a

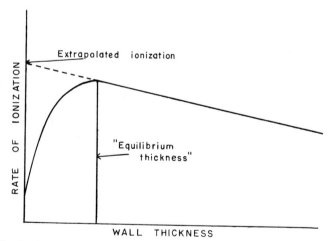

Fig 7-4.—Ionization in an air-filled cavity exposed to ^{60}Co radiation, expressed as a function of the thickness of the air-equivalent wall surrounding the cavity.

hypothetical element which attenuates photons at the same rate as the material.[9, 10] For photoelectric interactions, the effective atomic number $\overline{Z}$ of a mixture of elements is

$$\overline{Z} = {}^{2.94}\sqrt{a_1 Z_1{}^{2.94} + a_2 Z_2{}^{2.94} + \ldots + a_n Z_n{}^{2.94}} \qquad (7\text{-}16)$$

where $Z_1, Z_2, \ldots, Z_n$ are the atomic numbers of elements in the mixture and $a_1, a_2, \ldots, a_n$ are the fractional contributions of each element to the total number of electrons in the mixture.

Example 7-3.
Calculate $\overline{Z}$ for air. Air contains 75.5% nitrogen, 23.2% oxygen and 1.3% argon. Gram-atomic masses are: nitrogen 14.007, oxygen 15.999 and argon 39.948.

Number of electrons contributed by nitrogen to 1 gm air

$$= \frac{(1 \text{ gm})(0.755)(6.02 \times 10^{23} \text{ atom/gm-atomic mass})(7 \text{ electrons/atom})}{(14.007 \text{ gm/gm-atomic mass})}$$

$= 2.27 \times 10^{23}$ electrons

Number of electrons contributed by oxygen to 1 gm air

$$= \frac{(1 \text{ gm})(0.232)(6.02 \times 10^{23} \text{ atom/gm-atomic mass})(8 \text{ electrons/atom})}{(15.999 \text{ gm/gm-atomic mass})}$$

$= 0.70 \times 10^{23}$ electrons

Number of electrons contributed by argon to 1 gm air

$$= \frac{(1 \text{ gm})(0.013)(6.02 \times 10^{23} \text{ atom/gm-atomic mass})(18 \text{ electrons/atom})}{(39.948 \text{ gm/gm-atomic mass})}$$

$= 0.04 \times 10^{23}$ electrons

Total electrons in 1 gm air
$$= (2.27 + 0.70 + 0.04) \times 10^{23}$$
$$= 3.01 \times 10^{23} \text{ electrons}$$

$$a_1 \text{ for nitrogen} = \frac{2.27 \times 10^{23} \text{ electrons}}{3.01 \times 10^{23} \text{ electrons}} = 0.753$$

$$a_2 \text{ for oxygen} = \frac{0.70 \times 10^{23} \text{ electrons}}{3.01 \times 10^{23} \text{ electrons}} = 0.233$$

$$a_3 \text{ for argon} = \frac{0.04 \times 10^{23} \text{ electrons}}{3.01 \times 10^{23} \text{ electrons}} = 0.013$$

$$\overline{Z}_{air} = {}^{2.94}\sqrt{(0.753) \, 7^{2.94} + (0.233) \, 8^{2.94} + (0.013) \, 18^{2.94}}$$
$$= 7.64$$

The large distances in air required for electron equilibrium and collection of total ionization in a free air chamber may be replaced by smaller thicknesses of "air-equivalent material" with an effective atomic number of 7.64. Chambers with air-equivalent walls are known as *thimble chambers*. Usually, the walls are composed of bakelite $(C_{43}H_{38}O_7)^3$ coated with graphite. Most of the ion pairs collected within the air volume are produced by electrons released as photons interact with the air-equivalent walls of the chamber. Shown in Figure 7-4 is the ionization

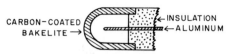

Fig 7-5. — Diagram of a thimble chamber with an air-equivalent wall.

in an air-filled cavity exposed to ^{60}Co radiation, expressed as a function of the thickness of the wall surrounding the cavity. Initially, the number of electrons entering the cavity increases with the thickness of the cavity wall. When the wall thickness equals the range of electrons liberated by incident photons, electrons from outer portions of the wall just reach the cavity and the ionization inside the cavity is maximum. The thickness of the wall should not be much greater than this *equilibrium thickness*, because the attenuation of incident x- and γ-ray photons increases with the thickness of the wall. The equilibrium thickness for the wall increases with the energy of the incident photons. In Figure 7-4, the slow decrease in ionization as the wall thickness is increased beyond the electron range reflects the attenuation of photons in the wall of the chamber. Extrapolation of this portion of the curve to a wall thickness of zero indicates the ionization that would occur within the cavity if photons were not attenuated by the surrounding wall.

A thimble chamber is illustrated schematically in Figure 7-5. Usually, the inside of the chamber wall is coated with carbon, and the central positive electrode is aluminum. The response of the chamber may be varied by changing the size of the collecting volume of air, the thickness of the carbon coating or the length of the aluminum electrode. Nevertheless, it is difficult to construct a thimble chamber with a response at all photon energies identical with that for a free air chamber. Usually, the response of a thimble chamber is compared at several photon energies to the response of a free air ionization chamber. By using the response of the free air chamber as a standard, calibration factors may be computed for the thimble chamber at different photon energies.

Condenser Chambers

As ion pairs produced by impinging radiation are collected, the potential difference is reduced between the central electrode and the wall of a thimble chamber. If a chamber with volume v is exposed to X R, the charge Q collected is

$$Q \text{ (coulombs)} = [X(R)]\left(2.58 \times 10^{-4} \frac{\text{coulombs}}{\text{kg-R}}\right)\rho\left(\frac{\text{kg}}{\text{cu m}}\right)v(\text{cu m})$$

$$= 2.58 \times 10^{-4} \, X\rho v$$

If the density of air is 1.29 kg/cu m,

$$Q = 3.33 \times 10^{-4} \, Xv$$

For a chamber with capacitance C in farads, the voltage reduction V across the chamber is

$$V = \frac{Q}{C} = \frac{3.33 \times 10^{-4} \, Xv}{C}$$

The voltage reduction per roentgen is

$$\frac{V}{X} = \frac{3.33 \times 10^{-4} \, v}{C} \tag{7-17}$$

where X is the exposure in roentgens and v is the volume of the chamber in cubic meters. The voltage drop per roentgen, defined as the *sensitivity* of the chamber, may be reduced by decreasing the chamber volume v or by increasing the chamber capacitance C. The chamber capacitance may be increased by connecting the thimble chamber permanently to a large capacitor. The combination is a condenser chamber (Fig 7-6). The capacitor consists of an inner layer of conducting carbon separated by a polystyrene insulator from an outer metal cylinder. The outer cylinder of the capacitor is connected to the inner wall of the thimble ionization chamber, and the positive electrode in the thimble is continuous with the carbon coating on the polystyrene insulator. The capacitance C of the entire chamber is

$$C = C_c + C_t$$

where C_c and C_t are the capacitances of the capacitor and thimble, respectively. Usually, C_c is much greater than C_t, and the sensitivity of a condenser chamber is reduced greatly from that for the thimble alone.

If an electrometer with capacitance C_e is used to measure the charge distributed over a condenser chamber with total capacitance C, then the sensitivity of the chamber may be defined as

$$\frac{V}{X} = \frac{3.33 \times 10^{-4} \, v}{C + C_e} \tag{7-18}$$

The sensitivity of most condenser chamber–electrometer units is defined in this manner.

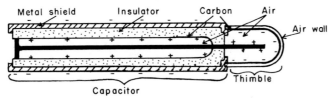

Fig 7-6. – Cross section of a typical condenser chamber.

Example 7-4

The capacitance of a 100-R condenser chamber is 50 $\mu\mu$F. The capacitance of the charger-reader used with the chamber is 10 $\mu\mu$F. The volume of the chamber is 0.46 cc. What is the sensitivity of the chamber? What reduction in voltage occurs when the chamber is exposed to 50 R?

$$\text{Sensitivity} = \frac{V}{X} = \frac{3.33 \times 10^{-4}\, v}{C + C_e} \tag{7-18}$$

$$= \frac{3.33 \times 10^{-4}\,(0.46\ \text{cc})(10^{-6}\ \text{cu m/cc})}{(50 + 10) \times 10^{-12}\ \text{F}}$$

$$= 2.55\,\frac{V}{R}$$

The reduction in voltage following an exposure of 50 R is

$$(50\ \text{R})\left(2.55\,\frac{V}{R}\right) = 128\ \text{V}$$

Condenser chambers frequently used in the United States are those developed by Glasser and Seitz[11] and manufactured primarily by Victoreen Instrument Company. Victoreen chambers with walls of different thicknesses and compositions are used to measure low-energy (4–35 keV), medium-energy (30–400 keV) and high-energy (400–1,300 keV) x-

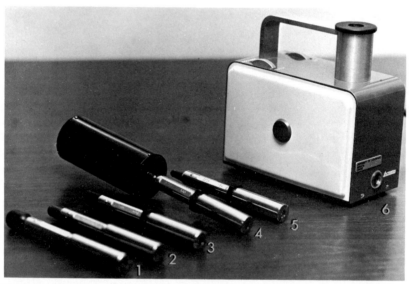

Fig 7-7.—Victoreen condenser chambers and a charger-reader electrometer. *(1)* 25 R, high-energy chamber; *(2)* 25 R, medium-energy chamber; *(3)* 250 R, low-energy chamber; *(4)* 0.25 R, medium-energy chamber; *(5)* 250 R, medium-energy chamber; and *(6)* charger-reader electrometer. (Courtesy of Victoreen Instrument Co.)

and γ-ray photons. A number of chambers with different sensitivities are available to measure medium- and high-energy x and γ rays. For example, a 100-R chamber exposed to 100 R furnishes a full-scale deflection of the electrometer. The volume of air in a 100-R chamber is about 0.46 cc, and the sensitivity of the chamber plus electrometer is about 2.5 V/R (Example 7-4). A 2.5-R, medium-energy chamber has an air volume of about 17 cc and a sensitivity of about 100 V/R. A charger-reader electrometer and a few Victoreen chambers are shown in Figure 7-7. Often, a condenser chamber together with its electrometer is referred to as an *R-meter*.

When a medium- or high-energy condenser chamber is exposed to radiation, the axis of the chamber should be oriented at a right angle to the direction of the incident photons. Low-energy chambers are designed to admit photons through a thin window at the end of the thimble and should be positioned parallel to the incident photons. During exposure, the metal cap of the chamber should be in place (Fig 7-7). The cap attenuates radiation impinging upon the condenser or "stem" portion of the chamber, and reduces the ionization occurring in the stem. The cap also shields the exposed tip of the central electrode, and greatly reduces the charge collected from irradiated air near the end of the chamber. Ionization in the stem, and that collected from irradiated air enclosed between the end of the chamber and the metal cap, is termed *stem ionization* or the *stem effect*. Correction for the stem effect may be as large as 4–5% for high-energy photons. The air within the central cavity of the stem also is ionized by photons that penetrate the stem. However, these ion pairs recombine and do not influence the measured exposure, because this region is shielded from the electric field.

Condenser chamber–electrometer units should be calibrated periodically by a standards or calibration laboratory, the manufacturer or the

TABLE 7-3.—TYPICAL CALIBRATION REPORT FOR VARIOUS
CHAMBERS OF VICTOREEN R-METER
(National Bureau of Standards Calibration, Victoreen R-Meter #892)

kVcp	EQUIVALENT INHERENT FILTER (mm)	ADDED FILTER (mm)	HVL (mm) OR ENERGY (keV)	CHAMBER MODEL	CHAMBER RANGE (R)	CORRECTION FACTOR
20	2.0 Be	0.0 Al	0.062 Al	651	250	0.98
50	2.0 Be	1.0 Al	0.87 Al	651	250	1.08
75	4.0 Al	0.0 Al	3.2 Al	131	100	1.06
100	4.0 Al	1.0 Al	5.2 Al	131	100	1.06
250	1.0 Al	{1.0 Cu 1.0 Al}	2.17 Cu	131	100	1.08
^{60}Co			1,250 keV	553	25	0.94°

°All of stem exposed.

user. A calibration report from the National Bureau of Standards is shown in Table 7-3 for different condenser chambers of a Victoreen R-meter.

A few precautions are necessary when a condenser chamber is used. If a chamber is not exposed to radiation, then charge placed on electrodes of the chamber should remain for a reasonable period of time. If some charge leaks from the chamber, then either the cause of leakage should be eliminated or measurements should be corrected for leakage. The chamber should be calibrated periodically and should be stored in an atmosphere of low humidity (e.g., a desiccator) to reduce the leakage of charge caused by accumulation of moisture. Always, condenser chambers must be handled gently and kept clean.

ELECTROMETERS

String Electrometers

A string electrometer used with Victoreen condenser chambers is illustrated schematically in Figure 7-8. The positive charge on the string support rod and platinum wire induces a negative charge on the deflection electrode. The deflection electrode attracts the platinum wire, and the wire moves a distance that depends upon the amount of charge distributed over the wire and the support rod. The movement of the shadow of the string across a scale is observed through a small microscope. With the condenser chamber inserted into the electrometer, the chamber,

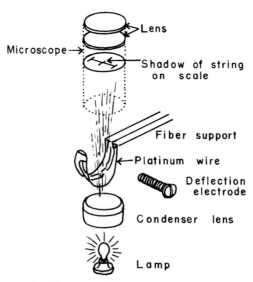

Fig 7-8.—Diagram of a Victoreen Model 570 string electrometer. (Courtesy of Victoreen Instrument Co.)

wire and support rod are charged until the shadow of the string falls upon zero on the scale. When the chamber is removed from the electrometer and exposed to radiation, ion pairs are collected and the charge is reduced on electrodes of the condenser chamber. When the chamber is reinserted into the electrometer, the reduction in charge is shared among the chamber, the platinum wire and the support rod. With the charge on the wire and rod reduced, the attraction is decreased between the wire and the deflection electrode and the wire moves upscale. The final position of the wire reflects the radiation exposure received by the chamber. By applying various correction factors, the exposure in roentgens may be computed.[12]

Other Electrometers

The condenser chambers discussed so far are detached from the electrometer during exposure. A variety of exposure-measuring devices are available in which the chamber remains connected to the electrometer by a shielded cable during exposure. While in the x-ray beam, the chamber may be made sensitive to radiation for a selected interval of time, and the exposure rate or cumulative exposure may be determined. A typical device of this type is illustrated in Figure 7-9. Shown in Figure 7-10 is an ionization chamber designed by the Department of Medical Physics of Memorial Hospital of New York especially for measurement of very low-energy (25 – 45 kVp) x-ray beams used for mammography.

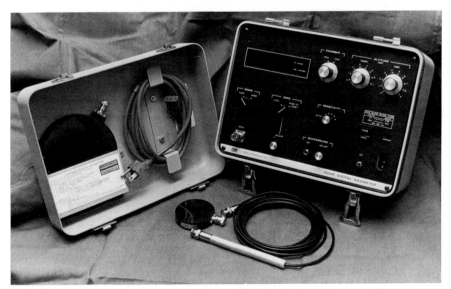

Fig 7-9.—A Keithley model 35020 Digital Dosimetry System. (Courtesy of Keithley Instruments, Inc.)

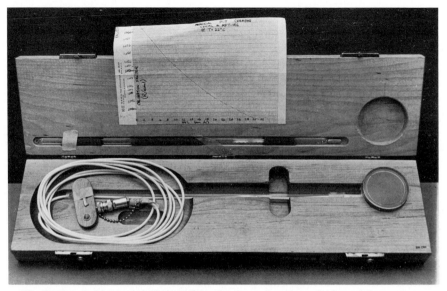

Fig 7-10.—A Memorial Hospital ionization chamber designed for measurement of mammographic x-ray beams. (Courtesy of the Southwestern Center for Radiological Physics, Denver, Colorado.)

EXTRAPOLATION CHAMBERS

Measurements with a condenser chamber are difficult to interpret if the chamber is at a location where the exposure rate changes rapidly with distance, because the measurements represent average exposure rates over the volume of the chamber. To determine the exposure rate accurately in such a location, a chamber with very small thickness is required. In the *extrapolation chamber*, the spacing between electrodes may be varied from a few centimeters to a fraction of a millimeter. The rate at which ion pairs are produced in the air between the electrodes is measured for different distances of separation of the electrodes. The ionization current per unit volume of air is plotted as a function of the distance between the electrodes, and the resulting curve is extrapolated to an electrode spacing of zero. The ionization current per unit volume at the intersection of the curve with the ordinate reflects the exposure rate at the exact location of the electrodes with zero separation distance (Fig 7-11).

Failla described the first extrapolation chamber in 1937.[13] Extrapolation chambers are used often to measure the rate at which air is ionized at the surface of a medium irradiated by x or γ rays. The *backscatter factor* is the ratio of this measurement (extrapolated to zero electrode spacing) to a measurement of the rate of ionization with the medium re-

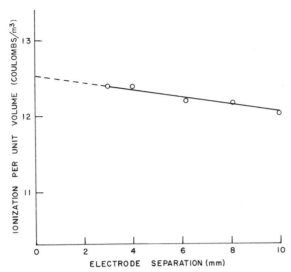

Fig 7-11.—Ionization per unit volume of an extrapolation chamber, plotted as. a function of the spacing between electrodes of the chamber. (From Stanton, L.: *Basic Medical Radiation Physics* [New York: Appleton-Century-Crofts, 1969].)

moved. Extrapolation chambers used for measurement of backscatter factors have two electrodes. One is a conducting layer of graphite deposited upon a very thin electrode placed on the surface of the medium. The second electrode is a thin conducting membrane which can be lowered toward the first electrode.

PROBLEMS

°1. The photon flux density is 10^9 photons/(sq m-sec) for a beam of gamma rays. One fourth of the photons have an energy of 500 keV and three fourths have an energy of 1.25 MeV. What is the energy flux density of the beam? If the photon flux density is constant, what is the energy fluence over an interval of 10 seconds?

°2. During an exposure of 75 R, how much energy is absorbed per kilogram of air?

°3. The energy absorption coefficient of air is 2.8×10^{-3} sq m/kg for photons of 1.0 MeV. What is the energy fluence required for an exposure of 100 R? What is the photon fluence for this exposure?

°4. How many ion pairs are produced in 1 cc of air during an exposure of 100 R?

°5. Water is 89% oxygen (gm-atomic mass = 15.999) and 11% hydrogen (gm-atomic mass = 1.008) by weight. Compute the effective atomic number of water.

°6. A thimble chamber with an air-equivalent wall receives an exposure of 60 R

°For those problems marked with an asterisk, answers are provided on the pages following the appendixes (see pp. 487–488).

in 1 minute. The volume of the chamber is 0.46 cc. What is the ionization current from the chamber?

°7. A condenser ionization chamber has a sensitivity of 2.5 V/R. The volume of the chamber is 0.46 cc. The capacitance of the chamber is six times the capacitance of the charger-reader. What is the capacitance of the chamber?

°8. A miniature ionization chamber has a sensitivity of 1 V/R. The chamber is discharged by 270 V during an exposure to x radiation. What exposure did the chamber receive?

9. A Victoreen condenser chamber receives identical exposures in New Orleans (sea level) and in Denver (5,000 ft above sea level). Is the deflection of the platinum wire lower or high in Denver? Why?

10. What is meant by the *energy dependence* of an air-wall thimble chamber?

REFERENCES

1. International Commission on Radiation Units and Measurements: *Radiation Quantities and Units*, ICRU Report 19 (Washington, D.C.: Government Printing Office, 1971).
2. Fano, U.: Gamma ray attenuation: I. Basic procedures, Nucleonics 11:8, 1953.
3. International Commission on Radiological Units and Measurements: *Physical Aspects of Irradiation*. Recommendations of the ICRU. National Bureau of Standards Handbook 85, 1964.
4. Berger, R.: The x- or gamma-ray energy absorption or transfer coefficient: Tabulation and discussion, Radiat. Res. 15:1, 1961.
5. Johns, H., and Cunningham, J.: *The Physics of Radiology* (3d ed.; Springfield, Ill.: Charles C Thomas, Publisher, 1969).
6. Lamperti, P., and Wyckoff, H.: NBS free-air chamber for measurement of 10–60 kV x rays, J. Res. Nat. Bur. Standards 69C:39, 1965.
7. Wyckoff, H., and Attix, F.: *Design of Free-Air Ionization Chambers*, National Bureau of Standards Handbook 64, 1957.
8. Meredith, W., and Massey, J.: *Fundamental Physics of Radiology* (Baltimore: Williams & Wilkins Co., 1968).
9. Mayneord, W.: The significance of the röntgen, Acta Unio Internat. Contra Cancrum 2:271, 1937.
10. Weber, J., and van den Berge, D.: The effective atomic number and the calculation of the composition of phantom materials, Br. J. Radiol. 42:378, 1969.
11. Glasser, O., and Seitz, V.: Method and apparatus for the measurement of radiation intensity, U.S. Patent 1,855,669, April 26, 1932.
12. Hendee, W.: *Medical Radiation Physics: Radiation Therapy* (in prep.).
13. Failla, G.: The measurement of tissue dose in terms of the same unit for all ionizing radiations, Radiology 29:202, 1937.

8 / Radiation Dose

ALTHOUGH THE ROENTGEN is used widely to describe the quantity of x- or γ-ray photons less than about 3 MeV, it is not used with photons of higher energy or with beams of charged or uncharged particles. For these radiations, other units of radiation quantity have been defined.[1] These units are used also with increasing frequency for x- and γ-ray photons less than 3 MeV.

UNITS OF RADIATION DOSE

The Rad

Chemical and biologic changes in tissue exposed to ionizing radiation depend upon the energy absorbed in the tissue from the radiation, rather than upon the amount of ionization that the radiation produces in air. To describe the energy absorbed in a medium from any type of ionizing radiation, the quantity of radiation should be described in units of *rads*. The rad (an acronym for radiation absorbed dose) is a unit of *absorbed dose*,* and represents the absorption of 10^{-2} J of energy per kilogram (or 100 ergs per gram) of absorbing material:

$$1 \text{ rad} = 10^{-2} \text{ J/kg} = 100 \text{ ergs/gm}$$

The absorbed dose D in rads delivered to a small mass m in kilograms is:

$$D \text{ (rad)} = \frac{E/m}{10^{-2} \text{ J/kg}} \qquad (8\text{-}1)$$

where E, the absorbed energy in joules, is:

the difference between the sum of the energies of all the directly- and indirectly-ionizing particles which have entered the volume and the sum of the energies of all those which have left it, minus the energy equivalent of any increase in rest mass that took place in nuclear or elementary particle reactions within the volume.[1]

This definition means that E is the total energy deposited in a small volume of irradiated medium, corrected for energy removed from the volume in any way.

*The rad is also a unit of kerma, defined as the sum of the initial kinetic energies of all charged particles liberated by indirectly ionizing particles (and photons) in a volume element, divided by the mass of matter in the volume element. Under conditions of charged-particle equilibrium with negligible energy loss by bremsstrahlung, kerma and absorbed dose are identical.

139

Example 8-1

If a dose of 5 rad is delivered uniformly to the uterus during a diagnostic x-ray examination, how much energy is absorbed by each gram of the uterus?

$$D = \frac{E/m}{10^{-2} \text{ J/kg-rad}}$$
$$E = 10^{-2}\,(D)(m) \tag{8-1}$$
$$= 10^{-2}\,(5 \text{ rad})\left(10^{-3}\,\frac{\text{kg}}{\text{gm}}\right)$$
$$= 5 \times 10^{-5} \text{ J/gm}$$

During an exposure of 1 R, the energy absorbed per kilogram of air is (chap. 7):

$$1 \text{ R} = 86.9 \times 10^{-4} \text{ J/kg in air}$$

Since 1 rad $= 10^{-2}$ J/kg,

$$1 \text{ R} = 0.869 \text{ rad in air}$$

The Gray

In the international (SI) system of units, the rad is replaced by the gray (Gy) defined as:

$$1 \text{ Gy} = 1 \text{ J/kg}$$

Since 1 rad $= 10^{-2}$ J/kg,

$$1 \text{ Gy} = 100 \text{ rad}$$

The Rem

Usually, chemical and biologic effects of irradiation depend not only upon the amount of energy absorbed in an irradiated medium but also upon the distribution of the absorbed energy within the medium. For equal absorbed doses, various types of ionizing radiation often differ in the efficiency with which they elicit a particular chemical or biologic response. The *relative biologic effectiveness (RBE)* describes the effectiveness or efficiency with which a particular type of radiation evokes a certain chemical or biologic effect. The relative biologic effectiveness is computed by comparing results obtained with the radiation in question to those obtained with a reference radiation (e.g., medium-energy x rays or ^{60}Co radiation):

$$RBE = \frac{\text{Dose of reference radiation required to produce a particular response}}{\text{Dose of radiation in question required to produce the same response}} \tag{8-2}$$

For a particular type of radiation, the *RBE* may vary from one chemical or biologic response to another. Listed in Table 8-1 are the results of

TABLE 8-1.—THE RBE OF ^{60}Co GAMMAS, WITH DIFFERENT
BIOLOGIC EFFECTS USED AS CRITERION FOR MEASUREMENT
(The RBE of 200-kV x rays is taken as 1.)

EFFECT	RBE OF ^{60}Co GAMMAS	REFERENCE
30-day lethality and testicular atrophy in mice	0.77	Storer et al.[2]
Splenic and thymic atrophy in mice	1	Storer et al.[2]
Inhibition of growth in Vicia faba	0.84	Hall[3]
LD$_{50}$ in mice, rat, chick embryo and yeast	0.82–0.93	Sinclair[4]
Hatchability of chicken eggs	0.81	Loken et al.[5]
HeLa cell survival	0.90	Krohmer[6]
Lens opacity in mice	0.8	Upton et al.[7]
Cataract induction in rats	1	Focht et al.[8]
L-cell survival	0.76	Till and Cunningham[9]

investigations of the relative biologic effectiveness of ^{60}Co radiation. For these data, the reference radiation is medium-energy x rays. From Table 8-1, it is apparent that the *RBE* for ^{60}Co gammas varies from one biologic response to the next.

The *RBE dose* in rem (acronym for roentgen equivalent in mammals) is the product of the *RBE* and the dose in rads.

$$RBE \text{ dose (rem)} = \text{Absorbed dose (rad)} \times RBE \qquad (8\text{-}3)$$

The ICRU has suggested that the concept of *RBE* dose should be limited to descriptions of radiation dose in radiation biology.[1]

Often, the effectiveness with which different types of radiation produce a particular chemical or biologic effect varies with the linear energy transfer *(LET)* of the radiation. The *dose-equivalent (DE)* is the product of the dose in rads and a *quality factor (QF)* which varies with the *LET* of the radiation:

$$DE \text{ (rem)} = D \text{ (rad)} \times QF \qquad (8\text{-}4)$$

TABLE 8-2.—RELATION BETWEEN SPECIFIC
IONIZATION, LINEAR ENERGY TRANSFER AND
QUALITY FACTOR*

AVERAGE SPECIFIC IONIZATION (IP/μ) IN WATER	AVERAGE LET (keV/μ) IN WATER	QF
100 or less	3.5 or less	1
100–200	3.5–7.0	1–2
200–650	7.0–23	2–5
650–1,500	23–53	5–10
1,500–5,000	53–175	10–20

*From Recommendations of the International Commission on Radiological Protection.[10]

TABLE 8-3.—QUALITY FACTORS FOR
DIFFERENT RADIATIONS*

TYPE OF RADIATION	QF
X rays, γ rays and β-particles	1.0
Neutrons and protons $\leq$ 10 MeV	10 (30 for irradiation of eyes)
α-Particles from natural radionuclides	10
Heavy recoil nuclei	20

*These data should be used only for purposes of radiation protection.[11]

The dose-equivalent reflects a recognition of differences in the effectiveness of different radiations to inflict overall biologic damage, and is used during computations associated with radiation protection. Quality factors are listed in Table 8-2 as a function of the *LET* and in Table 8-3 for different types or radiation. These quality factors should be used for the determination of shielding requirements and for the computation of radiation doses to personnel working with or near sources of ionizing radiation.

Example 8-2

A person receives an average whole body dose of 100 mrad from ^{60}Co gammas and 50 mrad from neutrons with an energy less than 10 MeV. What is the dose-equivalent to the person in mrems?

$$DE \text{ (mrem)} = [D \text{ (mrad)} \times QF]_{\text{gammas}} + [D \text{ (mrad)} \times QF]_{\text{neutrons}}$$
$$= (100 \text{ mrad})(1) + (50 \text{ mrad})(10)$$
$$= 600 \text{ mrem}$$

Example 8-3

A person accidentally ingests a small amount of tritium (beta $E_{\max} = 0.018$ MeV). The average dose to the gastrointestinal tract is estimated to be 500 mrad. What is the dose-equivalent in mrems?

From Table 8-3, the quality factor is 1.0 for tritium betas.

$$DE \text{ (mrem)} = D \text{ (mrad)} \times QF$$
$$= (500 \text{ mrad})(1.0)$$
$$= 500 \text{ mrem}$$

A *distribution factor (DF)* may be added to equation (8-4) to compensate for changes in the radiation response caused by a nonuniform distribution of radioactive nuclides within the body. Other terms may be added to equation (8-4) to describe the influence of additional factors upon the biologic response to radiation. Then equation (8-4) is written

$$DE \text{ (rem)} = D \text{ (rad)}(QF)(DF) \ldots \tag{8-5}$$

MEASUREMENT OF RADIATION DOSE

The absorbed dose to a medium describes the energy absorbed during exposure of the medium to ionizing radiation. A *dosimeter* responds to the energy that it absorbs from incident radiation. To be most useful, the dosimeter should absorb an amount of energy equal to that which would be absorbed in the medium that the dosimeter displaces. For example, a dosimeter used to measure radiation dose in soft tissue should absorb an amount of energy equal to that absorbed by the same mass of soft tissue. When this requirement is satisfied, the dosimeter is said to be *tissue-equivalent*. Few dosimeters are exactly tissue-equivalent, and most measurements of absorbed-dose in tissue should be interpreted with care.

Calorimetric Dosimetry

Almost all the energy absorbed from radiation is degraded eventually to heat. If an absorbing medium is insulated from its environment, then the rise in temperature of the medium is proportional to the energy absorbed. The temperature rise ΔT may be measured with a Wheatstone bridge and a thermistor.* A radiation calorimeter is an instrument used to measure radiation absorbed dose by detecting the increase in temperature of a mass of absorbing material.[12] The absorbed dose in the material is

$$D \text{ (rad)} = \frac{E}{m(10^{-2} \text{ J/kg-rad})} = \frac{4.186 \text{ (J/calorie) } s\Delta T}{(10^{-2} \text{ J/kg-rad})} \qquad (8\text{-}6)$$

where E is the energy absorbed in joules, m is the mass of the absorber in kilograms, s is the specific heat of the absorber in calories/kg C and ΔT is the temperature rise in Celsius (centigrade) degrees. For equation (8-6) to be correct, the absorbing medium must be insulated from its environment. To measure the absorbed dose in a particular medium, the absorber of the calorimeter must possess an atomic number similar to that of the medium. Graphite often is used as the absorbing medium in calorimeters designed to measure the absorbed dose in soft tissue. A calorimeter used to measure radiation absorbed dose is diagramed in Figure 8-1, A.

If the absorbing medium is thick and dense enough to absorb nearly all of the incident radiation, then the increase in temperature reflects the total energy delivered to the absorber by the radiation beam. Calorimeters that measure the total energy in a beam of radiation usually contain a massive lead absorber (Fig 8-1, B).

*A thermistor is a solid-state device with an electric resistance that changes rapidly with temperature. A Wheatstone bridge is an electric circuit used to measure small changes in electric resistance.

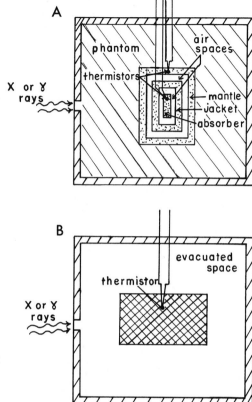

Fig 8-1.—Radiation calorimeters: **A,** for the measurement of absorbed dose in soft tissue; **B,** for the measurement of the total energy in a beam of radiation.

Example 8-4.

The specific heat of graphite is 170 calories /kg°C. What is the absorbed dose in a graphite block of a calorimeter if the temperature of the block increases by 0.2 Celsius degrees?

$$D = \frac{4.186\ s\Delta T}{10^{-2}}$$
$$= 4.186 \times 10^2\ (170\ \text{calories/kg°C})(0.2°\text{C})$$
$$= 14,200\ \text{rad}$$

Photographic Dosimetry

Photographic emulsions were used very early to detect ionizing radiation. The emulsion of a photographic film contains crystals of a silver halide embedded in a gelatin matrix. When the emulsion is developed, metallic silver is deposited in regions that were exposed to radiation. Unaffected crystals of silver halide are removed during fixation. The amount of silver deposited at any location depends upon many factors, including the amount of energy absorbed by the emulsion at that location. The transmission of light through a small region of film varies inversely with the amount of deposited silver. The transmission T is

$$T = \frac{I}{I_0}$$

where I represents the intensity of light transmitted through a small region of film and I_0 represents the light intensity with the film removed. The transmission may be measured with an optical densitometer. Curves relating transmission to radiation exposure, dose or energy fluence are obtained by measuring the transmission through films receiving known exposures, fluences or doses. If the problems described below are not insurmountable, the radiation exposure to a region of blackened film may be determined by measuring the transmission of light through the region and referring to the calibration curve.

Accurate dosimetry is difficult with photographic emulsions, for reasons including those listed below.[13]

1. The optical density of a film depends not only upon the radiation exposure to the emulsion, but also upon variables such as the energy of the radiation and the conditions under which the film is processed. For example, the optical density of a photographic film exposed to 40-keV photons may be as great as the density of a second film receiving an exposure 30 times greater from ^{60}Co gammas. Photographic emulsions are said to be "energy dependent," because their response to x- and γ-ray photons of various energies differs from the response of air or soft tissue. In most cases, calibration films used to relate optical density to the exposure in roentgens must be exposed to radiation identical to that for which dosimetric measurements are needed. This requirement often is difficult to satisfy, particularly when films are exposed in phantoms or in other situations where a large amount of scattered radiation is present.

2. Compared to air or soft tissue, the high-Z emulsion of a photographic film attenuates radiation rapidly. Errors caused by these differences in attenuation may be particularly severe when radiation is directed parallel to one film or perpendicular to a stack of films.

3. Differences in the thickness and composition of the photographic emulsion may cause the radiation sensitivity to vary from one film to another. Sometimes, variations in radiation sensitivity are noticeable across the surface of one film.

Chemical Dosimetry

Oxidation or reduction reactions are initiated when certain chemical solutions are exposed to ionizing radiation. The number of molecules affected depends upon the energy absorbed by the solution. Conse-

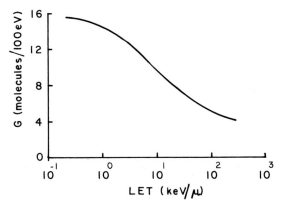

Fig 8-2. – Variation in G for the Fricke dosimeter with the *LET* of the radiation. (From International Commission on Radiological Units and Measurements: *Physical Aspects of Irradiation.* Recommendations of the ICRU. National Bureau of Standards Handbook 85, 1964.)

quently, the extent of oxidation or reduction is a reflection of the radiation dose to the solution. The chemical dosimeter used most widely is ferrous sulfate. For photons that interact primarily by Compton scattering, the ratio of the energy absorbed in ferrous sulfate to that absorbed in soft tissue equals 1.024, the ratio of the electron densities of the two media. For photons of higher and lower energy, the ratio of energy absorption increases above 1.024, because more energy is absorbed in the higher-$\overline{Z}$ ferrous sulfate.

The use of solutions of ferrous sulfate to measure radiation dose was described by Fricke and Morse in 1929.[14] A solution of ferrous sulfate used for radiation dosimetry sometimes is referred to as a *Fricke dosimeter*. Methods for preparing a Fricke dosimeter are discussed in NBS Handbook 85.[15] Although the Fricke dosimeter is reliable and accurate ($\pm$ 3%), it is relatively insensitive, and doses of 5,000–50,000 rad are required before the oxidation of Fe^{+2} to Fe^{+3} is measurable. The Fricke dosimeter has been recommended for calibration of high-energy electron beams used in radiation therapy.[16]

The yield of a chemical dosimeter such as ferrous sulfate is expressed by the G value:

$$G = \text{Number of molecules affected per 100 eV absorbed}$$

The G value for the oxidation of Fe^{+2} to Fe^{+3} in the Fricke dosimeter varies with the *LET* of the radiation (Fig 8-2). Many investigators have assumed that G is about 15.4 molecules/100 eV for a solution of ferrous sulfate exposed to high-energy electrons or x and γ rays of medium energy. After exposure to radiation, the amount of Fe^{+3} ion in a ferrous sulfate solution is determined by measuring the transmission of ultraviolet light (3,050 Å) through the solution. Once the number of affected molecules is known, the energy absorbed by the ferrous sulfate solution may be computed by dividing the number of molecules by the G value.

The radiation responses of many other solutions have been studied.[15] Occasionally, these solutions are used in place of ferrous sulfate. For example, cerous sulfate dosimeters sometimes are used to measure absorbed doses greater than 50,000 rad, the maximum dose measurable with aerated solutions of ferrous sulfate.

Example 8-5

A solution of ferrous sulfate is exposed to ^{60}Co gamma radiation. Measurement of the transmission of ultraviolet light (3,050 Å) through the irradiated solution indicates the presence of Fe^{+3} ion at a concentration of 0.0001M. What was the radiation dose absorbed by the solution?

For a concentration of 0.0001M, and with a density of 10^{-3} kg/ml for the ferrous sulfate solution, the number of Fe^{+3} ions/kg is

Number of Fe^{3+} ions/kg

$$= \frac{(0.0001 \text{ gm-mol-wt}/1{,}000 \text{ ml})(6.02 \times 10^{23} \text{ molecules/gm-mol-wt})}{(10^{-3} \text{ kg/ml})}$$

$$= 6.02 \times 10^{19} \frac{\text{molecules}}{\text{kg}}$$

For a G value of (15.4 molecules/100 eV) for ferrous sulfate, the absorbed dose in the solution is

$$D \text{ (rad)} = \frac{(6.02 \times 10^{19} \text{ molecules/kg})(1.6 \times 10^{-19} \text{ J/eV})}{(15.4 \text{ molecules}/100 \text{ eV})(10^{-2} \text{ J/kg-rad})}$$
$$= 6{,}300 \text{ rad}$$

Scintillation Dosimetry

Certain materials fluoresce or "scintillate" when exposed to ionizing radiation. The rate at which scintillations occur depends upon the rate of absorption of radiation in the scintillator. With a solid scintillation detector (e.g., thallium-activated sodium iodide), a light guide couples the scintillator optically to a photomultiplier tube. In the photomultiplier tube, light pulses from the detector are converted into electric pulses.

Scintillation detectors furnish a measurable response at very low dose rates and respond linearly over a wide range of dose rates. However, most scintillation detectors contain high-Z atoms, and low-energy photons are absorbed more rapidly in the detectors than in soft tissue or air. This *energy dependence* is the major disadvantage of using scintillation detectors to measure radiation exposure or dose to soft tissue. A few scintillation detectors have been constructed that are air-equivalent or tissue-equivalent over a wide range of photon energies.[15]

Thermoluminescence Dosimetry

Diagramed in Figure 8-3 are energy levels for electrons within crystals of LiF that contain trace amounts of impurities.* Electrons "jump" from the valence band to the conduction band by absorbing energy from ionizing radiation impinging upon the crystals. Some of the electrons return immediately to the valence band; others are "trapped" in intermediate energy levels supplied by impurities in the crystals. The number of electrons trapped in intermediate levels is proportional to the energy absorbed by the LiF phosphor during irradiation. Only rarely do electrons escape from the traps and return directly to the ground state. Unless energy is supplied for their release, almost all of the trapped electrons remain in the intermediate energy levels for months or years after irradiation. If the crystals are heated, energy is supplied to release the trapped electrons. Released electrons return to the conduction band, where they fall to the valence band. Blue-green light is released as the electrons return to the valence band. This light is directed upon the photocathode of a photomultiplier tube. Because the amount of light striking the photocathode is proportional to the energy absorbed in the LiF during irradiation, the signal from the photomultiplier tube increases with the radiation dose absorbed in the phosphor.

The signal from the photomultiplier tube may be amplified and recorded as a function of the heating time or temperature of the LiF phosphor. The resulting "glow curve" encloses an area proportional to the radiation dose (Fig 8-4). Thermoluminescence peaks that occur at low temperatures on the glow curve may be removed by annealing the LiF prior to use.[19]

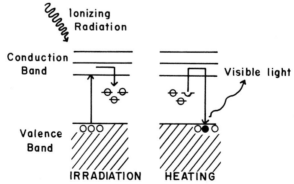

Fig 8-3.—Electron transitions occurring when thermoluminescent LiF is irradiated and heated.

*Thermoluminescence is more complex than this explanation implies. For a more thorough explanation, the reader should consult the literature.[17, 18]

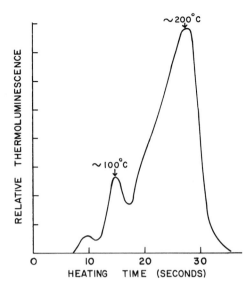

Fig 8-4.—Thermoluminescence glow curve of relative luminescence from LiF exposed to 100 R, plotted as a function of the heating time of the phosphor in seconds. Low-temperature peaks have been reduced by a standard annealing procedure.

For routine dosimetry, the signal from the photomultiplier tube is directed through an analog-digital converter and displayed as a digital count on a scaler (Fig 8-5). Optical filters between the heating pan and photomultiplier tube reduce the "background counts" contributed by infrared radiation from the heating pan.

The effective atomic number of dosimetric LiF (8.18) is close to that for soft tissue (7.4) and for air (7.65). Hence, for identical exposures to radiation, the amount of energy absorbed by LiF is very close to that absorbed by an equal mass of soft tissue or air. Small differences be-

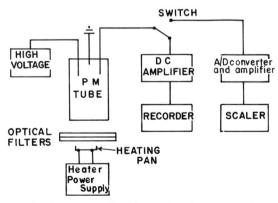

Fig 8-5.—Apparatus for measuring thermoluminescence from materials such as LiF and $Li_2B_4O_7$.

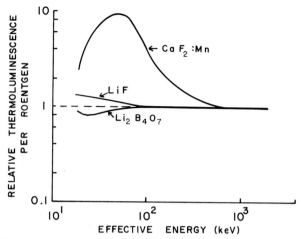

Fig 8-6.—Relative thermoluminescence from various materials per roentgen, plotted as a function of the effective energy of incident x- or γ-ray photons. Data have been normalized to the response per roentgen for ⁶⁰Co gammas.

tween the energy absorption in LiF and air are reflected in the "energy dependence" curve for LiF shown in Figure 8-6.

Thermoluminescence from dosimetric LiF is plotted in Figure 8-7 as a function of the exposure in roentgens. Between one and a few hundred roentgens, the response is linear with exposure; the response is "super-linear" above a few hundred roentgens. At least until very high exposure rates are reached, the response per unit exposure is independent of the exposure rate.[20] The response of irradiated LiF decreases (fades) slightly over the first 24 hr after exposure. Beyond 24 hr, the response remains almost constant for months. Lithium fluoride is used widely for the

Fig 8-7.—Thermoluminescence from dosimetric LiF as a function of the exposure in roentgens.

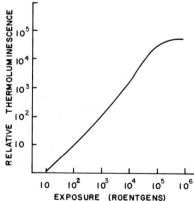

measurement of radiation dose within patients and phantoms, for personnel dosimetry and for many other dosimetric measurements. Dosimetric LiF may be purchased as loose crystals, solid extruded rod, solid chips, pressed pellets or as crystals embedded in a Teflon matrix.

Lithium borate ($Li_2B_4O_7$) exhibits a thermoluminescent response per unit exposure which decreases only slightly for photon energies less than about 100 keV (Fig 8-6). Irradiated lithium borate emits orange light when heated, and furnishes a glow curve comprised of two major peaks ($\sim$100 C and 180–220 C). The lower temperature peak fades rapidly after exposure of the phosphor, and usually is omitted from the measurement of thermoluminescence.

Thermoluminescent dosimeters composed of CaF_2:Mn are used frequently for personnel monitoring and, occasionally, for other measurements of radiation dose. Compared to LiF and $Li_2B_4O_7$, CaF_2:Mn phosphor is more sensitive to ionizing radiation; however, the response of this phosphor varies rapidly with the energy of x and γ radiation (Fig 8-6).[21]

Other Solid-State Dosimeters

Photoluminescent dosimeters are similar to thermoluminescent dosimeters except that ultraviolet light, rather than heat, causes the dosimeters to emit light (Fig 8-8). Most photoluminescent dosimeters are composed of silver-activated metaphosphate glass of either high-Z or low-Z composition. The response from both types of glass increases rapidly as the energy of incident x or γ rays is reduced. Shields have been designed to reduce the energy dependence of these materials.[22] For exposure rates up to at least 10^8 R/sec, the photoluminescent response of silver-activated metaphosphate glass is independent of exposure rate.[23] Chipping or scratching the surface of photoluminescent dosimeters reduces their sensitivity to radiation; consequently, these dosimeters must be handled carefully. Photoluminescent dosimeters are used occasionally for personnel monitoring and other dosimetric measurements.[21]

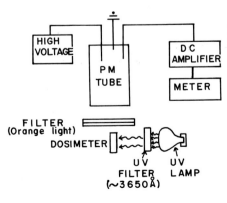

Fig 8-8. —Apparatus for measuring photoluminescence from Ag-activated metaphosphate glass.

Radiation-induced changes in the optical density of glasses and plastics have been used occasionally to measure radiation quantity. Changes in the optical density are determined by measuring the transmission of visible or ultraviolet light through the materials before and after exposure to radiation. Silver-activated phosphate glass and cobalt-activated borosilicate glass have been used as radiation dosimeters.[24] Some transparent plastics also have been used for dosimetric measurements.[21] Glass and plastic dosimeters are very insensitive to radiation, and high exposures are required to obtain a measurable response. Often, the change in light transmission of the dosimeter fades rapidly after exposure.

Erythema Dose

In early years, the amount of x radiation received by a patient was estimated by the redness of the patient's skin. The *total erythema dose* (TED) was defined as the amount of radiation that produced a slight reddening of the skin in 80% of the persons exposed. Because of the variable response of individuals to radiation, together with variations in the TED caused by changes in exposure rate and radiation quality, the TED was replaced rapidly with more explicit descriptions of radiation quantity.

PROBLEMS

*1. An organ with a mass of 10 gm receives a uniform dose of 10 rad. How much energy is absorbed in each gram of tissue in the tumor, and how much energy is absorbed in the entire tumor?

*2. A particular type of lesion recedes satisfactorily after receiving 5,500 rad from orthovoltage x rays. When the lesion is treated with ^{60}Co gamma radiation, a dose of 6,500 rad is required. Relative to orthovoltage x rays, what is the RBE of ^{60}Co radiation for treating this type of lesion?

*3. An individual who ingests a radioactive sample receives an estimated dose of 1,500 mrad to the testes: 1,100 mrad are delivered by betas and 400 mrad are delivered by gamma radiation. What is the dose to the testes in mrems?

*4. The specific heat of graphite is 170 calories/kg C. A uniform dose of 1,000 rad is delivered to a graphite block insulated from its environment. What is the rise in temperature of the block?

*5. With the assumption that $G = 15.4$, how many Fe^{+2} ions are oxidized if an absorbed dose of 15,000 rad is delivered to a 10 ml solution of ferrous sulfate? Assume that the density of ferrous sulfate is 10^{-3} kg/ml.

6. Explain clearly what is meant by the *energy dependence* of a radiation dosimeter.

---

*For those problems marked with an asterisk, answers are provided on the pages following the appendixes (see pp. 487–488).

REFERENCES

1. International Commission on Radiation Units and Measurements: *Radiation Quantities and Units*. ICRU Report 11 (Washington, D.C.: Government Printing Office, 1968).
2. Storer, J., et al.: Relative biological effectiveness of various ionizing radiations in mammalian systems, Radiat. Res. 6:188, 1957.
3. Hall, E.: Relative biological efficiency of x rays generated at 200 kVp and gamma radiation from cobalt 60 therapy unit, Br. J. Radiol. 34:313, 1961.
4. Sinclair, W.: Relative biological effectiveness of 22-MeVp x rays, cobalt 60 gamma rays and 200 kVp rays: 1. General introduction and physical aspects, Radiat. Res. 16:336, 1962.
5. Loken, M., et al.: Relative biological effectiveness of ^{60}Co gamma rays and 220 kVp x rays on viability of chicken eggs, Radiat. Res. 12:202, 1960.
6. Krohmer, J.: RBE and quality of electromagnetic radiation at depths in water phantom, Radiat. Res. 24:547, 1965.
7. Upton, A., et al.: Relative biological effectiveness of neutrons, x rays, and gamma rays for production of lens opacities; observations on mice, rats, guinea pigs and rabbits, Radiology 67:686, 1956.
8. Focht, E., et al.: The relative biological effectiveness of cobalt 60 gamma and 200 kV x radiation for cataract induction, Am. J. Roentgenol. 102:71, 1968.
9. Till, J., and Cunningham, J.: Unpublished data, cited in Johns, H., and Cunningham, J. (eds.): *The Physics of Radiology* (3d ed.; Springfield, Ill.: Charles C Thomas, Publisher, 1969), p. 720.
10. Recommendations of the International Commission on Radiological Protection: Br. J. Radiol., suppl. 6, 1955.
11. International Commission on Radiological Protection: *Radiation Protection*, Recommendations of the ICRP. Publ. 9 (New York: Pergamon Press, 1966).
12. Laughlin, J., and Genna, S.: Calorimetry, in Attix, F., and Roesch, W. (eds.): *Radiation Dosimetry* (2d ed.; New York: Academic Press, 1968), vol. 2, p. 389.
13. Ehrlich, M.: *Photographic Dosimetry of X and Gamma Rays*, National Bureau of Standards Handbook 57, 1954.
14. Fricke, H., and Morse, S.: The actions of x rays on ferrous sulfate solutions, Phil. Mag. 7:129, 1929.
15. International Commission on Radiological Units and Measurements: *Physical Aspects of Irradiation*. Recommendations of the ICRU. National Bureau of Standards Handbook 85, 1964.
16. The Subcommittee on Radiation Dosimetry (SCRAD) of the American Association of Physicists in Medicine: Protocol for the dosimetry of high energy electrons, Phys. Med. Biol. 11:505, 1966.
17. Cameron, J., Suntharalingam, N., and Kenney, G.: *Thermoluminescent Dosimetry* (Madison: University of Wisconsin Press, 1968).
18. Auxier, J., Becker, K., and Robinson, E. (eds.): *Proceedings Second International Conference on Luminescence Dosimetry*, CONF-680920 (Springfield, Va.: Clearinghouse for Federal Scientific and Technical Information, 1968).
19. Cameron, J., et al.: Thermoluminescent radiation dosimetry utilizing LiF, Health Phys. 10:25, 1964.
20. Karzmark, C., White, J., and Fowler, J.: Lithium fluoride thermoluminescence dosimetry, Phys. Med. Biol. 9:273, 1964.
21. Fowler, J., and Attix, F.: Solid State Integrating Dosimeters, in Attix, F.,

and Roesch, W. (eds.): *Radiation Dosimetry* (2d ed.; New York: Academic Press, 1968), vol. 2, p. 241.

22. Thornton, W., and Auxier, J.: Some x-ray and fast neutron response characteristics of Ag-metaphosphate glass dosimeters, ORNL-2912, 1960.

23. Tochilin, E., and Goldstein, N.: Energy and dose rate response of five dosimeter systems, Health Phys. 10:602, 1964.

24. Kreidl, N., and Blair, G.: Recent developments in glass dosimetry, Nucleonics 14(3):82, 1956.

9 / Radiation Quality

An X-RAY BEAM is not described completely by stating the exposure or dose it delivers to a small region within an irradiated medium. The penetrating ability of the radiation, often described as the *quality* of the radiation, also must be known before estimates may be made of the following.

1. The exposure or dose rate at other locations within the medium.
2. The differences in energy absorption between regions of different composition.
3. The biologic effectiveness of the radiation.

The spectral distribution for an x-ray beam depicts the relative number of photons of different energies in the beam. The quality of an x-ray beam is described explicitly by the spectral distribution. However, spectral distributions are difficult to measure or compute and are used only rarely to describe radiation quality. Usually, the quality of an x-ray beam is described by stating the half-value layer (HVL) of the beam, sometimes together with the potential difference (kVp) across the x-ray tube. Although other methods have been developed to describe the quality of an x-ray beam, the HVL is adequate for most clinical applications of x radiation.

HALF-VALUE LAYER

The half-value layer (HVL) or half-value thickness (HVT) of an x-ray beam is the thickness of a material that reduces the exposure rate of the beam to one-half. Although the HVL alone furnishes a description of radiation quality that is adequate for most clinical situations, the value of a second parameter (e.g., the peak potential difference across the x-ray tube or the homogeneity coefficient* of the x-ray beam) sometimes is stated with the HVL. Once the HVL of an x-ray beam is known, together with the exposure or dose rate at a particular location, the absorbed dose rate may be computed at other locations within an irradiated medium.

Half-value layers are measured with solid absorbers (more correctly, attenuators) such as thin sheets of aluminum, copper or lead of uniform

---

*The homogeneity coefficient of an x-ray beam is the quotient of the thickness of the attenuator required to reduce the exposure rate to one-half, divided by the thickness of attenuator required to reduce the exposure rate from one-half to one-fourth.

TABLE 9-1.—REQUIREMENTS FOR ATTENUATORS
USED TO MEASURE HALF-VALUE LAYER°

MATERIAL	ACCEPTABLE kV RANGE	USUAL kV RANGE	DENSITY (kg/cu m)	CHEMICAL PURITY (%)
Aluminum (Al)	10 kV – 20 MV	10 kV – 120 kV	2.70×10^3	>99.8
Copper (Cu)	35 kV – 8 MV	120 kV – 3.5 MV	8.93×10^3	>99.2
Lead (Pb)	350 kV – 50 MV	1 MV – 50 MV	11.35×10^3	>99.9

°Compiled from data in National Bureau of Standards Handbook 85.[1]

thickness. The ranges of tube voltage over which different attenuators are used are listed in Table 9-1, together with the density and chemical purity recommended for each type of attenuator.

Half-value layers may be measured by placing attenuators of different thickness but constant composition between the x-ray tube and an ionization chamber designed to measure radiation exposure. The distribution of photon energies changes as attenuators are added to an x-ray beam, and the response of the chamber should be independent of these changes. Measurements of HVL always should be made with narrow-beam geometry. Narrow-beam geometry (sometimes referred to as *good geometry*) ensures that the only photons that enter the chamber are primary photons that have been transmitted by the attenuator. Requirements for narrow-beam geometry are satisfied if the chamber is positioned far from the attenuator and if an x-ray beam with small cross-sectional area is measured. The cross-sectional area of the beam should be just large enough to deliver a uniform exposure over the entire sensitive

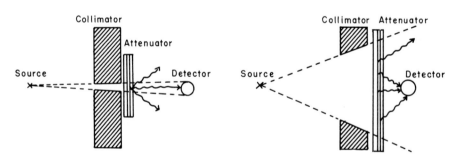

NARROW-BEAM GEOMETRY   BROAD-BEAM GEOMETRY

Fig 9-1.—Narrow-beam geometry is achieved by using a narrow beam and a large distance between the attenuator and the chamber used to measure radiation exposure. With narrow-beam geometry, few photons are scattered into the chamber by the attenuator. A significant number of photons are scattered into the chamber when attenuation measurements are made with broad-beam geometry.

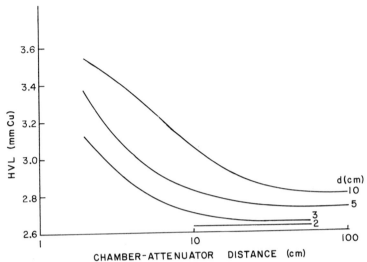

Fig 9-2. — Variation of the HVL with the diameter *d* of an x-ray beam at the attenuator, for various distances between the attenuator and the chamber. The x-ray beam was generated at 250 kVp and filtered by 2 mm Cu. The attenuator was placed 20 cm below the x-ray tube. The geometry improves with decreasing diameter of the x-ray beam and increasing distance between attenuator and chamber. (From International Commission on Radiological Units and Measurements: *Physical Aspects of Irradiation.* National Bureau of Standards Handbook 85, 1964.)

volume of the chamber. Conditions of narrow-beam and broad-beam *(poor)* geometry are depicted in Figure 9-1. Measurements of HVL under these conditions are compared in Figure 9-2. With broad-beam geometry, more photons are scattered into the detector as the thickness of the attenuator is increased. Consequently, HVL's measured with broad-beam geometry are greater than those measured under conditions of narrow-beam geometry.

Narrow-beam geometry may be achieved by placing the attenuator midway between the x-ray target and the chamber, with the chamber at least 50 cm from the attenuator. The area of the field should be no larger than a few square centimeters. Objects that might scatter photons into the chamber should be removed from the vicinity of the x-ray beam. Even greater accuracy can be attained by measuring the HVL for fields of different cross-sectional area and extrapolating the measured HVL's to a field size of zero.[2, 3] This procedure is not necessary for routine clinical dosimetry.

An attenuation curve for x rays in copper is shown in Figure 9-3. The HVL is 1.86 mm Cu for the x-ray beam described in the figure. A com-

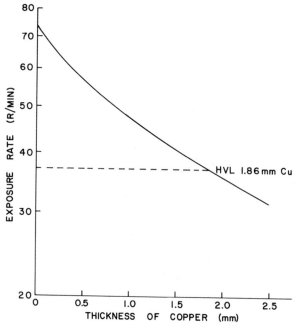

Fig 9-3. — Exposure rate for an x-ray beam as a function of the thickness of copper added to the beam. The HVL of the beam is 1.86 mm Cu.

plete attenuation curve is not required for routine dosimetry. Instead, thicknesses of the attenuator are identified that reduce the exposure rate to slightly more than half (50–55%) and slightly less than half (45–50%). These data are plotted on a semilogarithmic graph and connected by a straight line. The approximate HVL is given by the intersection of this straight line with a horizontal line drawn through the ordinate (y-axis) at one half of the exposure rate measured with no attenuator added to the beam.

TUBE VOLTAGE

For most purposes, the HVL furnishes an adequate description of the quality of an x-ray beam. However, the tube voltage sometimes is stated also. The tube voltage may be indicated by a meter on the console of the x-ray generator or by the position of the kilovolt peak selector switch or push-button array. A few methods are available for estimating the accuracy of the voltage indicated by the panel meter.

Sphere Gap Measurements

The potential difference across an x-ray tube may be measured directly with two polished metallic spheres. One sphere is connected to each high-voltage lead for the x-ray tube, and the distance between the spheres is reduced until an electric spark passes between them. When the spark occurs, the distance between the spheres, corrected for air density and humidity, reflects the potential difference across the x-ray tube.[4]

The high-voltage leads of newer, shockproof x-ray generators are enclosed within layers of insulating material and metallic braid. Consequently, special connectors are required to connect the metallic spheres to the high-voltage leads of these generators, and this method of high-voltage measurement is used only rarely.

Resistance-Tower Measurements

Coils of nickel-chromium wire with high electric resistance, connected in series to form a resistance tower, may be placed across the high-voltage leads to an x-ray tube. The resistance of the tower must be great enough to limit the current through the tower to 1 mA or less. The peak voltage across the x-ray tube is the product of the peak current through the tower and the resistance of the tower measured in ohms.

K-Fluorescence Measurements

The potential difference across a diagnostic x-ray tube may be determined by measuring the radiation scattered and transmitted by an attenuator placed in the x-ray beam.[5, 6] Two ionization chambers or scintillation detectors are placed as shown in Figure 9-4. Chamber *1* detects x radiation transmitted by the attenuator. Chamber *2* detects x radiation scattered by the attenuator and characteristic x rays emitted as primary photons interact in the attenuator. The low-Z filter in front of Chamber *2* absorbs most of the low-energy scattered radiation and L- and M-characteristic x rays emerging from the attenuator. Almost all of the K-characteristic x rays are transmitted by the filter.

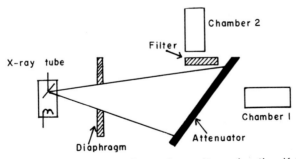

Fig 9-4.—Technique for measuring tube voltage by the K-fluorescence method. Chamber *1* detects x radiation transmitted by the attenuator. Chamber *2* detects scattered and characteristic x radiation from the attenuator. The low-Z filter absorbs most of the low-energy radiation from the attenuator.

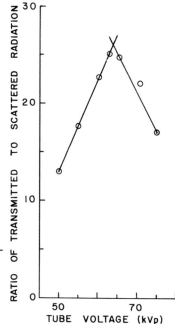

Fig 9-5.—Ratio of the response of Chamber *1* to the response of Chamber *2* for an erbium attenuator as a function of the tube voltage indicated on the generator console. The discontinuity occurs at an actual potential difference of 57.5 kVp across the x-ray tube. (From Davison, M., and Reckie, D.: Measurement of peak voltage of diagnostic x-ray generators, Phys. Med. Biol. 13:643, 1968.)

Initially, the ratio of the response of Chamber *1* to the response of Chamber *2* increases with the tube voltage. However, the attenuation of primary x rays increases sharply when these x rays are energetic enough to dislodge electrons from the K shell of atoms in the attenuator. At this tube voltage, the response of Chamber *1* is reduced because fewer x rays are transmitted by the attenuator. Also, K-characteristic x rays from the attenuator increase the response of Chamber *2*. Consequently, the ratio of the response of Chamber *1* to Chamber *2* decreases sharply, creating a discontinuity in the plot of the response ratio of the chambers as a function of the voltage indicated on the generator console. Results of measurements with an erbium attenuator in the x-ray beam are shown in Figure 9-5. The discontinuity in the curve occurs at 57.5 keV, the K-absorption edge of erbium. Hence, the potential difference was 57.5 kVp across the x-ray tube when the discontinuity was encountered. The voltage indicated by the meter on the generator console may be compared to this known voltage. By placing other attenuators with known absorption edges in the x-ray beam, the voltage indicated on the console may be plotted as a function of the potential difference known to exist across the x-ray tube. For any voltage indicated by the meter on the console, the actual potential difference across the x-ray tube may be determined from the curve.[7, 8]

A variation on this method uses a single semiconductor radiation detector to observe the K-fluorescence radiation from different scattering foils as the peak kilovoltage of the x-ray tube is varied. This method is capable of yielding peak kilovoltage measurements accurate to 1 kVp.[9]

Attenuation Measurements

The potential difference across a diagnostic x-ray tube may be estimated by exposing an ionization chamber or other detector to a heavily filtered x-ray beam from the tube.[10, 11] A second exposure is made after an aluminum or copper cap has been placed over the sensitive volume of the detector. The ratio of the chamber response with the aluminum or copper cap in place to that obtained without the cap reflects the potential difference across the x-ray tube.

Differential attenuation of the x-ray beam is the technique used in the Ardran-Crooks method for measurement of peak kilovoltage.[12, 13] This method uses an x-ray film cassette that contains a column of copper filters of various thicknesses above an x-ray film. Adjacent to the copper filters is an intensifying screen with a column of optical filters between the screen and film. After exposure, the developed film is examined for the copper filter image with an optical density equal to that of the adjacent optical filter image. The position within the columns of copper and optical filter images where the optical densities are matched is indicative of the peak kilovoltage across the x-ray tube.

EFFECTIVE ENERGY

The *effective energy* of an x-ray beam is the energy of photons in a monoenergetic beam that is attenuated at the same rate as the x-ray beam. For a beam of x rays with an exposure rate X_r, the rate of attenuation P is

$$P = \mu X_r$$

where μ is the total linear attenuation coefficient. The rate of attenuation P in a particular medium is given by the slope of the attenuation curve for the beam in the medium. Hence, the linear attenuation coefficient μ equals the slope P divided by the exposure rate X_r at the location on the attenuation curve where the slope is determined:

$$\mu = \frac{P}{X_r}$$

To determine the effective energy of an x-ray beam at a location denoted by X_r along the attenuation curve, the linear attenuation coefficient μ is computed by dividing the slope of the curve by the exposure rate X_r at the location chosen. Then, the energy is found for monoenergetic photons that have a linear attenuation coefficient equal to μ in the same medium. This energy is the effective energy of the x-ray beam at the location denoted by X_r. Attenuation coefficients of various media for photons of different energies are available in the literature.[2, 14]

Example 9-1

With reference to Figure 9-3, what is the effective energy of the x-ray beam before attenuation and after 50% attenuation?

From a tangent to the attenuation curve in copper at the point denoting 50% attenuation, the slope P of the curve is -9.5 mm^{-1}. The linear attenuation coefficient μ is obtained by dividing the slope by X_r (37.0 R/min).

$$\begin{aligned} \mu &= \frac{P}{X_r} \\ &= \frac{9.5 \text{ mm}^{-1}}{37.0} \\ &= 0.257 \text{ mm}^{-1} \\ &= 2.57 \text{ cm}^{-1} \end{aligned}$$

The mass attenuation coefficient μ_m is

$$\begin{aligned} \mu_m &= \frac{2.57 \text{ cm}^{-1}}{8.93 \text{ gm/cc}} \\ &= 0.288 \text{ sq cm/gm} \end{aligned}$$

Monoenergetic photons of 126 keV possess a mass attenuation coefficient of 0.288 sq cm/gm in copper.[14] Hence, the effective energy of the x-ray beam is 126 keV after 50% attenuation.

With no copper added to the x-ray beam, the slope P of the curve is -44.0 mm^{-1}. The linear attenuation coefficient is the slope of the curve divided by X_r (74.0 R/min):

$$\begin{aligned} \mu &= \frac{P}{X_r} \\ &= \frac{44.0 \text{ mm}^{-1}}{74.0} \\ &= 5.95 \text{ cm}^{-1} \end{aligned}$$

The mass attenuation coefficient μ_m is

$$\begin{aligned} \mu_m &= \frac{5.95 \text{ cm}^{-1}}{8.93 \text{ gm/cc}} \\ &= 0.666 \text{ sq cm/gm} \end{aligned}$$

Monoenergetic photons of 84 keV possess a mass attenuation coefficient of 0.666 sq cm/gm in copper.[14] Hence, the effective energy of the x-ray beam is 84 keV with no copper added.

The average effective energy of an x-ray beam is defined in Chapter 6 as the energy of monoenergetic photons that exhibit the same HVL as the x-ray beam. This concept of effective energy is not very useful for many purposes, because the effective energy may increase rapidly as the attenuation varies from 0% to 50%. The average effective energy is 100 keV for the x-ray beam described in Example 9-1.

VARIATION IN QUALITY ACROSS AN X-RAY BEAM

The exposure rate on the side of an x-ray beam nearest to the anode is less than the exposure rate on the cathode side, because x-rays on the anode side are attenuated by a greater thickness of target material before they emerge from the anode. This variation in exposure rate across an x-ray beam is termed the *heel effect* and is discussed in Chapter 4. The greater filtration on the anode side increases the HVL of the x-ray beam from the cathode to the anode side. The decrease in exposure rate from cathode to anode across an x-ray beam is less noticeable at depths within a patient, because the radiation on the anode side is more penetrating. Illustrated in Figure 9-6 are HVL's measured in air at various locations across an x-ray beam from a diagnostic x-ray tube.[15]

SPECTRAL DISTRIBUTION OF AN X-RAY BEAM

The spectral distribution for a beam of x- or γ-ray photons may be computed from an attenuation curve measured under conditions of good geometry.[1] One of a variety of curve-fitting techniques may be applied to the attenuation curve to obtain equations that are used to compute the spectral distribution. The accuracy of this method of obtaining a spectral distribution is limited by the accuracy of the curve-fitting technique and by the accuracy with which the attenuation curve is measured.

Most measurements of x- and γ-ray spectra are made with a scintillation or semiconductor detector. The height of a voltage pulse from one of

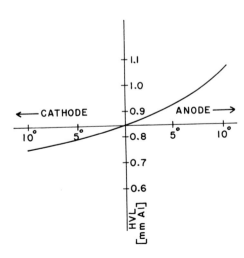

Fig 9-6. — Variation in HVL from cathode to anode across an x-ray beam of diagnostic quality. (From Kemp, L.: The physicist in the radiodiagnostic department, Br. J. Radiol. 19:304, 1946.)

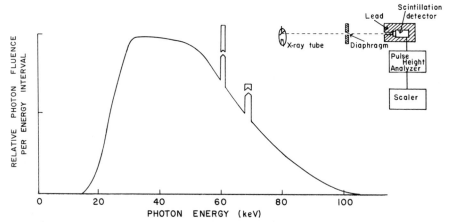

Fig 9-7.—Energy distribution of x-ray photons in a beam generated at 105 kVp and filtered by 2 mm Al. Equipment used to measure the spectra of primary x-rays is diagramed in the inset. (From Epp, E., and Weiss, H.: Experimental study of the photon energy spectrum of primary diagnostic x rays, Phys. Med. Biol. 11:225, 1966).

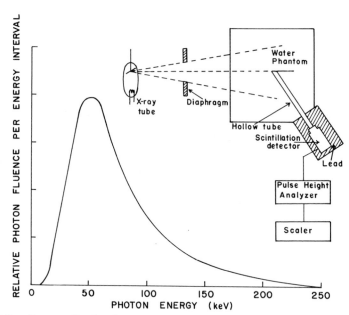

Fig 9-8.—Energy distribution of scattered radiation at 15 cm depth in a water phantom exposed to a 200 sq cm x-ray beam generated at 250 kVp. Equipment used to measure the spectra of scattered x-rays is diagramed in the inset. (From Hettinger, G., and Liden, K.: Scattered radiation in a water phantom irradiated by roentgen photons between 50 and 250 keV, Acta Radiol. 53:73, 1960.)

these detectors varies with the energy deposited in the detector by an x- or γ-ray photon. The pulses are sorted by height in a pulse height analyzer and counted in a scaler. The recorded counts are plotted as a function of pulse height to furnish a *pulse height distribution,* which reflects the energy distribution of photons impinging upon the detector. To portray the energy distribution accurately, the pulse height distribution must be corrected for statistical fluctuations in the energy distribution and for incomplete absorption of photons in the detector. Measured spectra for primary and scattered x rays are shown in Figures 9-7 and 9-8.

FACTORS INFLUENCING RADIATION QUALITY

The quality of an x-ray beam depends primarily on the energy of the electrons that strike the target of the x-ray tube and on the extent to which the x-ray beam is filtered after it emerges from the target.

Electron Energy

The energy of the electrons that impinge on the target of an x-ray tube is affected by (1) the waveform of the voltage supplied to the high-volt-

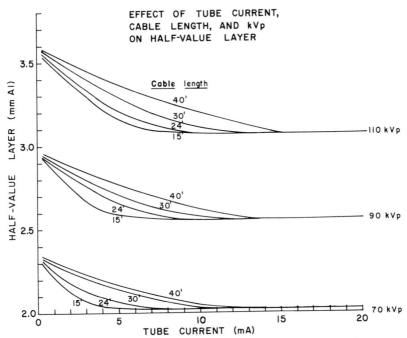

Fig 9-9.—Effect of the capacitance of high-voltage cables on the HVL of an x-ray beam of diagnostic quality. The effect on the HVL increases with the length of the cables. (From Trout, E., Kelley, J., and Lucas, A.: Influence of cable length on dose rate and half-value layer in diagnostic x-ray procedures, Radiology 74:255, 1960.)

age transformer, (2) the peak potential difference developed across the transformer and (3) the type of rectification used. The electron energy is influenced also by the cables between the high-voltage transformer and the x-ray tube, because the capacitance of these cables alters the waveform of the voltage applied to the x-ray tube. Illustrated in Figure 9-9 is the influence of cable capacitance on electron energy, as reflected in variations of the HVL of the x-ray beam.

Filtration

An x-ray beam traverses many attenuators before it reaches the object or patient to be irradiated. These attenuators include the glass envelope of the x-ray tube, the oil surrounding the x-ray tube, and the exit window in the tube housing. Collectively, these attenuators are referred to as the *inherent filtration* of the x-ray tube (Table 9-2). The *aluminum equivalent* for each component of inherent filtration is the thickness of aluminum that would reduce the exposure rate by an amount equal to the reduction provided by the component. The inherent filtration is approximately 0.90 mm Al equivalent for the tube described in Table 9-2, with most of the inherent filtration contributed by the glass envelope. The inherent filtration of most x-ray tubes is equivalent to about 1 mm Al.

In a particular medium, the probability that incident photons interact photoelectrically varies roughly as $1/E^3$, where E is the energy of the incident photons (chap. 6). Hence, lower-energy x rays are attenuated preferentially by material in the path of an x-ray beam. For example, the inherent filtration of an x-ray tube "hardens" (i.e., increases the HVL of) an x-ray beam emerging from the target. Additional hardening may be achieved by adding filters of various composition to the x-ray beam. Additional hardening of an x-ray beam almost always is desirable, because the added filtration removes low-energy x rays which, if left in the beam, increase the radiation dose to superficial tissues of a patient. These low-energy x rays do not contribute to the absorbed dose to a lesion in radiation therapy or to formation of a radiologic image in diagnostic radiology. A few filters used to increase the HVL of an x-ray beam are listed in

TABLE 9-2.—CONTRIBUTIONS TO INHERENT
FILTRATION IN TYPICAL DIAGNOSTIC
X-RAY TUBE*

COMPONENT	THICKNESS (mm)	ALUMINUM-EQUIVALENT THICKNESS (mm)
Glass envelope	1.4	0.78
Insulating oil	2.36	0.07
Bakelite window	1.02	0.05

*Derived from data of Trout.[16]

TABLE 9-3.—FILTERS USED TO HARDEN
AN X-RAY BEAM°

TUBE VOLTAGE	COMMON EXTERNAL FILTERS, ALIGNED IN ORDER FROM TARGET OUTWARD
10 kV – 120 kV	Al
120 kV – 400 kV	(Cu + Al) or (Sn + Cu + Al)
400 kV – 1 MV	Sn + Cu + Al
1 MV – 3 MV	Pb + Sn + Cu + Al
10 MV – 50 MV	None (other than beam-flattening filters)

°Compiled from data in National Bureau of Standards Handbook 85.[1]

Table 9-3. For diagnostic x-ray units, filters composed solely of aluminum usually are used.

Displayed in Figure 9-10 are energy distributions for x rays produced by 200-keV electrons and filtered by selected materials. The curve labeled *1 mm Al* represents a beam filtered by only the inherent filtration of the x-ray tube. By comparing curves labeled *1 mm Al* and *¼ mm Sn + 1 mm Al*, it is apparent that the tin filter removes lower-energy photons preferentially. A discontinuity in the curve labeled *¼ mm Sn + 1 mm Al* occurs at 29.3 keV, the K-absorption edge of tin. Photons with an energy less than 29.3 keV do not interact photoelectrically with K electrons in tin, and are transmitted by the tin filter with a probability greater than that for photons with an energy equal to or somewhat more than 29.3

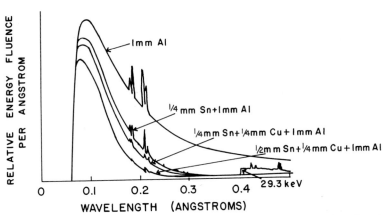

Fig 9-10.—Energy distribution for x rays from tungsten target bombarded by 200-keV electrons. The curves reflect different amounts of filtration added to the beam. The K-characteristic radiation is not drawn to scale. (From Johns, H., and Cunningham, J.: *The Physics of Radiology* [3d ed.; Springfield, Ill.: Charles C Thomas, Publisher, 1969].)

keV. Characteristic x rays—produced as primary x rays with an energy greater than 29.3 keV interact photoelectrically with K electrons in the tin filter—also contribute to the increased energy fluence below 29.3 keV.

The increased energy fluence below 29.3 keV may be reduced by placing a second filter of lower Z (e.g., copper) between the tin filter and the patient (Fig 9-10). Since the K-absorption edge of the second filter occurs at an energy less than 29.3 keV, x rays less than 29.3 keV are attenuated greatly by the second filter. However, photons with an energy less than the K edge of the second filter still may be transmitted with little attenuation. These x rays, together with K-characteristic x rays from the second filter, may be attenuated by a third filter (e.g., Al) of even lower atomic number. X rays transmitted by the third filter have little energy and are absorbed rapidly by air between the filter and the patient. Combination filters are used frequently with orthovoltage x-ray generators, because the increase in quality is gained with a minimum sacrifice of exposure rate.

The amount of filter to be added to an x-ray beam depends on the minimum exposure rate that can be tolerated and the quality that is desired for the beam. The exposure rate decreases as the beam is hardened, and a compromise between HVL and exposure rate may be required when a filter is selected. After a certain amount of filtration has been added to an x-ray beam, additional filtration may reduce the exposure rate without increasing the HVL significantly. This result suggests that more than the "optimum thickness" of filter has been added to the beam.

PROBLEMS

°1. Attenuation measurements for an x-ray beam from a 120-kVp x-ray generator yield the following results:

ADDED FILTRATION (mm Al)	PERCENT TRANSMISSION
1.0	60.2
2.0	41.4
3.0	30.0
4.0	22.4
5.0	16.9

Plot the data on semilogarithmic graph paper and determine:
  a. The first HVL.
  b. The second HVL.
  c. The homogeneity coefficient of the x-ray beam.
°2. A resistance tower of 5×10^8 ohms conducts a peak current of 150 μA when

°For those problems marked with an asterisk, answers are provided on the pages following the appendixes (see pp. 487–488).

connected across the high-voltage leads of a full-wave rectified, single-phase x-ray generator. What is the peak voltage applied to the x-ray tube?

°3. During K-fluorescence measurements of tube voltage with a platinum absorber (E_{BK} = 78.4 keV), the ratio of transmitted to scattered radiation varies as shown here:

TRANSMITTED RADIATION SCATTERED RADIATION	INDICATED TUBE VOLTAGE (kVp)
0.38	65
0.53	70
0.67	75
0.72	80
0.59	85
0.48	90

What is the tube voltage indicated by the meter when the actual voltage is 78.4 kVp across the x-ray tube?

4. Explain why combination filters should be used with the high-Z material nearest to the target and the low-Z material nearest to the patient. Would the quality of the x-ray beam change if the filter were reversed?

REFERENCES

1. International Commission on Radiological Units and Measurements: *Physical Aspects of Irradiation*. Recommendations of the ICRU. National Bureau of Standards Handbook 85, 1964.
2. Johns, H., and Cunningham, J.: *The Physics of Radiology* (3d ed.; Springfield, Ill.: Charles C Thomas, Publisher, 1969).
3. Trout, E., Kelley, J., and Lucas, A.: Determination of half-value layer, Am. J. Roentgenol. 84:729, 1960.
4. Young, M.: *Radiological Physics* (2d ed.; Springfield, Ill.: Charles C Thomas, Publisher, 1967).
5. Greening, J.: The measurement by ionizing methods of the peak kilovoltage across x-ray tubes, Br. J. Appl. Phys. 6:73, 1955.
6. Trout, E., Kelley, J., and Lucas, A.: Influence of cable length on dose rate and half-value layer in diagnostic x-ray procedures, Radiology 74:255, 1960.
7. Bloch, P., and Hale, J.: Calibration of potential of x-ray generators in the diagnostic energy region, Phys. Med. Biol. 11:577, 1966.
8. Davison, M., and Reckie, D.: Measurement of peak voltage of diagnostic x-ray generators, Phys. Med. Biol. 13:643, 1968.
9. Rauch, P., Chaney, E., Carson, P., and Hendee, W.: Absolute kilovoltage calibration of a diagnostic x-ray generator, Med. Phys. 2:1, 1975.
10. Newell, R., and Henny, G.: Inferential kilovoltmeter: Measuring x-ray kilovoltage by absorption in two filters, Radiology 64:88, 1955.
11. Morgan, R.: Physics of Diagnostic Radiology, in Glasser, O., et al. (eds.): *Physical Foundations of Radiology* (3d ed.; New York: Harper & Row, 1961), p. 117.
12. Ardran, G. M., and Crooks, H.: Checking diagnostic x-ray beam quality, Br. J. Radiol. 41:193, 1968.
13. Giarrantano, J., Waggener, R., Hevezi, J., and Shalek, R.: Comparison of voltage-divider, modified Ardran-Crooks cassette, and Ge (Li) spectrometer

methods to determine the peak kilovoltage (kVp) of diagnostic x-ray units, Med. Phys. 3:142, 1976.

14. Evans, R.: X-Ray and γ-Ray Interactions, in Attix, F., and Roesch, W. (eds.): *Radiation Dosimetry* (New York: Academic Press, 1968), vol. 1, p. 93.

15. Kemp, L.: The physicist in the radiodiagnostic department, Br. J. Radiol. 19: 304, 1946.

16. Trout, E.: The life history of an x-ray beam, Radiol. Technol. 35:161, 1963.

10 / Interaction of X and Gamma Rays in the Body

THE DOMINANT MODE of interaction of x- and γ-ray photons in a particular region of the body varies with the energy of the photons and with the effective atomic number and electron density (electrons per kilogram) of the region. For purposes of dosimetry, the body may be divided into regions of (1) fat, (2) muscle (or soft tissue excluding fat), (3) bone and (4) air-filled cavities. The effective atomic number, average density and electron density are listed in Table 10-1 for these constituents of the body.

F-FACTOR

As shown in Chapter 8, an exposure of 1 R provides an absorbed dose of 0.869 rad in air:

$$D_{air} \text{ (rad)} = 0.869 \, X \text{ (R)}$$

The dose to a medium such as soft tissue is related to the dose in air at the same location by the ratio of energy absorption in the medium to energy absorption in air:

$$D_{med} = D_{air} \frac{[(\mu_{en})_m]_{med}}{[(\mu_{en})_m]_{air}} \tag{10-1}$$

$$= 0.869 \frac{[(\mu_{en})_m]_{med}}{[(\mu_{en})_m]_{air}}(X) \tag{10-2}$$

In equation (10-2), $[(\mu_{en})_m]_{med}$ is the mass energy absorption coefficient of the medium for photons of the energy of interest. This coefficient describes the rate of energy absorption in the medium and $[(\mu_{en})_m]_{air}$ describes the rate of energy absorption in air. In equation (10-2), the expression may be simplified to

$$D_{med} = (f)(X) \tag{10-3}$$

where

$$f = 0.869 \frac{[(\mu_{en})_m]_{med}}{[(\mu_{en})_m]_{air}} \tag{10-4}$$

The expression denoted as f is known as the f-factor and varies with the nature of the absorbing medium and the energy of the radiation.

171

TABLE 10-1.—EFFECTIVE ATOMIC NUMBER,
PHYSICAL DENSITY AND ELECTRON DENSITY
FOR AIR, WATER AND BODY CONSTITUENTS

MATERIAL	EFFECTIVE ATOMIC NO.	DENSITY (kg/cu m)	ELECTRON DENSITY (ELECTRONS/kg)
Air	7.6	1.29	3.01×10^{26}
Water	7.4	1.00	3.34×10^{26}
Soft tissue	7.4	1.00	3.36×10^{26}
Fat	5.9–6.3	0.91	$3.34–3.48 \times 10^{26}$
Bone	11.6–13.8	1.65–1.85	$3.00–3.19 \times 10^{26}$

The f-factor is used to compute the absorbed dose D in rad in a medium receiving an exposure X in roentgens. The f-factor is plotted in Figure 10-1 for air, water, fat, muscle and compact bone as a function of photon energy. This plot is an explicit description of why high-contrast x-ray images are obtained with low-energy photons, and why image contrast is reduced at higher photon energies where interactions are primarily Compton scattering rather than photoelectric absorption.

For all photon energies for which the roentgen (and therefore the f-factor) is defined, an exposure of 1 R provides an absorbed dose of 0.869 rad in air. Consequently, the f-factor equals 0.869 for air and is independent of photon energy.

ATTENUATION OF X AND γ RAYS IN FAT

X- and γ-ray photons with energy less than about 35 keV interact in soft tissue primarily by the photoelectric effect, with a probability for interaction that varies roughly as Z^3. Compared to muscle and bone, fat

Fig 10-1.—The f-factor for conversion between roentgens and rads for air, water and different constituents of the body, plotted as a function of photon energy. Curves do not extend beyond 3 MeV, because the roentgen (and therefore the f-factor) is not applicable to photons of higher energy. Because of the varying composition of fat, the dotted curve for fat is only approximately correct.

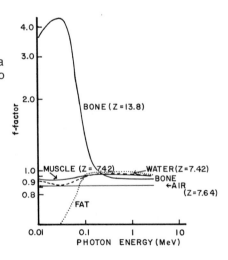

has a higher concentration by weight of hydrogen (~11%) and carbon (~ 57%) and a lower concentration of nitrogen (~1%), oxygen (30%) and high-Z trace elements (<1%).[1] Hence, the effective atomic number of fat (Z_{eff} = 5.9−6.3) is less than that for soft tissue (Z_{eff} = 7.4) or bone (Z_{eff} = 11.6−13.8), and low-energy photons are attenuated less rapidly in fat than in an equal mass of soft tissue or bone.[1, 2] The reduced attenuation in fat is reflected in a lower f-factor for photons of low energy in this body constituent (Fig 10-1).

X- and γ-ray photons of higher energy interact primarily by Compton scattering, with a probability that varies with the electron density of the attenuating medium but not with the atomic number. The electron density of hydrogen is about twice that of other elements, because the nucleus of hydrogen contains no neutrons. Since more hydrogen is present in fat than in other body constituents, more Compton interactions occur in fat than in an equal mass of muscle or bone. For photons of intermediate energy, therefore, the f-factor for fat exceeds that for other body constituents (Fig 10-1).

The f-factor cannot be defined rigorously for x- and γ-ray photons with energy greater than about 3 MeV, because the roentgen is not applicable to photons of higher energy. Consequently, f-factors in Figure 10-1 are plotted to only 3 MeV. The attenuation of x- and γ-ray photons in fat may be estimated from attenuation measurements in mineral oil or polyethylene, because the effective atomic numbers, densities and electron densities of these materials are close to those for fat.[3, 4]

ATTENUATION OF X AND γ RAYS IN SOFT TISSUE

The effective atomic number and density of body fluids and soft tissue, excluding fat, are almost identical to those for water, because soft tissue is roughly 75% water and body fluids are 85−100% water. Soft tissue often is simulated by a water-filled phantom or by Plexiglas, Mix D* or pressed wood (e.g., Masonite).

Hydrogen is absent from air, but contributes about 10% of the weight of muscle. Consequently, the electron density is greater for muscle than for air, and the f-factor for muscle exceeds that for air (Fig 10-1).

ATTENUATION OF X AND γ RAYS IN BONE

The effective atomic number and physical density (kg/cu m) are greater for bone than for soft tissue. Hence, x- and γ-ray photons are attenuated more rapidly in bone than in an equal volume (not necessarily mass) of soft tissue, and the absorbed dose is reduced to structures beyond

---

*Mix D has the following composition by weight: paraffin 60.8%, polyethylene 30.4%, magnesium oxide 6.4%, titanium dioxide 2.4%.[5]

bone. On the other hand, the absorbed dose to soft tissue adjacent to or enclosed within bone may be increased by photoelectrons liberated as photons interact with high-Z atoms (e.g., atoms of phosphorus and calcium) in bone.

Dose to Soft Tissue near an Interface
between Soft Tissue and Bone

Under conditions of electron equilibrium, the absorbed dose D in rad to compact bone is

$$D = (f)(X) \tag{10-3}$$

where X is the exposure in roentgens and f is the f-factor for compact bone exposed to photons of a particular energy (Fig 10-1). To compute the absorbed dose to soft tissue beyond the range of electrons escaping from bone, the f-factor for soft tissue is used in equation (10-3). The absorbed dose to soft tissue near bone is less than the absorbed dose in bone but greater than the absorbed dose in soft tissue beyond the range of electrons from bone. In tissue irradiated by diagnostic or orthovoltage x rays, the region of increased dose to soft tissue extends over a distance of 100 μ or less from an interface between soft tissue and bone. These transition zones of increased dose are illustrated in Figures 10-2 to 10-4 for x-ray beams of different qualities. Data in these figures were obtained with an ionization chamber and plastics designed to simulate bone and soft tissue.[6, 7]

The radiation dose delivered to soft tissue near an interface between

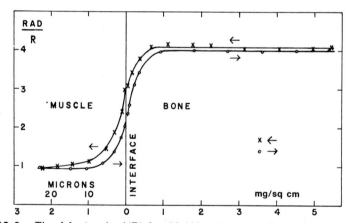

Fig 10-2.—The f-factor (rad/R) for 50-kVp, 0.08-mm Cu HVL x rays near an interface between soft tissue and bone. Arrows indicate the direction of the x-ray beam. (Figures 10-2 to 10-4 from Wingate, C., Gross, W., and Failla, G.: Experimental determination of absorbed dose from x rays near the interface of soft tissue and other material, Radiology 79:984, 1962.)

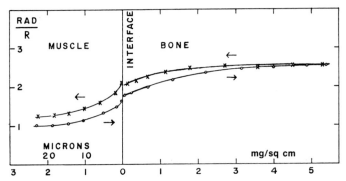

Fig 10-3.—The f-factor (rad/R) for 140-kVp, 0.70-mm Cu HVL x rays near an interface between soft tissue and bone. Arrows indicate the direction of the x-ray beam.

soft tissue and bone may be computed with an f-factor intermediate between those for soft tissue and bone. The f-factors for photons of different energies are plotted in Figure 10-5 as a function of the distance from the interface.

Dose to Soft Tissue within Bone

Soft tissue that occupies cavities within bone includes the soft-tissue components of the Haversian system. These components include osteocytes about 5 μ in diameter, connective tissue along the walls of Haversian canals, and blood vessels in the walls of the canals. Haversian canals vary from 50 to 100 μ in diameter. In trabecular bone, spaces occupied by bone marrow are relatively large, averaging about 400 μ across.

The absorbed dose in small (diameter <1 μ) inclusions of soft tissue within compact bone is close to that computed with equation (10-3) and

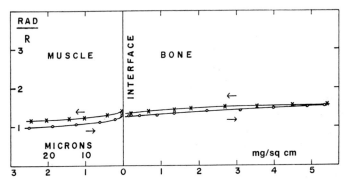

Fig 10-4.—The f-factors (rad/R) for 210-kVp, 2.1-mm Cu HVL x rays near an interface between soft tissue and bone. Arrows indicate the direction of the x-ray beam.

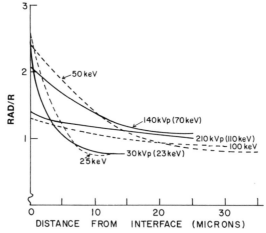

Fig 10-5. —Calculated and measured f-factors as a function of the distance in soft tissue from an interface between soft tissue and bone. (From Wingate, C., Gross, W., and Failla, G.: Experimental determination of absorbed dose from x rays near the interface of soft tissue and other material, Radiology 79:984, 1962; and Spiers, F.: Dosage in Bone, in *Clinical Dosimetry,* ICRU Report 10d. National-al Bureau of Standards Handbook 87, 1963.)

an f-factor for bone. The dose to larger (diameter >1 μ) soft-tissue inclu-sions is less than that estimated with equation (10-3) and an f-factor for bone. In larger inclusions, the absorbed dose varies from a maximum at the bone-tissue interface to a minimum at the center of the inclusion (Fig 10-6).

The absorbed dose across these larger inclusions is difficult to deter-mine. Average f-factors in Table 10-2 were computed by Spiers[8] for os-teocytes, for typical soft-tissue inclusions excluding bone marrow and for the soft-tissue lining of a typical Haversian canal. The average f-factors are highest for osteocytes because these components occupy very small cavities. Haversian canals, on the average, are much smaller than spaces in trabecular bone that contain bone marrow, and the average dose to bone marrow usually is not much greater than that delivered to soft tis-sue in the absence of bone. The increase in average absorbed dose in bone marrow spaces of different sizes is plotted in Figure 10-7 as a func-tion of the energy of incident photons. For marrow cavities of all sizes, the increase in dose is less than 50% of the dose to soft tissue without bone.

The probability of pair production increases with the atomic number of the attenuating medium. Consequently, the dose delivered by high-

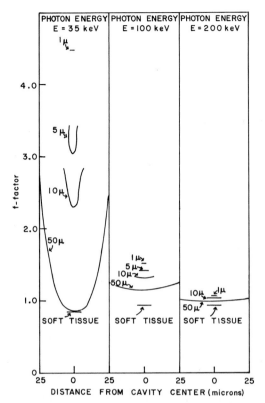

Fig 10-6. — The f-factor for photons of various energies, as a function of the distance from the center of cavities of different sizes. A layer of bone around the cavity provides electron equilibrium. (Figures 10-6 and 10-7 from Spiers, F.: Dosage in Bone, in *Clinical Dosimetry,* ICRU Report 10d. National Bureau of Standards Handbook 87, 1963.)

TABLE 10-2. — AVERAGE F-FACTORS FOR INCLUSIONS
OF SOFT TISSUE IN BONE*

PHOTON ENERGY (keV)	OSTEOCYTE 5 μ DIAMETER	TYPICAL SOFT TISSUE IN BONE	10 μ LINING OF 50 μ HAVERSIAN CANAL
25	2.80	1.73	1.50
35	3.12	2.05	1.76
50	3.25	2.27	1.89
75	2.40	1.85	1.60
100	1.52	1.36	1.26
200	1.05	1.03	1.02

*From Spiers.[8]

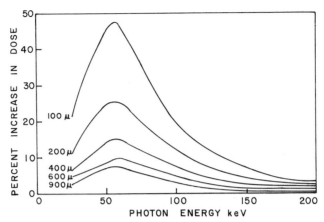

Fig 10-7.—Percent increase in average absorbed dose to bone marrow cavities, averaged over cavities of various sizes.

energy photons is greater in bone than in soft tissue. For example, the dose delivered by 10-MeV photons is about 15% greater in bone than in soft tissue receiving an identical exposure. Electrons released during pair-production interactions have an average range of about 2–3 cm in soft tissue and more than 1 cm in bone. For a thickness of bone less than that required for electron equilibrium, it is difficult to estimate the dose to bone and to soft-tissue inclusions within bone.

Dose to Soft Tissue beyond Bone

The dose delivered to soft tissue by x or γ rays is reduced by bone interposed between the soft tissue and the surface. The reduction in absorbed dose to soft tissue is influenced by:

1. The increased attenuation of primary photons in bone caused by the higher atomic number and density of this constituent of tissue.
2. Changes in the amount of radiation scattered to soft tissue beyond the location of bone. These changes depend upon many factors, including field size, quality of radiation and the distance between the bone and the soft tissue of interest.

Low-energy x- or γ-ray photons are attenuated primarily by photoelectric interactions, and the attenuation of these photons is much greater in bone than in an equal mass of soft tissue or fat. For photons of higher energy, Compton scattering replaces photoelectric absorption as the dominant interaction. The probability for Compton interaction depends on the electron density of the attenuating medium, but not on its atomic number. The electron density is slightly less for bone than for soft tissue or fat, and the energy absorbed per gram of bone is slightly less than the

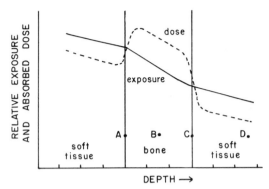

Fig 10-8. — Radiation exposure and absorbed dose plotted as a function of depth in soft tissue containing bone.

energy absorbed per gram of muscle or fat exposed to photons of intermediate energy. However, the physical density (kg/cu m) of compact bone is almost twice the density of fat or muscle. Therefore, the energy absorbed per unit volume of compact bone is almost twice that absorbed in an equal volume of fat or muscle exposed to an identical number of x- or γ-ray photons of intermediate energy.[*]

The effect of bone upon the radiation exposure and absorbed dose at various depths within a patient exposed to diagnostic or orthovoltage x rays is illustrated in Figure 10-8. The radiation exposure, which always is measured in a small volume of air, is reduced at locations B, C and D by bone interposed between the locations and the surface. The reduction in exposure at these locations reflects primarily the increased attenuation of photons in overlying bone. The dose absorbed in bone is increased at A, B and C, because the attenuation of diagnostic or orthovoltage x rays increases with the atomic number of the attenuating medium. The absorbed dose is reduced to soft tissue beyond bone because a greater number of photons are removed from the beam by the overlying bone.

HIGH-VOLTAGE ROENTGENOGRAPHY

Radiographic images obtained with x rays generated below about 100 kVp exhibit high contrast between soft tissue and bone. In a roentgenogram of the chest exposed to 80-kVp x rays (Fig 10-9, A), the image of

[*] In a radiograph obtained by exposure of film to high-energy photons (e.g., ^{60}Co γ rays), images of bone are displayed as regions of reduced optical density. Hence, the number of photons transmitted by bone is less than the number transmitted by an equal thickness of soft tissue. Although the energy absorbed per unit mass (absorbed dose) is less in bone than in soft tissue exposed to ^{60}Co γ rays, the transmission of photons through bone is less, because the physical density of bone is greater than that for soft tissue.

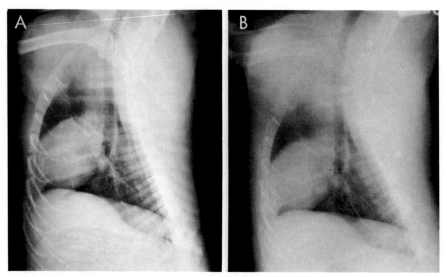

Fig 10-9. — Radiographs of the chest. **A,** 80 kVp, 1 mm Al filter; **B,** 140 kVp, 1 mm Cu filter.

bone obscures the visibility of the trachea. Shadows cast by bone may be reduced by increasing the voltage applied to the x-ray tube and by adding filtration to the x-ray beam. The radiograph in Figure 10-9, *B,* was obtained with x rays generated at 140 kVp and filtered by 1 mm Cu. The trachea, lung and retrocardiac markings are displayed more clearly in this radiograph than in *A.* A number of persons have suggested that radiographs obtained with x and γ rays greater than 1 MeV are useful for certain examinations, particularly chest radiography.[9-13]

High-voltage x-ray beams have been used in diagnostic radiology primarily for the study of air-filled structures such as the chest, larynx and paranasal sinuses, for myelography (introduction of air, gas or other contrast agent into the subarachnoid space of the spinal column) and pneumoencephalography (introduction of air, gas or other contrast agent into the subarachnoid space of the spinal column and into the ventricular system of the brain), and for study of the gastrointestinal tract with a contrast medium when retention of some tissue differentiation is desired in structures containing the contrast medium. Disadvantages of high-voltage radiography include (1) a reduction in contrast between adjacent soft tissues, (2) a reduction in radiographic detail caused by an increased amount of scattered radiation and (3) a reduction in the ability of grids to remove scattered radiation.

LOW-VOLTAGE ROENTGENOGRAPHY

X rays of very low energy often are used to delineate subtle differences in soft-tissue structures.[3, 4, 14-16] For example, mammography (examination of the breast) usually is performed with x rays generated at a tube voltage between 25 and 40 kVp and filtered lightly with aluminum or molybdenum. Long exposure times are required in mammography because: (1) the efficiency of x-ray production is extremely low at tube voltages between 25 and 40 kVp, (2) the inherent filtration of the tube reduces the exposure rate greatly, and (3) the beam is attenuated severely by the patient.

CONTRAST MEDIA

Many anatomical structures may be visualized more clearly with x rays if a material is introduced into the structures to increase or decrease the attenuation of x rays. These materials are referred to as *contrast agents* or *contrast media*. A few radiographic examinations that may be improved with contrast media are listed in Table 10-3. Many of the agents contain either iodine or barium for reasons that are apparent in Figure 10-10. For all photon energies included in this figure, the attenuation coefficient for iodine ($Z = 53$) greatly exceeds that for soft tissue ($Z_{eff} = 7.4$). Consequently, a structure containing an iodinated compound is clearly distinguishable from adjacent soft tissue. The attenuation coefficient for barium ($Z = 56$) is close to that for iodine, and is not included in Figure 10-10. The attenuation coefficient for iodine exceeds even the coefficient for lead between the K-absorption edges for iodine (33 keV) and lead (88 keV). Within this range of photon energies, x rays are attenuated more rapidly by iodine than by an equal mass of lead. Since most photons in a diagnostic x-ray beam possess an energy between 33 and 88 keV, iodinated compounds are better contrast agents, gram for gram, than would

TABLE 10-3.—A FEW CONTRAST AGENTS USED IN
RADIOGRAPHIC EXAMINATIONS

EXAMINATION	COMPOUND	CONTRAST ELEMENT
Adult intravenous pyelography	Sodium iothalamate	Iodine
Upper gastrointestinal series	Barium sulfate	Barium
Intravenous cholangiography	Meglumine iodipamide	Iodine
Sinus tract	Meglumine diatrizoate	Iodine
Oral cholecystography	Iopanoic acid	Iodine
Myelography	Iophendylate	Iodine
Myelography	Air	
Pneumoencephalography	Air	

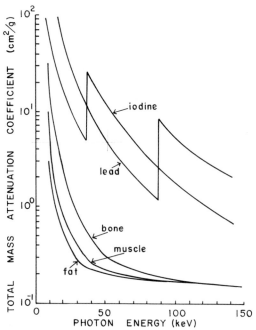

Fig 10-10.—Attenuation coefficients for fat, muscle, bone, iodine and lead as a function of photon energy.

be compounds containing lead or other high-Z elements, even if the toxicity of these compounds did not prohibit their use. Compounds containing iodine or barium are relatively nontoxic and may be used in a wide variety of roentgenographic examinations. One advantage of barium over iodine compounds is their miscibility into solutions of higher physical density.

Air may be introduced into certain locations (e.g., the subarachnoid space of the spinal column and the ventricular system of the brain) to displace tissues and fluids that interfere with the visualization of anatomical structures of interest. The density of air is very low, and x rays are transmitted through the air-filled cavities with little attenuation. Hence, the introduction of air improves the visualization of structures in, or adjacent to, air-filled cavities.

PROBLEMS

1. Referring to Figure 10-1, discuss why x rays generated at low voltage are used to distinguish between fat and muscle.
2. Referring to Figure 10-10, explain why iodine and barium are used in contrast agents.

3. Why is air an effective contrast agent if the effective atomic number of air (Z_{eff} = 7.65) is near that for muscle (Z_{eff} = 7.4)?
4. Discuss the advantages and disadvantages of high-voltage radiography.
5. Plot curves similar to those in Figure 10-8 for a diagnostic x-ray beam penetrating successive layers of muscle, fat, muscle, bone and muscle.
6. Would 250-kVp x rays or ^{60}Co γ rays be preferable for the treatment of a soft-tissue lesion that invades bone?

REFERENCES

1. Ter-Pogossian, M.: *The Physical Aspects of Diagnostic Radiology* (New York: Harper & Row, 1967).
2. Meredith, W., and Massey, J.: *Fundamental Physics of Radiology* (Baltimore: Williams & Wilkins Co., 1968).
3. Stanton, L., et al.: Physical aspects of breast radiography, Radiology 81:1, 1963.
4. Stanton, L., and Lightfoot, D.: Obtaining proper contrast in mammography, Radiology 81:1, 1963.
5. Jones, D., and Raine, H.: Letter to the editor, Br. J. Radiol. 22:549, 1949.
6. Wingate, C., Gross, W., and Failla, G.: Experimental determination of absorbed dose from x rays near the interface of soft tissue and other material, Radiology 79:984, 1962.
7. Shonka, F., Rose, J., and Failla, G.: Conducting plastics equivalent to tissue, air and polystyrene, Proceedings of the Second International Conference on the Peaceful Uses of Atomic Energy 21:184, 1958.
8. Spiers, F.: Dosage in Bone, in *Clinical Dosimetry*, ICRU Report 10d. National Bureau of Standards Handbook 87, 1963, Appendix II.
9. Beique, R.; Rotenberg, A., and Maguire, G.: Heavy filtration in diagnostic radiology, SRW News 26:52, 1965.
10. McDonnell, G.: Megavoltage diagnostic radiography, Radiology 80:279, 1963.
11. Vogler, H.: High-voltage technique, Gevaert News 9:3, 1963.
12. Tuddenbam, W., et al.: Super-voltage and multiple simultaneous roentgenography—a new technique for the examination of the chest, Radiology 63:184, 1954.
13. Deans, B.: Megavoltage radiography, J. Coll. Radiol. Australia 6:130, 1962.
14. Karcher, K.: 10 years of technical development in mammography, Electromedica 1:6, 1967.
15. Stanton, L., and Lightfoot, D.: The selection of optimum mammography technic, Radiology 83:442, 1964.
16. Kirka, C.: X-ray tube considerations for mammography, Cathode Press 18, 1961.

11 / Detection of Radiation from Low-Activity Sources

DESCRIBED IN THIS CHAPTER are a variety of radiation detectors that respond to alpha, beta and gamma radiation from radioactive sources of relatively low activity.

IONIZATION CHAMBERS

Ion pairs (IP) are produced as energy is deposited in a medium by ionizing radiation. If a gas is used as the attenuating medium, the ion pairs may be collected by charged electrodes placed in the medium. The ion pairs migrate toward the charged electrodes with a "drift velocity" that depends on the type and pressure of the gas between the electrodes and on the potential difference and distance between the electrodes. In a gas-filled ionization chamber, the voltage between the electrodes is increased until all ion pairs produced by the impinging radiation are collected. However, the voltage remains below that required to produce additional ion pairs as the ion pairs produced by radiation interactions migrate to the collecting electrodes. Consequently, the electrodes receive only ion pairs that result directly from interactions of ionizing radiation with gas in the chamber.

An ionization chamber designed to detect radiation from radioactive sources of low activity consists of parallel-plate or coaxial electrodes in a volume occupied by a filling gas. A parallel-plate chamber resembles the free air ionization chamber which serves as a calibration standard in most countries for ionization chambers used to calibrate x- and γ-ray beams used in radiation therapy.[1] A coaxial chamber is composed of a central electrode in the form of a straight wire or wire loop which is charged positively with respect to the surrounding cylindrical case (Fig 11-1). The entrance of radiation into the chamber results in an electric current or voltage pulses produced as ion pairs are collected by the electrodes.

Pulse-Type Ionization Chambers

Consider a 1.75-MeV alpha particle traversing the collecting volume of an ionization chamber. If the gas in the collecting volume is air, then the alpha particle loses an average energy of 33.7 eV for each ion pair produced. If the kinetic energy of the alpha particle is dissipated com-

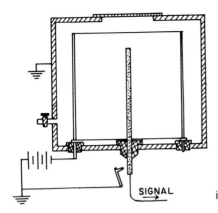

Fig 11-1. — A simple coaxial ionization chamber.

SIGNAL

pletely within the collecting volume, then $(1.75 \times 10^6 \text{ eV})/(33.7 \text{ eV/IP}) = 5 \times 10^4$ ion pairs are produced. Electrons liberated by the radiation migrate rapidly to the central electrode (anode) and reduce the positive charge of this electrode. Usually, electrons are collected within a microsecond after their liberation. The heavier, positively charged ions migrate more slowly toward the negative case (cathode) of the chamber. As the positive ions approach the case, they induce a negative charge on the case, which masks the total reduction in voltage between the electrodes. Hence, the total reduction in voltage between the electrodes is not attained until all positive ions within the chamber have been neutralized. Usually, a few hundred microseconds are required to neutralize the positive ions. In most pulse-type ionization chambers, only that portion of the reduction in voltage that is created by the collection of electrons is utilized in forming a voltage pulse.

Example 11-1

What size voltage pulse is produced when a 1.75-MeV alpha particle is absorbed totally within an air-filled ionization chamber with a capacitance of 10 picofarad? (10 picofarad = 10×10^{-12} farad)

A 1.75-MeV alpha produces 5×10^4 IP = 5×10^4 electrons plus 5×10^4 positive ions.

$$Q = (5 \times 10^4 \text{ electrons})(1.6 \times 10^{-19} \text{ coulomb/electron}) = 8 \times 10^{-15} \text{ coulomb}$$

The voltage pulse produced is

$$V = \frac{Q}{C} \text{ where } C = 10 \times 10^{-12} \text{ farad}$$
$$V = \frac{8 \times 10^{-15} \text{ coulomb}}{10 \times 10^{-12} \text{ farad}}$$
$$= 8 \times 10^{-4} \text{ V}$$
$$= 0.8 \text{ mV}$$

In a pulse-type chamber designed to produce voltage pulses by the rapid collection of electrons, no interference with the migration of these electrons can be tolerated. Gases such as oxygen, water vapor and the halogens have an affinity for electrons. These gases should not be present in the collecting volume of an ionization chamber. Other gases, such as helium, neon, argon, hydrogen, nitrogen, carbon dioxide and methane, form negative ions only rarely by combining with electrons. These gases are used often as filling gases in ionization chambers.

The average kinetic energy of beta particles (negatrons and positrons) is less than that of most alpha particles. Furthermore, the specific ionization is $1/100 - 1/1,000$ less for negatrons and positrons than for alpha particles. Usually, alpha particles expend their entire kinetic energy by interacting with the gas in the collecting volume of an ionization chamber; negatrons and positrons usually strike the wall of the chamber before dissipating all of their kinetic energy. For these reasons, voltage pulses produced as beta particles traverse an ionization chamber are much smaller than those produced by alpha particles. Pulses produced by x and γ rays are even smaller. Ionization chambers usually are operated in the pulse mode for the detection of alpha particles; other radiations with lower specific ionization usually are measured by operation of the chamber in the current mode.

Current-Type Ionization Chambers

Electrons collected by the anode of an ionization chamber constitute a direct current which may be amplified and measured with a conventional DC meter. In general, this approach is unsatisfactory because instability and zero-drift are introduced by the DC amplifier and accurate measurements are difficult to achieve.

Small currents from an ionization chamber may be measured more accurately with a vibrating reed (dynamic capacitor) electrometer. The vibrating reed electrometer consists of a capacitor with one moving plate which oscillates at a frequency of $200 - 500$ Hz. The signal from the ionization chamber is converted by the dynamic capacitor into an alternating current which may be amplified with an AC amplifier. An AC amplifier is not subject to the problems of instability and zero-drift encountered with a DC amplifier. The amplified alternating current may be measured to within $\pm 0.05\%$ precision by one of two methods, referred to as the *voltage-drop method* and the *rate-of-charge method*.

With the voltage-drop method, the amplified alternating current is rectified and directed through a precision resistance. The voltage developed across the resistance is proportional to the current. With the rate-of-charge method, the current is rectified and collected by a precision capacitor. The rate of collection of electric charge on the plates of the ca-

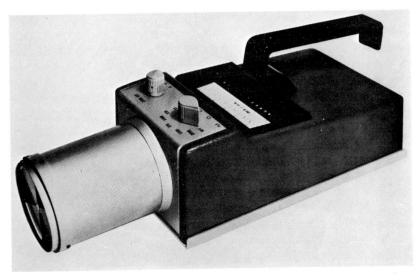

Fig 11-2.—A "cutie pie" portable survey meter. The scale of the meter is calibrated to read directly in units of mR/hr, with a range switch which decreases the sensitivity of the meter by factors of 10. (Courtesy of Baird-Atomic, Inc.)

pacitor is proportional to the current. The rate-of-charge method may be used with currents smaller than those measured by the voltage-drop method. The voltage-drop method without current amplification is used in portable survey meters such as the "cutie pie" (Fig 11-2).

Example 11-2*

A 0.001-μCi sample of $^{14}CO_2$ is contained within a current-type ionization chamber. The ionization current is converted to alternating current and is measured by the voltage-drop method, using a precision resistance of 10^{12} ohms. Assuming that all the energy of the beta particles from ^{14}C is deposited in the gas, and that the AC signal is not amplified, what voltage is developed across the precision resistance?

$$(0.001 \ \mu\text{Ci})[3.7 \times 10^4 \text{ disintegrations/(sec-}\mu\text{Ci)}] = 37 \text{ disintegrations/sec}$$

The average energy of beta particles from ^{14}C is 0.045 MeV = 45×10^3 eV. The average energy dissipated per second in the counting volume is

$$(37 \text{ disintegrations/sec})(45 \times 10^3 \text{ eV/disintegration}) = 16.6 \times 10^5 \text{ eV/sec}$$

The number of electrons released per second is

$$\frac{16.6 \times 10^5 \text{ eV/sec}}{33.7 \text{ eV/IP}} = 4.9 \times 10^4 \text{ IP/sec} = 4.9 \times 10^4 \text{ electrons/sec}$$

*Examples 11-2 and 11-3 are modified from data of Chase and Rabinowitch.[2]

The charge liberated per second is

$$(4.9 \times 10^4 \text{ electrons/sec})(1.6 \times 10^{-19} \text{ coulomb/electron})$$
$$= 7.8 \times 10^{-15} \text{ coulomb/sec}$$
$$1 \text{ coulomb/sec} = 1 \text{ A}$$
$$7.8 \times 10^{-15} \text{ coulomb/sec} = 7.8 \times 10^{-15} \text{ A}$$

The voltage drop V across a resistance is the product of the resistance in ohms and the current in amperes:

$$V = IR$$
$$V = (7.8 \times 10^{-15} \text{ A})(10^{12} \text{ ohms})$$
$$= 7.8 \times 10^{-3} \text{ V}$$
$$= 7.8 \text{ mV}$$

Example 11-3

Repeat Example 11-2, finding the rate of change in voltage across the plates of a precision 10-picofarad capacitor.

The rate of flow of charge is 7.8×10^{-15} coulombs/sec. Since $V = Q/C$, where C is the capacitance, the rate of change of voltage $V_r = Q_r/C$, where Q_r is the rate of flow of charge:

$$V_r = \frac{7.8 \times 10^{-15} \text{ coulombs/sec}}{10 \times 10^{-12} \text{ farad}}$$
$$= 7.8 \times 10^{-4} \text{ V/sec}$$
$$= (7.8 \times 10^{-4} \text{ V/sec})(60 \text{ sec/min})$$
$$= 46.8 \times 10^{-3} \text{ V/min}$$
$$= 47 \text{ mV/min}$$

In Figure 11-3, the ionization current is plotted as a function of the voltage applied across the electrodes of an ionization chamber. At low voltages, the electrons and positive ions are not attracted strongly to the electrodes and some of the ion pairs are lost by recombination. The attraction for ion pairs increases with the voltage between the electrodes, and a smaller fraction of the ion pairs recombine. When the voltage between the electrodes exceeds the *saturation voltage*, the electrodes collect all ion pairs produced by the radiation. The saturation voltage for a particular ionization chamber depends upon the design of the chamber, the shape and spacing of the electrodes, and the type and pressure of the gas in the chamber. No increase in ionization current is observed as the electrode voltage is raised a few hundred volts above saturation, because all ion pairs produced by the radiation are collected. This region of voltage is referred to as the *ionization chamber plateau*. The ionization current increases abruptly at the end of the plateau. This amplification of the signal reflects the production of additional ion pairs, as electrons liberated by the incident radiation gain energy on their way to the anode.

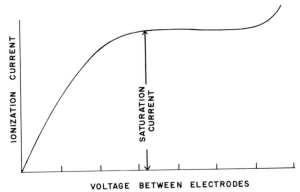

VOLTAGE BETWEEN ELECTRODES

Fig 11-3.—Ionization current from an ionization chamber, plotted as a function of the voltage between electrodes. Recombination of ion pairs occurs at voltages below that which furnishes a saturation current. At high voltages, the signal is amplified by ionization produced as electrons are accelerated toward the anode.

Ionization chambers are operated at a voltage less than that which causes signal amplification. At any particular voltage, the ionization current produced by an alpha-emitting sample is much greater than that produced by a sample that emits beta particles. The reduced signal for the beta-emitting sample reflects the reduced ionization produced by beta particles.

Uses of Ionization Chambers

Radiation from solid, liquid and gaseous samples may be measured with an ionization chamber and vibrating-reed electrometer.[3] The activity of liquid samples prepared for administration to patients often is determined by placing the vial or syringe containing the sample into a well-type ionization chamber referred to as an *isotope calibrator* (Fig 11-4). Gaseous samples may be counted by filling an ionization chamber with the radioactive gas. For example, ionization chambers may be used to measure the amount of $^{14}CO_2$ in air expired by patients metabolizing compounds labeled with ^{14}C.

Portable survey instruments such as that depicted in Figure 11-2 are used frequently in nuclear medicine to monitor exposure rates in the vicinity of radioactive sources and patients receiving therapeutic quantities of radioactive material. A neutron detector may be constructed by filling an ionization chamber with BF_3 gas or by coating the wall of an ionization chamber with lithium or boron. Ionization is produced within the chamber by alpha particles and recoil nuclei which are liberated during interactions of neutrons with the lithium or boron.

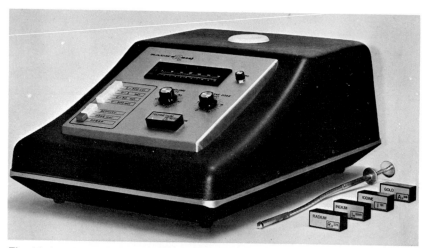

Fig 11-4.—Well-type ionization chamber and electrometer (isotope calibrator) used to measure the activity of a radioactive sample prior to administration of the sample to a patient. The volume of the sample to be administered is computed from the measured activity, often automatically by the isotope calibrator. (Courtesy of RADX Corp.)

PROPORTIONAL COUNTERS

The small signals from an ionization chamber must be amplified greatly before they are measured. Because of the introduction of electronic noise and instability, amplification by electric circuits is difficult to achieve without distortion of the signal. This problem may be reduced if the signal is amplified within the counting volume of the chamber. If the potential difference between the electrodes of a chamber is raised beyond a certain voltage, electrons liberated by radiation traversing the chamber are accelerated to a velocity great enough to produce additional ionization. Most of the additional ionization occurs near the anode of the chamber. As a result, many $(10^6 - 10^7)$ electrons and positive ions are collected by the electrodes for a much smaller number $(10^3 - 10^5)$ of ion pairs produced directly by radiation entering the chamber. This process is referred to as *gas amplification* or the *Townsend effect*. The *amplification factor* for the chamber is the ratio of the total number of ion pairs produced within the chamber to the number liberated directly by radiation entering the chamber. The amplification factor depends upon the construction of the chamber and upon the type of gas enclosed within the chamber. The amplification factor varies from 10^2 to 10^4 for most proportional counters, providing a signal (approximately 1 mV) that requires only a small amount of external amplification.

The number of ion pairs produced in a gas-filled chamber is plotted in

Figure 11-5 as a function of the voltage applied across the electrodes. The voltage between electrodes must be regulated closely, because the amplification factor is affected greatly by small changes in voltage. In the *proportional region*, the amount of charge collected by the electrodes increases with the number of ion pairs produced initially by the imping-ing radiation. Consequently, the size of the signal from a proportional chamber increases with the amount of ionization produced by radiation that traverses the chamber.

Example 11-4

An alpha particle produces 10^5 IP in a proportional chamber with an amplifica-tion factor of 10^3. How many ion pairs are collected by the electrode?

With an amplification factor of 10^3, 1,000 IP are collected for every ion pair liberated by the incident radiation. The total number of ion pairs collected is

$$(10^5 \text{ IP})(10^3) = 10^8 \text{ IP}$$

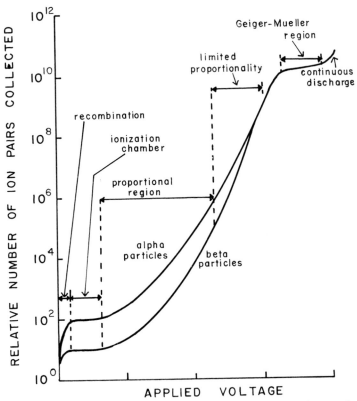

Fig 11-5. — Relationship between the total number of ion pairs produced in a gas-filled detector and the high voltage between electrodes of the detector.

Example 11-5

Repeat the calculation in Example 11-4 for a beta particle that produces 10^3 IP within the chamber.

For an amplification factor of 10^3,

$$(10^3 \text{ IP})(10^3) = 10^6 \text{ IP}$$

At voltages higher than the proportional region, alpha particles and other densely ionizing radiations initiate ionization of most of the atoms of gas in the vicinity of the anode. If the chamber is operated at a voltage in this region, then the number of ion pairs collected is not proportional strictly to the ionization produced directly by the radiation. Hence, this voltage region is referred to as the *region of limited proportionality*. Proportional chambers are not operated routinely in the region of limited proportionality.

If signals below a selected size are rejected by a "discriminator" inserted between the proportional chamber and the device used to record signals, then signals produced by alpha particles may be recorded and signals produced by beta particles may be rejected. In this manner, the recording device may reflect only alpha particles from a source that emits both alpha and beta particles. If the voltage across the chamber is increased until the signals produced by beta particles also are large enough to be transmitted by the discriminator, then both alpha particles and beta particles may be recorded. The beta particles alone are "counted" by subtracting the alpha counts measured at a lower voltage from the alpha-plus-beta counts measured at a higher voltage.

A characteristic curve for a proportional chamber is shown in Figure

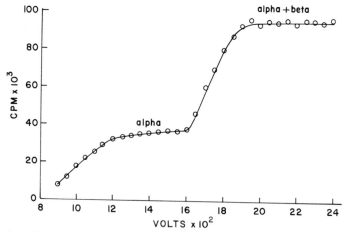

Fig 11-6. — Characteristic curve for a proportional flow counter and P-10 gas.

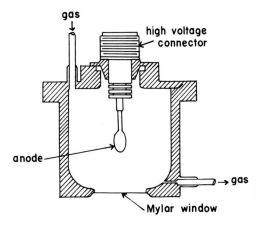

gas

high voltage
connector

anode

Mylar window

Fig 11-7. — End-window proportional flow counter for routine counting of radioactive samples.

→ gas

11-6. Alpha particles only are counted if the detector is operated at a voltage along the alpha plateau. The count rate produced by background radiation is very low when the chamber is operated at a low voltage. Both alphas and betas are counted if the voltage is increased to the beta plateau. For a well-designed proportional detector, the slope of the beta plateau should not exceed 0.2%/100 V.* Proportional counters are used only rarely for the detection of gamma radiation from radioactive sources of low activity, because the efficiency of the chambers is very low for these sparsely ionizing radiations. Proportional counters are useful with x-ray beams of high intensity, however, and are used widely in x-ray spectrometers.[4]

For proportional counting of radioactive samples, a chamber similar to that diagramed in Figure 11-7 may be used. The anode is a rod or loop of thin wire. Frequently, radiation is admitted into the chamber through a very thin window (e.g., 150 μg/sq cm of Mylar or split mica) which is permeable to counting gas in the chamber. Hence, the chamber must be flushed continuously with counting gas, and the detector is referred to as a *flow counter*. A flow counter must be purged with counting gas prior to operation, because the amplification factor of the detector is reduced by oxygen and nitrogen present in air. In a windowless flow counter, the radioactive sample is sealed within the chamber while radiation from the sample is detected. Radioactive gases may be counted by mixing the

*The slope of the plateau may be computed by

$$\text{Slope } (\%/100 \text{ V}) = \frac{2[(\text{CPM})_2 - (\text{CPM})_1] \, 10^4}{[(\text{CPM})_2 + (\text{CPM})_1](V_2 - V_1)}$$

where $(\text{CPM})_2$ is the count rate at voltage V_2 on the plateau, and $(\text{CPM})_1$ is the count rate at voltage V_1 on the plateau.

gases with counting gas and introducing the mixture into the chamber. The voltage required for operation of the detector on the alpha or beta plateau is dependent on the type of counting gas used. If methane is used, then the beta plateau for most detectors is in the region of 3,000–3,500 V. With "P-10 gas," a mixture of 90% argon and 10% methane, the beta plateau occurs between 2,000 and 2,500 V.

Because of its rapid response to ionizing events, the multiwire proportional chamber has been investigated as an imaging device for nuclear medicine.[5, 6] By raising the pressure of the counting gas to 10 atm or more, the sensitivity of the chamber to γ rays can be improved. The γ-ray sensitivity also can be improved by placing high-Z foils in front of the chamber to convert incoming photons to photoelectrons and Compton electrons. Although the intrinsic resolution of multiwire proportional chambers is excellent, the resolution achievable in practice has been comparable to that for other nuclear medicine imaging devices.

GEIGER-MUELLER TUBES

If the potential difference between the electrodes of a gas-filled detector exceeds the region of limited proportionality (Fig 11-5), then the interaction of a charged particle or x- or γ-ray photon within the chamber

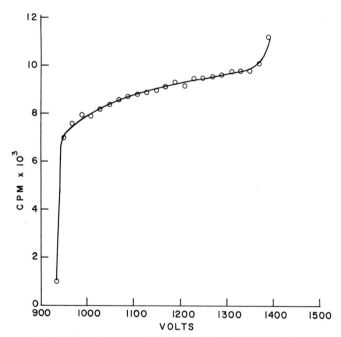

Fig 11-8. — Characteristic curve for a G-M detector.

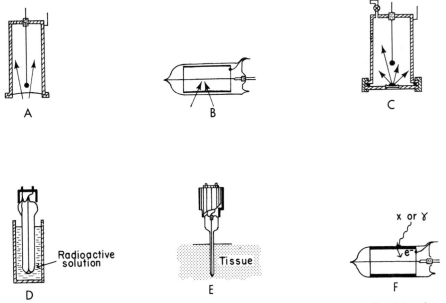

Fig 11-9.—Various Geiger-Mueller detectors: **A,** end-window; **B,** side-window; **C,** windowless flow; **D,** thin-wall dipping tube; **E,** needle probe; **F,** heavy-metal wall.

initiates an *avalanche of ionization*, which represents almost complete ionization of the counting gas in the vicinity of the anode. Because of this avalanche process, the number of ion pairs collected by the electrodes is independent of the amount of ionization produced directly by the impinging radiation. Hence, the voltage pulses (usually 1–10 V) emerging from the detector are similar in size and independent of the type of radiation that initiates the signal. The range of voltage over which signals from the detector are independent of the type of radiation entering the detector is referred to as the *Geiger-Mueller region* or *G-M region*. For detectors operating in this voltage region, the amplification factor is 10^6-10^8.

In Figure 11-8, the number of pulses (or counts) recorded per minute is plotted as a function of the voltage across the electrodes of a G-M detector exposed to a radioactive source. No counts are recorded if the voltage is less than the starting voltage, because voltage pulses formed by the detector are too small to pass the discriminator and enter the scaler. As the voltage is raised slightly above the starting voltage, some of the pulses are transmitted by the discriminator and recorded. At the *plateau threshold voltage*, all pulses are transmitted to the scaler. Increasing the voltage beyond the plateau threshold does not increase the count rate significantly. Consequently, relatively inexpensive high-voltage supplies that are not exceptionally stable may be used with a G-M detector, Usually, G-M detectors are operated at a voltage about one third of the way up the plateau. In Figure 11-8, for example, an operating voltage of 1,150 V might be selected for the detector. The voltage range encompassed by the plateau varies with the construction of the G-M detector and with the counting gas used.

Atoms of counting gas near the anode may be ionized spontaneously if the voltage applied to the detector is raised beyond the Geiger-Mueller plateau. This region of voltage is referred to as the *region of spontaneous discharge* or *region of continuous discharge*, because the counting gas may be ionized in the absence of radiation. A Geiger-Mueller tube may be damaged permanently by the application of voltages higher than the Geiger-Mueller plateau.

A few G-M detectors are illustrated in Figure 11-9. The anode is a thin wire of tungsten or stainless steel in the center of the detector. The anode is surrounded by a metal or glass cathode which is coated internally with a conducting layer of graphite or evaporated metal. The efficiency of a G-M detector for high-energy x and γ rays may be increased to 6–8% by coating the cathode with a heavy metal, such as bismuth or lead. The end-window G-M detector (Fig 11-9, A) is used often for assay of radioactive samples. Usually, the window is constructed from split mica with a thickness of a few mg/sq cm. The thin window admits alpha particles and low-energy beta particles into the counting volume. Ultrathin Mylar windows between 100 and 200 μg/sq cm thick are available, but they must be used with a flow counter and a continuous supply of counting gas, because windows this thin are permeable to the counting gas.

Detectors with thin walls are used primarily with portable survey meters (Fig 11-9, B). The walls are metal or glass and are about 30 mg/sq cm thick. These detectors may be made very small (e.g., 2 mm outer diameter) and have been used to detect beta radiation in the circulating blood.[7] With the windowless flow detector (C), the radioactive sample is sealed inside the chamber while it is counted. The thin-wall dipping tube (D) may be inserted into a radioactive solution. With the needle probe detector (E), the sensitive volume occupies the tip of a long, thin probe. These detectors may be used to locate radioactive material concentrated in tissues within the body. The chamber with a high-Z wall (F) is used primarily for the detection of x and γ rays.

When an ionizing event is initiated in a G-M detector, an avalanche of electrons is created along the entire length of the anode. The residual positive ions require 200 μsec or longer to migrate to the cathode. During the time required for migration of the positive ions, the detector will not respond fully to additional radiation that enters the counting volume.

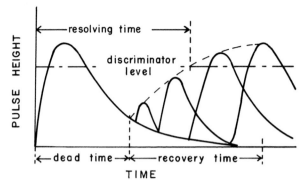

Fig 11-10.—Diagram illustrating the formation of a voltage pulse in a G-M detector as a function of time after an ionizing event.

The curve in Figure 11-10 depicts the response of the detector as a function of time after an ionizing event. During the "dead time," the detector is completely unresponsive to additional radiation. An ionizing event occurring within the "recovery time" produces a voltage pulse that is smaller than normal. The "resolving time" is the time between an ionizing event and a second event that furnishes a pulse large enough to pass the discriminator.

Positive ions that approach the cathode of a G-M detector dislodge electrons from the wall of the chamber. As these electrons combine with the positive ions, ultraviolet and x-ray photons are released. Some of these photons strike the chamber wall and release electrons that cause

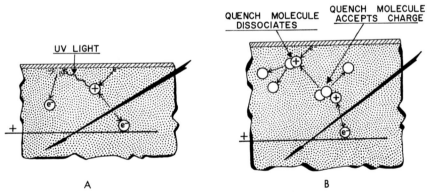

Fig 11-11.—**A,** self-perpetuating discharge of a G-M detector caused by bombardment of the cathode by ultraviolet and x-ray photons which are released as positive ions are neutralized. **B,** molecules of quench gas accept the charge of positive ions and dissociate when neutralized near the cathode. In this way, the self-perpetuating discharge is prevented.

the chamber to remain discharged. If this secondary release of electrons is permitted to occur, the detector will be unresponsive to radiation after the first ionizing event. Self-perpetuating discharge of a G-M detector is diagramed in Figure 11-11, *A*.

Various methods have been devised to "quench" the self-perpetuating discharge of G-M detectors. The most common method is to add a small concentration (about 0.1%) of a selected gas to the counting gas. The gases used most often as "internal quench agents" are polyatomic organic gases (e.g., amyl acetate or ethyl alcohol vapor) or halogens (e.g., Br_2 or Cl_2). Their effect is shown in Figure 11-11, *B*. As the positive ions move toward the cathode, they collide with and transfer charge to molecules of quench gas. The charged molecules of quench gas migrate to the cathode and dislodge electrons from the chamber wall. Energy released as the dislodged electrons combine with the charged molecules causes the dissociation of molecules of the quench gas. The dissociation is irreversible with a polyatomic organic gas, and the useful life is $10^8 - 10^{10}$ pulses for a G-M detector quenched with one of these agents. Halogen-quenched tubes have an infinite useful life, theoretically, because the molecules recombine after dissociation.

The counting gas used routinely in G-M detectors is an inert gas such as argon, helium or neon. "Geiger gas" used in flow counters is composed of 99% helium and about 1% butane or isobutane. For G-M tubes

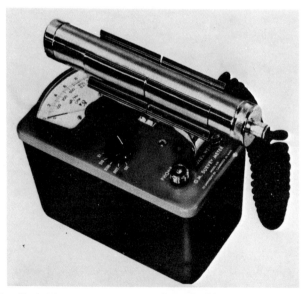

Fig 11-12.—Portable survey meter equipped with an end-window G-M tube. (Courtesy of Baird-Atomic, Inc.)

quenched with an organic gas, the plateau should be 200–300 V long and should have a slope not greater than 1–2%/100 V. Halogen-quenched tubes have a shorter plateau (100–200 V) and a plateau slope of 3–4%/100 V.

The detection efficiency of a Geiger-Mueller counter is about 1% for x and γ rays and nearly 100% for alpha and beta particles that enter the counting volume. Of course, many alpha and low-energy beta particles are absorbed by the window of the detector. Windowless flow counters often are used to detect these particles. Shown in Figure 11-12 is a survey meter equipped with an end-window G-M tube for detecting the presence of radioactive contamination.

SOLID SCINTILLATION DETECTORS

Gas-filled chambers are not efficient detectors for x and γ radiation, because most of the x- and γ-ray photons pass through the low-density gas without interacting. The probability of x- and γ-ray interaction is increased if a solid detector with a high density and atomic number is used. Atoms of a solid are immobile, however, and an interaction cannot be registered by the collection of electrons and positive ions. Instead, the interaction must be detected by some alternate method. In a scintillation crystal, light is released as radiation is absorbed. The light impinges upon a photosensitive surface in a photomultiplier tube. Electrons released from this surface constitute an electric signal. Scintillation detectors may be used to detect particulate radiation as well as x- and γ-ray photons. For example, liquid scintillators are used often to detect low-energy beta particles.

Principles of Scintillation Detection

When an x or γ ray interacts within a scintillation crystal, electrons are raised from one energy state to a state of higher energy. The number of electrons raised to a higher energy level depends upon the energy deposited in the crystal by the incident x- or γ-ray photon. Light is released as these electrons return almost instantaneously to the lower energy state. In most scintillation detectors, about 20–30 photons of light are released for every kiloelectron volt of energy absorbed. The photons of light are transmitted through the transparent crystal and are directed upon the photosensitive cathode (photocathode) of a photomultiplier tube. If the wavelength of light striking the photocathode matches the spectral sensitivity of this photosensitive surface, then electrons are ejected. The number of electrons is multiplied by various stages (dynodes) of the photomultiplier tube, and a signal is provided at the photomultiplier anode which may be amplified electronically and counted. The size of the signal at the anode is proportional to the energy dissipated in the detector by the incident radiation.

Scintillation Crystals

Gamma rays from radioactive samples often are detected with a scintillation crystal. Usually, alkali halide crystals are used because the probability of photoelectric interactions is increased by the presence of the high-Z halide component. Sodium iodide is the alkali halide used most frequently, although crystals of cesium iodide and potassium iodide are available at higher cost. Crystals of sodium iodide up to 9 in. in diameter by 9 in. thick or 20 in. in diameter by 0.5 in. thick are available commercially. Smaller crystals (e.g., 2 in. in diameter by 2 in. thick) are used routinely for the assay of gamma-emitting samples. The efficiency of a crystal for detecting x- and γ-ray photons increases with the size of the crystal.

To be used as a scintillation detector, an alkali halide crystal must be "activated" with an impurity. The impurity usually is thallium iodide at a concentration of about 0.1%, and the crystals are denoted as NaI(Tl), CsI(Tl) or KI(Tl).

Highly purified organic crystals (e.g., anthracene and *trans*-stilbene) are used to detect beta particles. The atomic number of these crystals is relatively low, and the probability is reduced that beta particles will be scattered out of the detector after only part of their energy has been dissipated. The sensitivity of an anthracene or *trans*-stilbene detector to γ rays is low, particularly if the crystal is thin. Consequently, beta particles may be detected with limited interference from γ rays.[8, 9]

Mounting Scintillation Crystals

Sodium iodide crystals are hygroscopic and must be protected from moisture. If exposed to moisture, a NaI(Tl) crystal turns yellow and absorbs much of the radiation-induced fluorescence. The yellow color probably reflects the release of free iodine. Crystals are mounted in a dry atmosphere and are sealed to prevent the entrance of moisture. A light pipe of Lucite, clear glass or quartz sometimes is attached to the side of the crystal nearest the photocathode. Other surfaces of the crystal are coated with a light-reflecting material (e.g., Al_2O_3, MgO or aluminum foil). The crystal may be enclosed within an aluminum canister, perhaps $1/32$ in. thick. The canister prevents moisture from reaching the crystal and ambient light from reaching the photocathode. The crystal or light pipe is coupled to the glass face of the photomultiplier tube with a transparent viscous medium such as silicone fluid.

Photomultiplier Tubes

A photomultiplier tube is diagramed in Figure 11-13. The photocathode usually is an alloy of cesium and antimony, often mixed with sodium and potassium (i.e., a *bialkali* photocathode), from which an acceptable

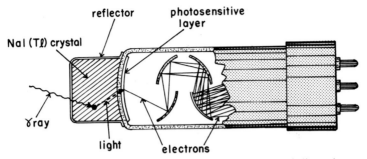

Fig 11-13. — A sodium iodide crystal and photomultiplier tube.

number of electrons are released per light photon absorbed. The spectral sensitivity of the alloy must match the wavelength of light emerging from the crystal. The spectral sensitivity of a photocathode with an "S-11 response" is compared in Figure 11-14 to the emission spectrum of light from irradiated NaI(Tl). Only 10–30% of the light photons that strike the photocathode cause the ejection of electrons. These electrons are accelerated to the first dynode, a positively charged electrode positioned a short distance from the photocathode. For each electron absorbed by the first dynode, three or four electrons are ejected and accelerated to the second dynode, where more electrons are released. Since photomultiplier tubes contain 6 to 14 dynodes, with a potential difference of 100–150 V between successive dynodes, 10^6–10^8 electrons reach the anode for each electron liberated from the photocathode. The amplification of the signal is very dependent upon the potential difference between dynodes, and the high-voltage supply for dynodes must be very stable.

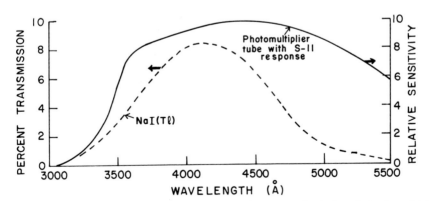

Fig 11-14. — The emission spectrum of NaI(Tl) is matched closely to the spectral sensitivity of a photomultiplier tube with an S-11 response.

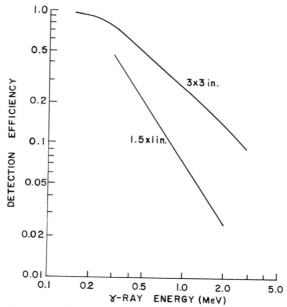

Fig 11-15. — Detection efficiency of 3 × 3 in. and 1.5 × 1 in. NaI(Tl) crystals, plotted as a function of the energy of incident γ rays. The radioactive sources were positioned 7 cm from the 1.5 × 1 in. crystal and 9.3 cm from the 3 × 3 in. crystal. (From Lazar, N., Davis, R., and Bell, P.: Peak efficiency of NaI, Nucleonics 14(4):52, 1956.)

Electrons collected by the anode are converted to a voltage pulse with an amplitude of a few millivolts to a few volts. This voltage pulse is delivered to the preamplifier, which often is mounted on the photomultiplier tube.

Energy Dependence of NaI(Tl) Detectors

The detection efficiency of a NaI(Tl) scintillation detector decreases with increasing energy of impinging γ rays (Fig 11-15). The efficiency of a scintillation detector for detection of γ rays may be improved by using a larger crystal and by improving the "counting geometry." For example, a crystal into which the radioactive sample may be inserted (i.e., a well detector) may furnish a detection efficiency greater than that provided by a crystal that receives at best no more than half the γ rays from a radioactive source.

LIQUID SCINTILLATION DETECTORS

With a solid scintillation detector such as a NaI(Tl) crystal, the radioactive sample is positioned outside the detector. In liquid scintillation counting, the radioactive sample is mixed intimately with the scintillat-

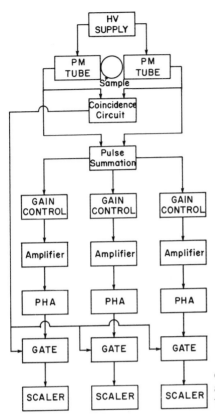

Fig 11-16. — A liquid scintillation counter with two photomultiplier tubes and a coincidence circuit to reduce the background count rate.

ing material, and attenuation by materials between the radioactive sample and the scintillating material is reduced to a minimum.[10-12] Consequently, the detection efficiency is high for radiations with very short range, including weak beta particles such as those from ^3H ($E_{max} = 0.018$ MeV), ^{14}C ($E_{max} = 0.156$ MeV) and ^{35}S ($E_{max} = 0.168$ MeV). Usually, light from the mixture of scintillator and radioactive sample is directed toward at least two photomultiplier tubes. The signal from each photomultiplier tube is transmitted by a preamplifier and amplifier to a coincidence circuit (Fig 11-16). The coincidence circuit transmits a voltage pulse to the scaler only if a pulse is received simultaneously from both photomultiplier tubes.

Except for very low energy particles and photons, radiation emitted by the sample usually produces a signal in each photomultiplier tube, and a pulse passes to the scaler for most disintegrations of the sample. However, spurious pulses generated by "thermal noise" in the photomultiplier tubes or preamplifiers are received by the coincidence circuit from one direction only, and a pulse is not passed to the scaler. In this manner, the coincidence circuit reduces the background count rate. Without this circuit, the background count rate would be intolerably high. In older liquid scintillation counters, the scintillation mixture, photomultiplier tubes and preamplifiers were cooled to a few degrees above zero to help eliminate spurious counts. Newer photomultiplier tubes do not require refrigeration.

The scintillating solution or "cocktail" consists of the radioactive sample, a solvent, a primary fluor or solute and, if necessary, a secondary fluor. Solvents used include toluene, xylene and dioxane. Toluene and xylene molecules transfer energy efficiently from the sites of interaction of the radiation to the molecules of fluor in the scintillation mixture. Dioxane transfers energy with reduced efficiency, but exhibits a higher solubility for water-soluble samples.

Molecules of the primary fluor release light upon receipt of energy from the solvent molecules. Usually, the primary fluor comprises about 0.5% of the scintillation cocktail. Primary fluors used most often include 2,5-diphenyloxazole (PPO), 2,5,-bis-2-(5-T-butyl-benzoxazolyl)-thiophene (BBOT), p-terphenyl and 2-phenyl-5-biphenyloxadiazole (PBD). Because of its lower cost, PPO (fluorescence peaked at 3,800 Å) is the primary fluor used for most liquid scintillation procedures. For certain samples, BBOT (fluorescence peaked at 4,350 Å) and PBD (fluorescence peaked at 3,700 Å) may be preferred.

The wavelengths of light emitted by the scintillation cocktail must correspond to the spectral sensitivity of the photocathodes of the photomultiplier tubes. Some photomultiplier tubes with quartz windows are sensitive to the light emitted by primary fluors. With many photomultiplier tubes, however, a secondary fluor must be added to the scintillation solution. The secondary fluor is termed a *wavelength shifter*, because light of longer wavelength is emitted by the scintillation solution when the secondary fluor is present. The concentration of the secondary fluor is about 0.1%. Common secondary fluors include 1,4-bis-2-(5-phenyloxazolyl)-benzene (POPOP) and 1,4-bis-2-(4-methyl-5-phenyloxazolyl)-benzene (dimethyl-POPOP).

Introduction of the sample into the scintillation mixture may interfere with the transfer of energy among solvent molecules. To lessen this interference, materials such as naphthalene and anisole may be added to the scintillation cocktail. Frequently, materials are added to the cocktail to increase the solubility of radioactive samples in the scintillation mixture. Examples of these solubilizing agents include the hydroxide of Hyamine 10-X (hyamine), ethanolic potassium hydroxide, aqueous potassium hydroxide and a number of "solubilizers," which are available commercially. In a liquid scintillation counter, the size of the voltage

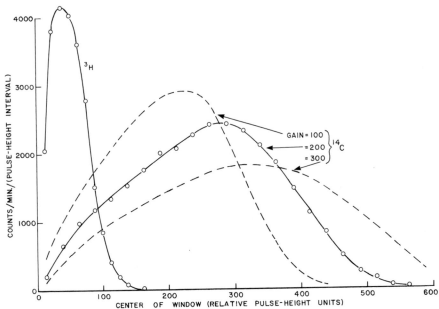

Fig 11-17. — Liquid scintillation spectra for beta particles from ³H (E_{max}=0.018 MeV) and ¹⁴C (E_{max}=0.156 MeV). The dashed curves illustrate the effects of the amplifier gain upon the ¹⁴C spectrum.

pulse depends on the energy dissipated in the scintillation cocktail by a photon or particle emitted by the radioactive sample. The number of pulses of different sizes is shown in Figure 11-17 for beta-emitting samples of ³H and ¹⁴C. By adjusting upper and lower discriminators, one isotope may be counted in the presence of the other. For a number of reasons, these spectra do not correspond exactly to the energy distribution of the emitted particles.

Interference with the production or transmission of light in a liquid scintillation solution is termed *quenching*. Quenching always is present in liquid scintillation counting, and is caused by:

1. Interference with the mechanism of energy transfer contributed by the sample or other components of the cocktail. This mode of interference is termed *chemical quenching*.
2. Absorption of light by colored materials in the sample. This mode of interference is called *color quenching*.
3. Passive interference with the mechanism of energy transfer resulting from dilution of the scintillation mixture by the sample or other material. This mode is termed *dilution quenching*.
4. Absorption of light by the scintillation vial, fingerprints on the vial, etc. This mode of interference is termed *optical quenching*.

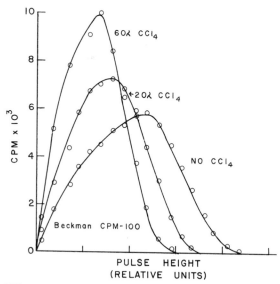

Fig 11-18. — Effects of quenching on the liquid scintillation spectrum for ^{14}C. The quenching agent is CCl_4.

Quenching shifts the spectrum for any isotope toward pulses of smaller size. Shown in Figure 11-18 are spectra for a ^{14}C-labeled sample dissolved in a scintillation cocktail and quenched with different amounts of carbon tetrachloride, a chemical quench agent.

The count rate for a particular sample must be corrected for quenching before the disintegration rate of the sample can be determined. Three methods for quench correction have been developed. With the *internal spike method* (internal standard method), a cocktail is counted before and after a small quantity of "unquenched" material has been added to the sample. The unquenched material and the sample are labeled with the same radioactive isotope. The count rate without the unquenched material is subtracted from the count rate with the unquenched material. The counting efficiency is the difference in count rate divided by the disintegration rate for the unquenched material. With the *channels ratio method* for quench correction, a sample is counted in two separate "counting windows" or "channels," which are defined by upper, lower and intermediate discriminators. The ratio of the count rates in the two channels varies with the amount of quenching in the cocktail. By reference to a calibration curve of counting efficiency versus the ratio of count rates, the counting efficiency for a particular sample may be determined. With the *external standard method* for quench correction, the sample is counted before and after a gamma-emitting source (e.g., ^{137}Cs, radium or ^{133}Ba) has been positioned adjacent to the scintillation vial. The increase in count rate obtained with the source near the vial varies with the amount of quenching in the sample. The counting efficiency is determined by referring to a calibration curve of counting efficiency versus the ratio of count rates before and after the gamma-emitting source has been positioned adjacent to the scintillation vial.

Samples that are not soluble in a liquid scintillation cocktail may be counted by *suspension counting*. Gelling agents such as aluminum stearate, Cab-O-Sil and Thixcin furnish suspensions of radioactive samples in various counting solutions. Techniques have been developed for counting insoluble samples such as filter paper, paper chromatograms and Millipore filter disks. Scintillating beads sometimes are used when liquid or gaseous samples are counted by liquid scintillation.

SEMICONDUCTOR RADIATION DETECTORS

Semiconductor detectors are being used with increasing frequency for the detection of charged particles and photons emitted by radioactive nuclei. Semiconductor detectors exhibit many desirable properties, including: (1) a response that varies linearly with the energy deposited in the detector and does not depend upon the type of radiation that deposits the energy; (2) a negligible absorption of energy in the entrance window of the detector; (3) excellent energy resolution; (4) the formation of pulses with fast rise times; and (5) small size.

The mechanism of response of a semiconductor detector resembles that for an ionization chamber. Ionization produced within the sensitive volume of the detector is converted to a voltage pulse which is amplified and counted. The size of the voltage pulse is proportional to the energy expended in the detector by the incident radiation. Compared to an ionization chamber, the voltage pulse is larger and reflects more accurately the energy deposited in the detector. Also, the rise-time of the pulse is shorter because the ionization is collected more rapidly.

In most gases, an average energy of 30–40 eV is expended per ion pair produced. An ion pair is produced in a silicon semiconductor detector for each 3.5 eV deposited by incident radiation; in a germanium detector, only 2.94 eV are required to produce an ion pair. Compared to an ionization chamber, therefore, many more ion pairs are produced in a semiconductor detector for a given amount of energy absorbed.

Response of Semiconductor Detectors

A semiconductor radiation detector is similar to a transistor and is diagramed in Figure 11-19. The *p*-type region is composed of a semiconducting element* (e.g., germanium or silicon) "doped" with an *electron acceptor impurity* with fewer valence electrons. For example, a *p*-type

---

*A semiconducting element is an element with an electric resistance that decreases rapidly with increasing temperature.

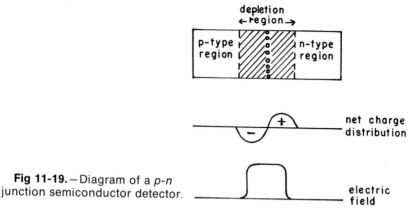

Fig 11-19. — Diagram of a *p-n* junction semiconductor detector.

semiconductor may be obtained by doping tetravalent germanium with trivalent boron, indium or gallium. The *n*-type region is comprised of germanium doped with an *electron donor impurity* such as antimony or lithium. Electrons flow from the *n*-type region to the *p*-type region and establish an electric field across the junction between the two regions. The region in the vicinity of the junction is termed the *depletion region* and may be increased in width by applying a *reverse bias* across the junction (positive potential to the *n*-type region, negative potential to the *p*-type region). The width of the depletion region may be increased also by a process known as *lithium drifting* to produce a Ge(Li) or Si(Li) detector. If a charged particle or x- or γ-ray photon loses energy within the depletion region, electrons are released from the valence band and attracted to the positive electrode (the *n*-type region). In the valence band, electrons move closer to the positive terminal by jumping to holes left by the released electrons. Other electrons fill the holes left by the jumping electrons. In this manner, holes migrate toward the negative terminal as if they were positively charged particles. The migration of positive holes in the valence band constitutes a current similar to that provided by electrons moving in the conducting band to the positive terminal. In fact, electrons released from the valence band, together with the positive holes left behind, constitute the ion pairs for a semiconductor detector.

If a potential difference is applied across a pure semiconductor, a current is produced even if the semiconductor is not exposed to ionizing radiation. This current is the sum of: (1) a *bulk current* that is dependent on the resistance of the semiconductor and the number of electron-hole pairs produced by thermal excitation; and (2) a current caused by *charge leakage* at the surface of the semiconductor. These currents interfere with the identification of signals produced as radiation interacts within the detector. The bulk current is reduced with the *p-n* junction described above, and this barrier to current flow is required in a semiconductor radiation detector. The *p-n* junction reduces the bulk current in silicon to an acceptable level at room temperature. Even with a *p-n* junction, however, the bulk current in a germanium detector is too great at room temperature. Consequently, germanium semiconductor detectors must be operated at reduced temperature. Germanium detectors usually are mounted in a cryostat and are maintained at the temperature of liquid nitrogen (-190 C). The surface-leakage current is reduced in germanium and silicon by special techniques for constructing the detectors.

The size *V* of a voltage pulse from a semiconductor detector equals the charge *Q* collected by the electrodes, divided by the capacitance *C* of the depletion region.* The charge *Q* equals *Ne*, where *N* is the number of electron-hole pairs produced and *e* is the charge of the electron; that is, the size of the voltage pulse is proportional to the energy lost in the detector by the incident radiation. The size of the pulse is not dependent on the specific ionization of the radiation, because the ion pairs are swept away immediately and cannot recombine. Consequently, the response of the detector depends on the energy deposited in the detector but not on the type of radiation that deposits the energy.

The energy required to produce an ion pair in a semiconductor detector is only about one tenth of the energy required in a gas, and the voltage pulse from a semiconductor detector is about ten times larger than the pulse from a gas-filled ionization detector. For example, a 1-MeV alpha particle absorbed completely in the depletion region of a silicon semiconductor detector produces about $[10^6 \text{ eV}/(3.5 \text{ eV/IP})] = 3 \times 10^5$ ion pairs. The same particle produces only about $[10^6 \text{ eV}/(33.7 \text{ eV/IP})] = 3 \times 10^4$ ion pairs in an air-filled ionization chamber. The estimated percent standard deviation $\%\hat{\sigma}/N$ (chap. 12) for the pulse is

$$\frac{\%\hat{\sigma}}{N} = \frac{100}{\sqrt{\text{Pulse size}}}$$

For the semiconductor detector, $\%\hat{\sigma}/N$ is 0.18 for the pulse produced by a 1-MeV alpha particle. For the gas-filled detector, $\%\hat{\sigma}/N$ is 0.58. Consequently, the range of pulse heights produced by the absorption of a given amount of energy is much narrower for a semiconductor detector than for a gas-filled ionization chamber, and the resolution of the semiconductor detector is much better. A similar analysis is applicable to the com-

---

*The capacitance *C* of a semiconductor detector may be computed with the expression

$$C = 1.44 \frac{A}{W}$$

where *A* is the area of the junction and *W* is the width of the depletion region.

parison of a semiconductor detector to a scintillation detector. Often, the maximum resolution obtainable with a semiconductor detector is limited by the preamplifier rather than by the detector.

Properties of Semiconductor Detectors

The efficiency of semiconductor detectors is nearly 100% for particulate radiations and relatively high for low-energy x and γ rays. The effi-

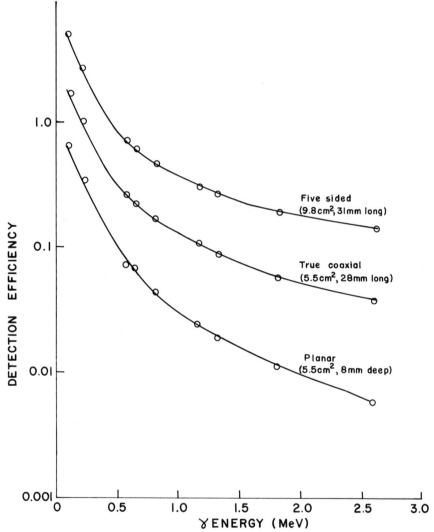

Fig 11-20.—Detection efficiency of three different germanium [Ge(Li)] semiconductor detectors. (Courtesy of H. Fiedler, O. Tench and Canberra Industries, Inc.)

ciency for detecting high-energy x- and γ-ray photons is lower, because the depletion regions of the detectors are small. The atomic number is greater for germanium ($Z = 32$) than for silicon ($Z = 14$), and the gamma-detection efficiency is higher. The efficiency of three germanium detectors is plotted in Figure 11-20 as a function of the γ-ray energy.

Applications of Semiconductor Detectors

Because of their excellent energy resolution, semiconduction detectors are used widely for x- and γ-ray spectrometry and for similar laboratory measurements. These detectors have also been used for fluorescence scanning, in which quantitative estimates of iodine in the thyroid are obtained by measurement of iodine x rays released as the thyroid is exposed to low-energy x or γ radiation.[13] Some effort has been directed toward extension of semiconductor detectors to imaging applications in nuclear medicine. These efforts have been handicapped by the high cost and small size of semiconductor detector matrices constructed for imaging purposes.[14, 15]

PROBLEMS

*1. For a G-M detector operated with a voltage on the G-M plateau:
    a. Is the pulse produced by an α-particle larger than a pulse produced by a β-particle?
    b. Do the size and shape of the pulse vary with the length of the anode? With the diameter of the detector?
    c. Does the size of the pulse vary with the voltage?

*2. Should a G-M detector be used to measure the exposure rate in the vicinity of a storage safe for radioactive nuclides?

3. What type of radiation detector would you recommend for:
    a. Detection of γ-rays from ^{131}I in a patient's thyroid?
    b. Detection of β-particles from ^{3}H-thymidine dissolved in water?
    c. Detection of β-particles from ^{14}C in a gaseous sample of CO_2?
    d. Detection of α-particles from a plated source of ^{210}Po?
    e. Detection of radioactive contamination on a workbench in a laboratory where ^{32}P is used? In a laboratory where ^{3}H is used?
    f. Measurement of the exposure rate in the vicinity of a patient with a radium implant?
    g. ^{131}I in aqueous solution with ^{32}P?
    h. A mixture of ^{51}Cr and ^{131}I in blood?

*4. A γ-ray from ^{241}Am (60 keV) is absorbed completely in a NaI(Tl) crystal. The photomultiplier tube has 10 dynodes, with each dynode providing an electron multiplication factor of 3. About 80% of the light from the crystal is absorbed by the photocathode, which has a photocathode efficiency (number of electrons emitted per light photon absorbed) of 0.05. Assuming that 30 photons of light are produced in the NaI(Tl) crystal per kiloelectron volt of energy absorbed, compute the number of electrons received at the anode of the photomultiplier tube.

*For those problems marked with an asterisk, answers are provided on the pages following the appendixes (see pp. 487–488).

°5. An α-particle from ^{210}Po (5.30 MeV) is absorbed completely in an air-filled, pulse-type ionization chamber. Assuming a capacitance of 40 picofarad, compute the size of the voltage pulse.

6. Compare the efficiency and resolution of a semiconductor detector and a scintillation detector exposed to γ rays. Why are the efficiency and resolution different?

REFERENCES

1. Hendee, W.: *The Physics of Therapeutic Radiology* (in prep.).
2. Chase, G., and Rabinowitch, J.: *Principles of Radioisotope Methodology* (3d ed.; Minneapolis: Burgess Publishing Co., 1967).
3. Boag, J.: Ionization Chambers, in Attix, F., and Roesch, W. (eds.): *Radiation Dosimetry* (2d ed.; New York: Academic Press, 1966).
4. O'Kelley, G.: *Detection and Measurement of Nuclear Radiation*, NAS-NS3105 (Washington, D.C.: Office of Technical Services, 1962), p. 81.
5. Reynolds, R., Snyder, R., and Overton, T.: A multiwire proportional chamber positron camera: Initial results, Phys. Med. Biol. 20:136, 1975.
6. Lim, C., et al.: A multiwire proportional chamber positron camera: Preliminary imaging device, J. Nucl. Med. 16:546, 1975.
7. Wang, C., and Willis, D.: *Radiotracer Methodology in Biological Science* (Englewood Cliffs, N.J.: Prentice-Hall, Inc., 1965).
8. Robertson, J., and Lynch, J.: The luminescent decay of various crystals for particles of different ionization density, Proc. Phys. Soc. London 77:751, 1961.
9. Ramm, W.: Scintillation Detectors, in Attix, F., and Roesch, W. (eds.): *Radiation Dosimetry* (2d ed.; New York: Academic Press, 1966).
10. Rapkin, E.: Samples for Liquid Scintillation Counting, in Hine, G. (ed.): *Instrumentation in Nuclear Medicine* (New York: Academic Press, 1967), vol. 1, p. 182.
11. Horrocks, D.: Liquid Scintillation Counting, in Scott, A. F. (ed.): *Survey of Progress in Chemistry* (New York: Academic Press, 1968).
12. Hendee, W.: *Radioactive Isotopes in Biological Research* (New York: John Wiley & Sons, Inc., 1973).
13. Esser, P., and Lister, D.: A new apparatus for fluorescent scanning: A moving x-ray tube, J. Nucl. Med. 18:640, 1977.
14. Strauss, M., et al.: Performance of a coaxial germanium gamma-ray detector, J. Nucl. Med. 15:1196, 1974.
15. Hoffer, P., Beck, R., and Gottschalk, A.: *Semiconductor Detectors in the Future of Nuclear Medicine* (New York: Society of Nuclear Medicine, 1971).

12 / Accumulation and Analysis of Nuclear Data

Signals from radiation detectors described in Chapter 11 may be transmitted to a variety of electronic circuits for analysis and display. Some of the more common circuits and their applications are discussed in this chapter. Data displayed by different output devices must be interpreted in terms of their statistical significance and their relationship to the activity and modes of decay of the radioactive sample. Also considered in this chapter are some of the difficulties encountered during this interpretation.

COUNTING SYSTEMS

Counting systems are assembled by combining various electronic circuits and display devices. A general purpose counting system is outlined in Figure 12-1. Each component of this system is discussed separately in the following sections.

Preamplifiers

Almost all radiation detectors exhibit low capacitance and high impedance. Signals from these detectors are distorted and attenuated severely if they are transmitted by coaxial cable directly from the detector to an amplifier some distance away. To reduce this distortion and attenuation, a preamplifier may be inserted near the detector. If the preamplifier matches the impedance of the detector to that of the amplifier, then the cable joining the two components may be several feet long. Preamplifiers are used also to "clip" and "shape" the voltage pulse from the detector to meet the specifications of the amplifier. Provided the amplifier is not too far away, a preamplifier is not required with a G-M detector, because pulses from this detector are relatively large.

The *cathode-follower preamplifier* (or *emitter-follower preamplifier*) is a voltage-sensitive circuit used primarily to match the impedance of a detector with that of an amplifier. The term *preamplifier* is misleading when applied to the cathode-follower circuit, because the voltage pulse from the detector is not amplified by the circuit. In fact, the gain of the cathode follower is slightly less than 1.*

---

*Gain = $\dfrac{\text{Size of output signal}}{\text{Size of input signal}}$

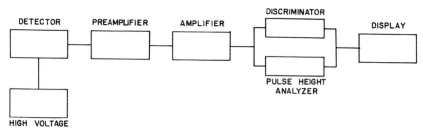

Fig 12-1. — Block diagram for components of a general purpose counting system.

A *charge-sensitive preamplifier* is used with a semiconductor detector. The charge sensitivity of this circuit is the ratio of the size of the voltage pulse from the circuit to the amount of charge collected by the detector.

Amplifiers

An amplifier is used to increase the size and vary the shape of signals from the detector or preamplifier. An amplifier may be either *voltage sensitive* or *charge sensitive,* depending on the type of signal received at the input terminal. The increase in signal size is described as the *amplifier gain,* which is the ratio of the height of the voltage pulse leaving the amplifier to the size of the signal received at the input terminal of the amplifier. Depending on the type of detector and the characteristics of circuits in the counting system, an amplifier gain of 10–50,000 may be required for a particular counting system.

The pulse furnished by an amplifier is plotted in Figure 12-2 as a function of time. The *pulse rise time* is the time required for the pulse amplitude to increase from 10% to 90% of its maximum amplitude. The *pulse decay time* is the time required for the pulse to decrease from maximum amplitude to 10% of maximum. The rise time of an amplifier should be less than the time required to collect the ion pairs or light produced during interaction of a particle or photon in the detector. The amplifier pulse should be terminated rapidly to prevent the amplifier from summing successive pulses from the detector. The *integration time* of an amplifier is the time required to form an output pulse. The integration time represents a compromise between the time required for complete collection of a signal from the detector and the time that causes a significant number of successive pulses to combine. The integration time is about 1 μsec for an amplifier used with a NaI(Tl) scintillation detector.

Large input pulses and high rates of pulse reception of input pulses may cause the characteristics of an amplifier to change. For example, a few output pulses may be distorted after a very large pulse (e.g., a pulse produced by interaction of a cosmic ray) has been received by the ampli-

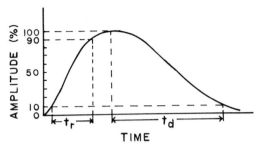

Fig 12-2.—Pulse delivered by an amplifier. The amplitude may be either voltage or instantaneous current. The pulse rise time t_r and pulse decay time t_d are shown.

fier. This distortion of output pulses is termed *pulse-amplitude overloading. Count-rate overloading* refers to distortions in pulse shape caused by the delivery of pulses to the amplifier at too high an input rate. Pulse-amplitude overloading and count-rate overloading may distort data displayed by the output device.[1]

Pulses are amplified linearly in most amplifiers used in counting circuits. Linear amplification may be disadvantageous, however, if pulses from the detector are variable in size over a wide range. For these applications, an amplifier with logarithmic gain may be useful. The size of a pulse from a logarithmic amplifier is proportional to the logarithm of the size of the input pulse. With a logarithmic amplifier, a wide range of input pulses may be amplified without pulse-amplitude overloading and without the rejection of very small pulses.

Pulse Height Analyzers

With a detector such as a scintillation or semiconductor detector, the height of a voltage pulse from the amplifier is proportional to the energy expended in the detector by a charged particle or x- or γ-ray photon. A typical train of pulses from an amplifier connected to a scintillation or semiconductor detector is depicted in Figure 12-3. These pulses may be sorted by a pulse height analyzer to yield a pulse height spectrum that reflects the distribution in energy lost in the detector by incident pho-

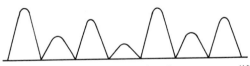

Fig 12-3.—Train of voltage pulses emerging from an amplifier which follows a preamplifier and a scintillation detector or a semiconductor detector. The height of each pulse reflects the energy expended in the detector by an incident photon or particle.

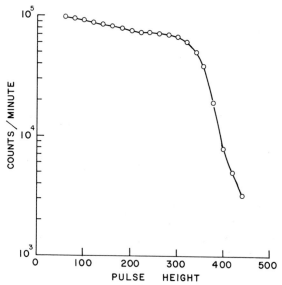

Fig 12-4.—Integral pulse height spectrum for ^{131}I, measured with a 2 × 2 in. NaI(Tl) well crystal.

tons or particles. Two techniques, *differential sorting* and *integral sorting*, are used for pulse height analysis.

For integral sorting, a single discriminator in the pulse height analyzer is varied from a position where all pulses are transmitted to the display device to a position where all pulses are rejected. Shown in Figure 12-4 is an integral spectrum for ^{131}I. At any value of pulse height on the x-axis, the height of the curve denotes the number of pulses that are large enough to pass by the input discriminator and reach the display device.

A differential pulse height analyzer is composed basically of two discriminators connected to an anticoincidence circuit. The discriminators transmit pulses above a certain minimum size. In Figure 12-5, for example, the lower discriminator transmits pulses larger than size V_1 and the upper discriminator transmits pulses larger than size V_2. Pulses from the

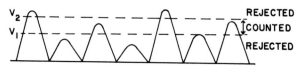

Fig 12-5.—Diagram of a series of voltage pulses impinging on discriminators V_1 and V_2 of a differential pulse height analyzer. Pulses with height between V_1 and V_2 are counted. Pulses with height less than V_1 are rejected by both discriminators, and pulses with height greater than V_2 are rejected by an anticoincidence circuit.

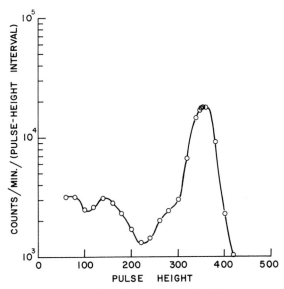

Fig 12-6. — Differential pulse height spectrum for ^{131}I, measured with a 2 × 2 in. NaI(Tl) well crystal. The peak in the spectrum represents pulses produced by total absorption of 364 keV γ rays in the scintillation crystal.

amplifier are applied simultaneously to both discriminators. Pulses too small ($<V_1$) to be transmitted by either discriminator are rejected and are not transmitted to the anticoincidence circuit. Pulses of size between V_1 and V_2 are transmitted by the lower discriminator only and are delivered to one input terminal of the anticoincidence circuit. Pulses large enough ($>V_2$) to be transmitted by both discriminators are delivered simultaneously to both input terminals of the anticoincidence circuit. The anticoincidence circuit transmits a pulse to the display device when it receives a pulse at one input terminal only. A pulse is not transmitted to the display device when signals are received simultaneously at both input terminals. Consequently, the display device registers only the number of pulses of size between V_1 and V_2. The range of pulse sizes registered by the display device may be varied by changing the settings V_1 and V_2 of the lower and upper discriminators. These settings may be labeled on the pulse height analyzer as "lower discriminator" and "upper discriminator," "E_1" and "E_2," or "lower level" and "upper level." Occasionally, the lower and upper discriminators of a pulse height analyzer are not adjustable (e.g., in some scintillation cameras). With this type of analyzer, differential pulse height analysis may be achieved by changing the range of pulse sizes emerging from the detector or by varying the amplification of the pulses in the amplifier. These changes may be accomplished by varying the high voltage of the photomultiplier tube or by changing the gain of the amplifier.

In a pulse height analyzer with discriminators that can be adjusted independently of each other, the range of pulse sizes transmitted to the anticoincidence circuit may be affected severely by small fluctuations in voltage applied to the discriminators. To reduce this dependence on voltage stability, the upper discriminator may be arranged to "ride" on the lower discriminator. In this manner, a constant difference in pulse heights may be maintained between the discriminators. The lower discriminator may be termed "lower level," "threshold," "E" or "baseline," and the difference in pulse size between the two discriminators may be referred to as "window width," "window," "slit width" or "ΔE." The position of the lower discriminator determines the minimum size of pulses transmitted to the display device, and the width of the window determines the increment of pulse sizes transmitted. As the window width is reduced, fewer pulses are transmitted to the display device, but the resolution of the pulse height spectrum is increased (see chap. 13). A differential pulse height spectrum for ^{131}I is shown in Figure 12-6.

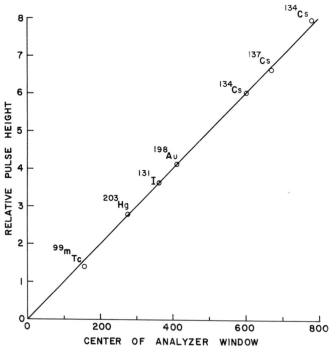

Fig 12-7.—Average size of pulses transmitted by a pulse height analyzer, plotted as a function of the position of the center of the analyzer window.

Most pulse height analyzers may be operated in either the integral or differential mode. In the differential mode, some analyzers may be operated with independent lower and upper discriminators, or with a variable lower discriminator and a dependent window.

The *linearity* of a pulse height analyzer describes the relationship between the position of the lower discriminator (or middle of the window) and the size of pulses transmitted to the display device. For a counting system with linear amplification, a straight line should be obtained if the average size of pulses admitted to the display device is plotted as a function of the position of the lower discriminator or center of the analyzer window (Fig 12-7). The maximum departure from a straight line is termed the *integral nonlinearity* and is less than 1% in a satisfactory counting system. Zero offset describes the positive or negative displacement from the origin of a curve such as that in Figure 12-7.

Scalers and Timers

A scaler is used to record or count the number of pulses received from an amplifier or pulse height analyzer. In all modern scalers, this number can be read directly from the display; that is, a count of 4,431 is displayed as the number 4431.

In some scaler-timer systems, electromechanical timers driven by a synchronous motor are used. The timer either may indicate elapsed counting time or may stop the accumulation of counts by the scaler after a preset counting time. Electronic timers are more accurate than electromechanical timers and are used in most counting systems. These timers consist of a scaler pulsed by a constant-frequency oscillator. Elapsed or preset time may be displayed visually or printed automatically.

High-Voltage Supplies

The specifications for a high-voltage supply for a counting system vary with the detector used. For example, a high-voltage supply for a G-M tube or a semiconductor detector need not be so stable as that for a scintillation detector, because the signal from a G-M or semiconductor detector is affected little by fluctuations in applied voltage. On the other hand, the signal from a scintillation detector may vary by as much as 10% for a 1% change in high voltage. The stability of a high-voltage supply may be affected by changes in temperature, fluctuations in line voltage or variations in the resistance (load) across the output terminals.

Rate Meters

Rate meters may be grouped into two categories; analog and digital. Pulses entering an analog rate meter result in the accumulation of charge on a capacitor, with the accumulated charge leaking through a resistance R. The charge on the capacitor increases until the rate of accumulation

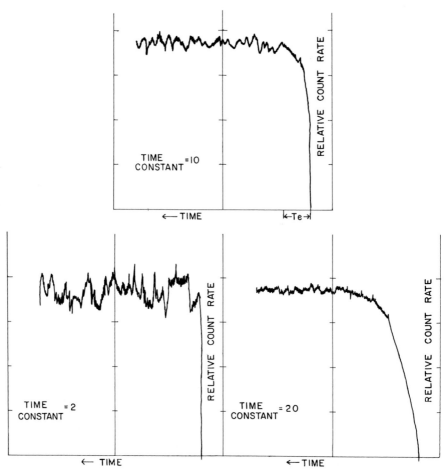

Fig 12-8.—Top, graph of meter position of an analog rate meter changing from a lower to a higher count rate. The equilibrium time T_e for the rate meter is shown. **Bottom left,** rapid response and high sensitivity to statistical fluctuations in count rate are provided by a short time constant. **Bottom right,** data "smoothing" but a slow response is furnished by a long time constant.

equals the rate of leakage. When accumulation and leakage are equal, the voltage across the resistance-capacitance (RC) circuit is proportional to the average rate at which pulses are delivered to the rate meter. This voltage is displayed by a meter calibrated in units of count rate.

The product of the resistance and capacitance of an RC circuit is referred to as the *time constant* for the circuit; that is, the time constant = RC. The time required to achieve equilibrium between charge accumulation and leakage varies with the input pulse rate and with the time constant. The *equilibrium time* is the time required for the meter of an analog rate meter to increase from zero count rate to within one standard deviation of the equilibrium count rate. The equilibrium time T_e is:

$$T_e = RC\{0.5 \ln[2N(RC)] + 0.394\} \qquad (12\text{-}1)$$

where RC is the time constant for the rate meter and N is the equilibrium count rate.[2] The equilibrium time indicates the speed of response of an analog rate meter (Fig 12-8).

The equilibrium time is decreased if the time constant for the rate meter is reduced. When this is done, however, the rate meter is more sensitive to statistical fluctuations in count rate. Most rate meters offer a choice of time constants. The time constant chosen is a compromise between data smoothing obtained with a long time constant and rapid response to changing count rates provided by a short time constant.

The count-rate display of most rate meters is linear, and may be changed, usually by factors of 10, by a range switch on the control panel of the rate meter. A few rate meters furnish a logarithmic display of count rate. A range switch is unnecessary on a logarithmic meter because many decades of count rate are included on the meter. The count rate on a logarithmic rate meter is difficult to read and interpolate, and this type of rate meter should be used only when a highly accurate display of the count rate is not required. For example, logarithmic rate meters often are used with portable survey meters. Some rate meters may be used in either the linear or the logarithmic mode.

A digital rate meter usually consists of a timer and a "buffered scaler." The scaler accumulates counts over a preset interval of time, then transfers the accumulated counts to the buffer. Almost instantly, the scaler resets to zero and again begins to accumulate counts. The counts stored in the buffer may be displayed visually, printed or recorded on magnetic tape, transmitted to a computer, or used to modulate the brightness of the light image from a cathode-ray tube. Although the response of a digital rate meter lags slightly behind changes in count rate, the lag does not vary with the actual count rate.

Multichannel Analyzers

To determine the number of pulses of different sizes impinging upon a single-channel pulse height analyzer, counts must be recorded for selected intervals of time while the window of the analyzer is moved incrementally from the smallest to the largest pulse size encountered. This procedure is tedious and imprecise, because each pulse height "channel" is sampled independently and for only a short time. Also, pulse height spectra for isotopes with short half-lives are difficult to measure with a single-channel analyzer. With a multichannel analyzer, pulses in each of a large number of pulse height channels are counted simultaneously. With a single channel analyzer and a counting time of 1 minute per channel, more than 100 minutes are required to sample a pulse height distribution that is divided into 100 parts. With a 100-channel analyzer, the same data may be collected in 1 minute. Multichannel analyzers are available commercially with approximately 100, 400, 1,000, 4,000 and more channels.

In the multichannel analyzer, a pulse from the amplifier is fed to an analog-digital converter (ADC). Within the ADC, charge is stored in a capacitor in proportion to the amplitude of the incoming pulse. After receipt of the pulse, the capacitor is discharged to a certain fraction of its original charge, while an oscillator emits pulses at a constant rate. The number of pulses emitted by the oscillator reflects the amplitude of the original pulse fed to the ADC. The number of oscillator pulses determines the location in the magnetic core memory where a binary number is increased by 1 to reflect receipt by the ADC of a pulse of specified magnitude. Each storage location in the magnetic core memory corresponds to a specific pulse amplitude, and the binary number stored at each location reflects the number of pulses of a specific amplitude received by the ADC during the counting period. These numbers can be displayed graphically on the screen of a cathode-ray tube or other display device to portray the pulse height spectrum for the radionuclide. By arithmetic manipulation of data stored in the multichannel analyzer, the pulse height spectrum can be corrected for background counts, the presence of more than one radionuclide in the sample, or other influences.

STATISTICS OF COUNTING

The moment of decay of a particular radioactive nucleus is not predictable. Furthermore, the moment of decay is not influenced by the history of the nucleus (i.e., the period of time over which the nucleus has not decayed) or by its environment or treatment. This unpredictability is described as the *random nature of radioactive decay*. Because radioactive nuclei decay randomly, data obtained for radioactive samples must be interpreted with an understanding of probability and statistics.

Precision and Accuracy

The error of a measurement is the difference between the measured value and the "true value" for the measurement. The two categories of error are *determinate errors* and *indeterminate errors*. Determinate errors (sometimes termed *systematic errors*) result from factors such as inadequate experimental design, malfunctioning equipment and incomplete correction for extraneous influences. The influence of determinate errors upon experimental results may be reduced by better instrumentation and thorough planning and execution of an experiment. Indetermi-

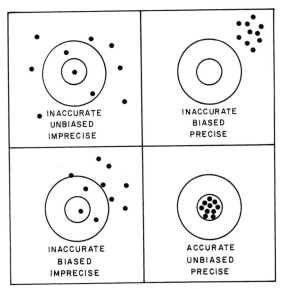

Fig 12-9. — Precision, bias and accuracy.

nate errors (sometimes termed *random errors*) are those that cannot be reduced by eliminating or correcting extraneous factors. In experiments with radioactive materials, the random nature of radioactive decay often is the most significant indeterminate error.

The *precision* of a series of measurements describes the range or spread of the individual measurements from the average value for the series. Precision describes the reproducibility of the measurements and improves with a reduction in the influence of indeterminate error upon the measurements. The *accuracy* of a series of measurements is not described by the precision of the measurements, because accuracy is achieved only if the measured values agree with the true value. To increase accuracy, the influence of both indeterminate and determinate errors must be reduced. The contribution of determinate error to a reduction in the loss of accuracy in a set of measurements is termed the *bias* of the measurements. The distinction between precision, accuracy and bias is illustrated in Figure 12-9.

Poisson Distribution

If a radioactive sample with a relatively long half-life is counted many times, a graph is obtained similar to that in Figure 12-10. If the number of times the sample is counted is very large, then the probability of obtaining a particular count may be estimated as the number of times the

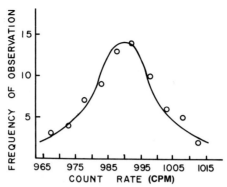

Fig 12-10.—Data for a ^{137}Cs source that provided a count rate of about 1,000 CPM. A count of 10,000 was accumulated for each measurement. The results of 100 measurements were plotted as a function of the number of times that the count rate fell within successive increments of 5 (i.e., between 975 and 980, or 980 and 985, etc.). The Poisson curve of the best fit is drawn through the data points. (From Low, F.: Basic Considerations in Nuclear Instrumentation, in Hine, G. [ed.]: *Instrumentation in Nuclear Medicine* [New York: Academic Press, 1967], vol. 1.)

particular count is obtained divided by the total number of times the sample is counted. This probability is described accurately by the equation

$$p_n = \frac{r^n e^{-r}}{n!}$$

where p_n is the probability of obtaining a count n, and r is the true average count for the sample. The term $n!$ (*n*-factorial) equals $(n)(n-1)(n-2) \ldots (2)(1)$. The probability p_n is termed the *Poisson probability density* and radioactive decay is said to follow a *Poisson probability law*. The true average count or *true mean* for the sample cannot be measured, and must be assumed to equal the average measured count or estimated mean $\hat{r}$. Often, $\hat{r}$ is referred to as the *sample mean*.

$$p_n = \frac{\hat{r}^n e^{-\hat{r}}}{n!} \tag{12-2}$$

Example 12-1

What is the probability of obtaining a count of 12 when the average count is 15?

$$p_n = \frac{\hat{r}^n e^{-\hat{r}}}{n!} \tag{12-2}$$

$$p_{12} = \frac{(15)^{12}e^{-15}}{12!}$$

$$= \frac{(129.7 \times 10^{12})(30.6 \times 10^{-8})}{(4.79 \times 10^{8})}$$

$$= 0.0829$$

The probability is 0.0829 (or 8.29%) that a count of 12 will be obtained when the average count is 15. Mathematical tables in the *Handbook of Chemistry and Physics* (Chemical Rubber Co.) contain solutions to arithmetic expressions such as those in this example.

Normal Distribution

If a large number of counts is accumulated for a radioactive sample, then the Poisson distribution curve of frequency of occurrence versus counts is approximated closely by a Gaussian distribution curve, and the data are described reasonably well by the equation for a *Gaussian* or *normal probability density function*. Illustrated in Figure 12-11 is the approach of a Poisson probability density curve to that for a normal

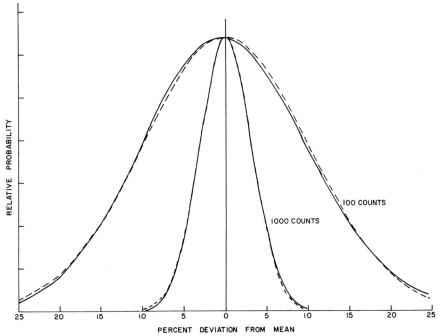

Fig 12-11.—Probability of observing a particular count, plotted for 100 measurements and 1,000 measurements. Dotted curves illustrate normal probability density functions and solid curves illustrate Poisson probability density functions. Curves have been normalized to equal heights at the mean.

probability density. The equation for the normal probability density g_n is

$$g_n = \frac{1}{\sqrt{2\pi\hat{r}}} e^{-(n - \hat{r})^2/2\hat{r}}$$

(12-3)

where g_n is the probability of observing a count n when the true count (estimated as the average count) is $\hat{r}$.

Example 12-2

Using equation (12-3), estimate the probability of obtaining a count of 12 when the true or average count is 15.

$$g_n = \frac{1}{\sqrt{2\pi\hat{r}}} e^{-(n - \hat{r})^2/2\hat{r}}$$

$$= \frac{1}{\sqrt{2\pi(15)}} e^{-(12 - 15)^2/2(15)}$$

$$= 0.103\ e^{-0.3}$$

$$= 0.0764$$

METHODS TO DESCRIBE PRECISION: STANDARD DEVIATION

The *standard deviation* for a series of measurements describes the precision or reproducibility of the measurements. The standard deviation σ is

$$\sigma = \sqrt{r}$$

where r is the true mean and the data are distributed according to the Poisson probability law. If the true mean is estimated as the average value $\hat{r}$ for a series of measurements, then the estimated standard deviation $\hat{\sigma}$ for the measurements is

$$\hat{\sigma} = \sqrt{\hat{r}}$$

and equation (12-3) may be rewritten as

$$g_n = \frac{1}{\hat{\sigma}\sqrt{2\pi}} e^{-(n - \hat{\sigma}^2)^2/2\hat{\sigma}^2}$$

If only one measured value n is available, then the standard deviation may be estimated as $\sqrt{n}$ by assuming that the value n represents the true mean.

In a normal distribution, 68.3% of all measured values fall within one standard deviation on either side of the mean, 95.5% within two standard deviations and 99.7% within limits of three standard deviations.

The standard deviation σ may be computed exactly with equation

TABLE 12-1. – DATA FOR EXAMPLE 12-3

n_i (COUNTS)	$n_i - \hat{r}$ (DEVIATION)	$(n_i - \hat{r})^2$
43,440	−510	260,100
43,720	−230	52,900
44,130	180	32,400
43,760	−190	36,100
44,390	440	193,600
43,810	−140	19,600
44,740	790	624,100
43,750	−200	40,000
44,010	60	3,600
43,750	−200	40,000

(12-4) for a set of actual measurements distributed according to the normal probability law:

$$\sigma = \sqrt{\frac{\sum\limits_{i=1}^{N} (n_i - \hat{r})^2}{N - 1}} \tag{12-4}$$

In this equation, N is the number of measurements from which the sample mean $\hat{r}$ is determined and n_i represents the individual measurements. The quantity $(N - 1)$ is termed the *number of degrees of freedom*.

Example 12-3

Determine the standard deviation for the set of measurements in Table 12-1.

$$\text{Mean} = \hat{r} = 43{,}950$$
$$\sum (n_i - \hat{r})^2 = 1{,}302{,}400$$

$$\sigma = \sqrt{\frac{\sum (n_i - \hat{r})^2}{N - 1}}$$

$$= \sqrt{\frac{1{,}302{,}400}{10 - 1}}$$

$$= 380$$

The mean may be expressed as $43{,}950 \pm 380$, where 380 is understood to be one standard deviation.

Precision of Count Rates

The estimated standard deviation $\hat{\sigma}_c$ of a count rate is

$$\hat{\sigma}_c = \frac{\hat{\sigma}}{t}$$

where $\hat{\sigma}$ is the estimated standard deviation of a count n, and where the average count rate is determined by dividing the count n by the counting time t. Since

$$\hat{\sigma} = \sqrt{n}$$

$$\hat{\sigma}_c = \frac{\sqrt{n}}{t}$$

The count n is the average count rate c multiplied by the counting time t.

$$\hat{\sigma}_c = \frac{\sqrt{ct}}{t}$$

$$= \sqrt{\frac{c}{t}}$$

Hence, the estimated standard deviation of a count rate (average or instantaneous) is the square root of the count rate divided by the counting time.

Accumulation of Errors

If the precision of numbers A and B is denoted by standard deviations σ_A and σ_B, then the standard deviations of the results of arithmetic operations involving A and B may be computed with expressions in Table 12-2.

Example 12-4

What is the net count and standard deviation for a sample if the count is 400 ± 22 for the sample plus background, and the background count is 64 ± 10?

$$\text{Sample net count} = (A - B) \pm \sqrt{\sigma_A^2 + \sigma_B^2}$$
$$= (400 - 64) \pm \sqrt{(22)^2 + (10)^2}$$
$$= 336 \pm 24 \text{ counts}$$

Example 12-5

From repeated counts of a radioactive sample, the average sample plus background count was 232 ± 16. The counting time for each count was 2.0 ± 0.1 minute. What are the average (sample plus background) count rate and the estimated standard deviation?

Average (sample plus background) count rate

$$= \frac{\text{Average (sample plus background)}}{\text{Time}}$$

$$= \left(\frac{A}{B}\right)\left[1 \pm \sqrt{\left(\frac{\sigma_A}{A}\right)^2 + \left(\frac{\sigma_B}{B}\right)^2}\right]$$

$$= \left(\frac{232}{2.0}\right)\left[1 \pm \sqrt{\left(\frac{16}{232}\right)^2 + \left(\frac{0.1}{2.0}\right)^2}\right]$$

$$= 116 \pm 10 \text{ CPM}$$

TABLE 12-2.—RESULTS OF ARITHMETIC OPERATIONS
WITH NUMBERS A AND B
(The precision of A and B is described by the standard
deviations σ_A and σ_B.)

ARITHMETIC OPERATION	FIRST NUMBER	SECOND NUMBER	RESULT ± STANDARD DEVIATION
Addition	$(A \pm \sigma_A)$	$+ (B \pm \sigma_B)$	$(A + B) \pm \sqrt{\sigma_A{}^2 + \sigma_B{}^2}$
Subtraction	$(A \pm \sigma_A)$	$- (B \pm \sigma_B)$	$(A - B) \pm \sqrt{\sigma_A{}^2 + \sigma_B{}^2}$
Multiplication	$(A \pm \sigma_A)$	$\times (B \pm \sigma_B)$	$(AB)[1 \pm \sqrt{(\sigma_A/A)^2 + (\sigma_B/B)^2}]$
Division	$(A \pm \sigma_A)$	$\div (B \pm \sigma_B)$	$(A/B)[1 \pm \sqrt{(\sigma_A/A)^2 + (\sigma_B/B)^2}]$

Example 12-6

A 10-minute count of sample plus background yields 10,000 counts, and a 6-minute count of background alone yields 1,296 counts. What are the net sample count rate and its standard deviation?

$$\text{Sample plus background count rate} = \frac{10{,}000 \text{ counts}}{10 \text{ min}} = 1{,}000 \text{ CPM}$$

$$\text{Background count rate} = \frac{1{,}296 \text{ counts}}{6 \text{ min}} = 216 \text{ CPM}$$

$$\begin{aligned}\hat{\sigma}_c \text{ for sample plus background count rate} &= \sqrt{\frac{c}{t}} = \sqrt{\frac{1{,}000 \text{ CPM}}{10 \text{ min}}} \\ &= 100 \text{ CPM}\end{aligned}$$

$$\begin{aligned}\hat{\sigma}_c \text{ for background count rate} &= \sqrt{\frac{c}{t}} = \sqrt{\frac{216 \text{ CPM}}{6 \text{ min}}} \\ &= 36 \text{ CPM}\end{aligned}$$

$$\begin{aligned}\text{Net sample count rate} &= (A - B) \pm \sqrt{\sigma_A{}^2 + \sigma_B{}^2} \\ &= (1{,}000 - 216) \pm \sqrt{(100)^2 + (36)^2} \\ &= 784 \pm \sqrt{11{,}176} \\ &= 784 \pm 106\end{aligned}$$

OTHER METHODS FOR DESCRIBING PRECISION

In addition to the standard deviation, a number of other methods are used to describe the precision of data. Only a brief explanation of these methods is provided here; the reader is referred to standard texts on probability and statistics for a more complete explanation.

Probable error (PE) may be used in place of the standard deviation to describe the precision of data. The probability is 0.5 that any particular measurement will differ from the true mean by an amount greater than the *PE*; $PE = 0.6745\sigma$.

9/10 error may be used in place of the standard deviation to describe the precision of data. The probability is 0.1 that any particular measurement will differ from the true mean by an amount greater than the 9/10 error.

95/100 error is similar to the 9/10 error, except that the probability is 0.05 that the difference between a particular measurement and the true mean is greater than the 95/100 error.

Confidence limits may be used to estimate the precision of a number, when repeated measurements are not made. For example, if a result is stated as $A \pm a$, where $\pm a$ are limits of the 95% confidence interval, then it may be said with "95% confidence" that a second measurement of A would be between $A - a$ and $A + a$.

Fractional standard deviation (σ/r) may be used in place of the standard deviation to describe the precision of data. If r represents the true mean, then $\sigma = \sqrt{r}$, and the fractional standard deviation (σ/r) is $1/\sqrt{r}$. For example, σ for the number 10,000 is 100, and the fractional standard deviation is $100/10,000 = 0.01$. The *percent standard deviation* $(\%\sigma)$ is the fractional standard deviation multiplied by 100. In the example above, $\%\sigma = 1$. The percent standard deviation $(\%\sigma_c)$ of a count rate c is

$$\%\sigma_c = 100 \sqrt{\frac{1}{ct}} \tag{12-5}$$

where c is the average count rate measured over a time t.

Example 12-7

For a count rate of 1,000 CPM, what counting time is necessary to achieve a percent standard deviation of 1%?

$$\%\sigma_c = 100 \sqrt{\frac{1}{ct}}$$

$$1\% = 100 \sqrt{\frac{1}{(1,000 \text{ CPM}) \, t}}$$

$$\frac{1}{(1,000)t} = (100)^2 = 10,000$$

$$t = \frac{10,000}{1,000} = 10 \text{ min}$$

Standard deviation σ_m *of the mean* yields an estimate of the precision of the mean of a set of measurements. For N individual measurements constituting a mean, $\sigma_m = \sigma/N$, where σ is the standard deviation of the individual measurements.

SELECTED STATISTICAL TESTS

A number of statistical tests may be applied to measurements of radioactive samples. A few of these tests are described briefly in this section.

TABLE 12-3. – CUMULATIVE NORMAL FREQUENCY DISTRIBUTION

t-VALUE	p	t-VALUE	p
0.0	1.000	2.5	0.0124
0.1	0.920	2.6	0.0093
0.2	0.841	2.7	0.0069
0.3	0.764	2.8	0.0051
0.4	0.689	2.9	0.0037
0.5	0.617	3.0	0.00270
0.6	0.548	3.1	0.00194
0.7	0.483	3.2	0.00136
0.8	0.423	3.3	0.00096
0.9	0.368	3.4	0.00068
1.0	0.317	3.5	0.00046
1.1	0.272	3.6	0.00032
1.2	0.230	3.7	0.00022
1.3	0.194	3.8	0.00014
1.4	0.162	3.9	0.00010
1.5	0.134	4.0	0.0000634
1.6	0.110	4.1	0.0000414
1.7	0.090	4.2	0.0000266
1.8	0.072	4.3	0.0000170
1.9	0.060	4.4	0.0000108
2.0	0.046	4.5	0.0000068
2.1	0.036	4.6	0.0000042
2.2	0.028	4.7	0.0000026
2.3	0.022	4.8	0.0000016
2.4	0.016	4.9	0.0000010

Student's t Test

This is a method for testing for the significance of the difference between two measurements. The t-value for the difference between two measurements n_1 and n_2 is

$$t\text{-value} = \frac{|n_1 - n_2|}{\sqrt{\sigma_1^2 + \sigma_2^2}} \qquad (12\text{-}6)$$

where σ_1 and σ_2 are the standard deviations for the measurements n_1 and n_2, and the vertical bars enclosing $n_1 - n_2$ indicate that the absolute or positive value of the difference is used for the computation. With the computed t-value and Table 12-3, the probability may be determined that the difference in the numbers is simply statistical in nature and is not a real difference between dissimilar samples.

Example 12-8

Livers excised from two rabbits given ^{99m}TcS intravenously were counted for 1 minute. The net count rate was 1,524 ± 47 CPM for the first liver and 1,601 ± 49 CPM for the second. Is the difference significant?

$$t\text{-value} = \frac{|n_1 - n_2|}{\sqrt{\sigma_1^2 + \sigma_2^2}}$$

$$= \frac{|1,524 - 1,601|}{\sqrt{(47)^2 + (49)^2}}$$

$$= \frac{77}{68}$$

$$= 1.13$$

From Table 12-3, the probability p is 0.259 (or 25.9%) that the difference is attributable to random variation of the count rate for similar samples. The probability is $1 - 0.259 = 0.741$ that the difference between the samples is significant.

Values of p greater than 0.01 or 0.05 seldom are considered indicative of a significant difference in values between measurements.

Efficient Distribution of Counting Time

In this method, the estimated standard deviation of the net count rate for a radioactive sample is reduced to a minimum. The reduction is achieved by distributing the counting time in a certain manner between sample and background (equation 12-7). England and Miller[3] have prepared useful graphs for the selection of counting times and the number of counts that must be accumulated to provide a desired precision for the net sample count:

$$\frac{(t)_{s+b}}{(t)_b} = \sqrt{\frac{(c)_{s+b}}{(c)_b}} \tag{12-7}$$

where

$(t)_{s+b}$ = Counting time for sample plus background.
$(t)_b$ = Counting time for background.
$(c)_{s+b}$ = Estimated count rate for sample plus background.
$(c)_b$ = Estimated count rate for background.

Example 12-9

The count rate for a radioactive sample is estimated at 3,500 CPM, uncorrected for background. The background count rate is about 50 CPM. A total counting time of 10 minutes is available. What interval of time should be used to count the sample, and what interval of time should be alloted to background?

$$\frac{(t)_{s+b}}{(t)_b} = \sqrt{\frac{(c)_{s+b}}{(c)_b}}$$

$$= \sqrt{\frac{3,500}{50}}$$

$$= 8.35$$

Also, $(t)_{s+b} + (t)_b = 10$ min
Hence, $8.35\,(t)_b + (t)_b = 10$ min
$(t)_b = 1.07$ min
$(t)_{s+b} = (10.00 - 1.07)$ min
$= 8.93$ min

The sample might be counted for 9 minutes and the background for 1 minute.

Chi-Square (χ^2) Test

The chi-square test is used to determine the goodness of fit of measured data to a Poisson probability density function. From a series of repeated measurements and equation (12-8), the value of χ^2 may be computed:

$$\chi^2 = \frac{1}{\hat{r}} \sum_{i=1}^{N} (n_i - \hat{r})^2 \tag{12-8}$$

where n_i represents each of N individual measurements and $\hat{r}$ is the sample mean. From the computed value of χ^2, the number of degrees of freedom $(N - 1)$ and data in Table 12-4, a probability p may be determined. Values for p less than 0.1 or 0.05 suggest that the data are distributed over a wider range of values than that expected for data that follow a Poisson probability law. Values for p greater than 0.9 or 0.95 suggest that the data are confined to a smaller range of values than that predicted by the Poisson probability density function.

Example 12-10

A series of 25 measurements on a radioactive sample provides a mean of 950 and a value of 17,526 for

$$\sum_{i=1}^{N} (n_i - \hat{r})^2$$

Do the data appear to be distributed according to a Poisson probability density function?

$$\chi^2 = \frac{1}{\hat{r}} \sum_{i=1}^{N} (n_i - \hat{r})^2$$

$$= \frac{1}{950}\,(17,526)$$

$$= 18.5$$

With $N - 1$ or 24 degrees of freedom, this value for χ^2 falls between probabilities of 0.9 and 0.5 and suggests that the data are distributed according to a Poisson probability density function.

TABLE 12-4. – TABLE OF CHI-SQUARE

DEGREES OF FREEDOM $(N - 1)$	0.99	0.95	0.90	0.50	0.10	0.05	0.01
			THERE IS A PROBABILITY OF THAT THE CALCULATED VALUE OF CHI-SQUARE WILL BE EQUAL TO OR GREATER THAN				
2	0.020	0.103	0.211	1.386	4.605	5.991	9.210
3	0.115	0.352	0.584	2.366	6.251	7.815	11.345
4	0.297	0.711	1.064	3.357	7.779	9.488	13.277
5	0.554	1.145	1.610	4.351	9.236	11.070	15.086
6	0.872	1.635	2.204	5.348	10.645	12.592	16.812
7	1.239	2.167	2.833	6.346	12.017	14.067	18.475
8	1.646	2.733	3.490	7.344	13.362	15.507	20.090
9	2.088	3.325	4.168	8.343	14.684	16.919	21.666
10	2.558	3.940	4.865	9.342	15.987	18.307	23.209
11	3.053	4.575	5.578	10.341	17.275	19.675	24.725
12	3.571	5.226	6.304	11.340	18.549	21.026	26.217
13	4.107	5.892	7.042	12.340	19.812	22.362	27.688
14	4.660	6.571	7.790	13.339	21.064	23.685	29.141
15	5.229	7.261	8.547	14.339	22.307	24.996	30.578
16	5.812	7.962	9.312	15.338	23.542	26.296	32.000
17	6.408	8.672	10.085	16.338	24.769	27.587	33.409
18	7.015	9.390	10.865	17.338	25.989	28.869	34.805
19	7.633	10.117	11.651	18.338	27.204	30.144	36.191
20	8.260	10.851	12.443	19.337	28.412	31.410	37.566
21	8.897	11.591	13.240	20.337	29.615	32.671	38.932
22	9.542	12.338	14.041	21.337	30.813	33.924	40.289
23	10.196	13.091	14.848	22.337	32.007	35.172	41.638
24	10.856	13.848	15.659	23.337	33.196	36.415	42.980
25	11.534	14.611	16.473	24.337	34.382	37.382	44.314
26	12.198	15.379	17.292	25.336	35.563	38.885	45.642
27	12.879	16.151	18.114	26.336	36.741	40.113	46.963
28	13.565	16.928	18.939	27.336	37.916	41.337	48.278
29	14.256	17.708	19.768	28.336	39.087	42.557	49.588

Figure of Merit

This test is used to determine which of two counting techniques provides greater precision. If Technique 1 furnishes a sample net count rate c_1 and a background count rate b_1, and Technique 2 furnishes a sample net count rate c_2 and a background count rate b_2, then the technique that provides better precision may be determined with equation (12-9):

$$\text{Figure of merit} = \left(\frac{c_1}{c_2}\right)^2 \left(\frac{c_2 + 2b_2}{c_1 + 2b_1}\right) \tag{12-9}$$

If the figure of merit exceeds 1, then Technique 1 furnishes better precision. Technique 2 is preferred if the figure of merit is less than 1.

If the sample net count rates are high compared to background, then equation (12-9) reduces to

$$\text{Figure of merit} = \frac{c_1}{c_2}$$

If the net count rates for the sample are low compared to background, then equation (12-9) reduces to

$$\text{Figure of merit} = \frac{c_1^2/b_1}{c_2^2/b_2}$$

and the preferred technique is that which yields the highest ratio of (sample net count rate)^2/(background count rate).

Example 12-11
A series of samples may be counted with either of two counting systems. System 1 provides an estimated net count rate of 85 CPM for the sample and a count rate of 25 CPM for background. For System 2, the sample and background count rates are estimated to be 126 CPM and 43 CPM, respectively. Which counting system provides better precision?

$$\text{Figure of merit} = \left(\frac{c_1}{c_2}\right)^2 \left(\frac{c_2 + 2b_2}{c_1 + 2b_1}\right) \tag{12-9}$$
$$= \left(\frac{85}{126}\right)^2 \left[\frac{126 + 2(43)}{85 + 2(25)}\right]$$
$$= 0.71$$

Counting System 2 is preferred.

PRECISION OF RATE METER MEASUREMENTS
The precision of a rate meter reading is improved if the pulse rate from the detector is averaged over a longer interval of time. The estimated standard deviation $\hat{\sigma}_c$ of a rate meter reading c in counts per second is

$$\hat{\sigma}_c = \sqrt{\frac{c}{2(RC)}} \tag{12-10}$$

where RC is the time constant of the rate meter in seconds. The percent estimated standard deviation $\%\hat{\sigma}_c$ is

$$\%\hat{\sigma}_c = 100 \sqrt{\frac{1}{2c(RC)}}$$

Example 12-12

A rate meter with a time constant of 2 seconds displays an equilibrium count rate of 1,000 CPM. What are the estimated standard deviation $\hat{\sigma}_c$ and the percent estimated standard deviation $\%\hat{\sigma}_c$?

$$\hat{\sigma}_c = \sqrt{\frac{c}{2(RC)}}$$

$$= \sqrt{\frac{(1,000/60)}{2(2 \text{ sec})}}$$

$$\simeq 2 \text{ CPS}$$

$$\%\hat{\sigma}_r = 100 \sqrt{\frac{1}{2c(RC)}}$$

$$= 100 \sqrt{\frac{1}{2(1,000/60)(2 \text{ sec})}}$$

$$\%\hat{\sigma}_c = 12$$

DETERMINATE ERRORS IN MEASUREMENTS OF RADIOACTIVITY

The count rate measured for a radioactive sample reflects the rate of decay of atoms in the sample. However, the influence of a number of determinate errors must be known before the activity of the sample can be determined from the measured count rate. The influence of these errors must be included in an expression for the relationship between the sample activity A and the measured count rate $(c)_{s+b}$ (equation 12-11).

$$A = \frac{(c)_{s+b}}{\{[1 - (c)_{s+b}]\tau\} \, EfGBf_cf_wf_s} - (c)_b \qquad (12\text{-}11)$$

where corrections to the background count rate are assumed to be negligible.

$(c)_{s+b}$ = (Sample plus background) count rate in counts per minute.
$(c)_b$ = Background count rate in counts per minute.
τ = Resolving time in minutes.
E = Detector efficiency.
f = Fractional emission of source.
G = Geometry correction.
B = Backscatter correction.
f_c = Sidescatter correction.
f_w = Correction for attenuation in detector window, air, sample covering, etc.
f_s = Correction for self-absorption.

These corrections are discussed in the following sections.

Background Count Rate

A counting system used to measure radiation from a radioactive sample almost always indicates the presence of small amounts of radiation when the radioactive sample is removed. The residual radiation (background) originates from a number of sources, including (1) cosmic radiation; (2) radioactive materials, such as ^{226}Ra, ^{14}C and ^{40}K in the earth, the human body and in walls of buildings, etc.; (3) radioactive materials stored or used nearby; (4) radioactive materials used in devices such as watches and instrument dials; (5) radioactive contamination of the counting equipment, laboratory benches, etc.; and (6) radioactive fallout (this source contributes no more than 1–2% to the total background radiation). Usually, radiation detectors are surrounded by lead or other shielding material to reduce the background count rate. Other methods to reduce background include the use of pulse height analyzers and coincidence or anticoincidence circuits.

Resolving Time

The *resolving time* of a radiation detector is the interval of time required between successive interactions in the detector for the interactions to be recorded as independent events. Compared to other common radiation detectors, the resolving time of a G-M detector is very long (100–300 μsec). The resolving time of a G-M detector may be measured by the "paired-source method."[4] The resolving time of any detector may be measured with an oscilloscope with which pulses from the detector can be displayed. Sequential measurements of the count rate for a short-lived radioactive nuclide also may be used to determine resolving time.[5] The count rate c_0, corrected for the loss of counts caused by resolving time, is

$$c_0 = \frac{c}{1 - c\tau} \tag{12-12}$$

where c is a measured count rate in counts per minute and τ is the resolving time in minutes. The coincidence loss is the difference between the uncorrected count rate c and the corrected count rate c_0.

Detector Efficiency

The efficiency of a radiation detector is the quotient of the number of particles or photons that interact within the detector divided by the number of particles or photons that enter the detector. The efficiency of most G-M and proportional detectors is close to 1 for alpha and beta particles and about 0.01 for x and γ rays. The efficiency of a NaI(Tl) crystal for the detection of x and γ rays varies with the size of the crystal and with the energy of the x or γ rays.

Fractional Emission

The fractional emission of a radioactive sample is the fractional number of decays that result in the emission of the type of radiation detected. For example, suppose that γ rays (0.393 MeV) from ^{113m}In are detected.

Since the coefficient of internal conversion is 0.55 for ^{113m}In, the number of decays that furnish a γ ray of 0.393 MeV is $1/(1 + 0.55) = 0.645$. Hence, the fractional emission is 0.645 for γ rays from ^{113m}In.

Detector Geometry

The *geometry correction* is the ratio of the number of particles or photons emitted in the direction of a radiation detector to the total number of particles or photons emitted by a radioactive sample. Usually, the detector is said to "subtend" a certain solid angle Ω measured in steradians. A sphere subtends a solid angle of 4π steradians, and the geometry correction G is

$$G = \frac{\Omega}{4\pi}$$

The expressions 2π *geometry* and 4π *geometry* are used to describe counting conditions where half or all of the radiation emitted by the source is intercepted by the detector.

The geometry correction varies with the radius d of the detector and with the distance h between the detector and the source. The correction is described in Figure 12-12 and in equation (12-13) for point and disk sources of radioactive material:

Point source: $G = 0.5\left(1 - \dfrac{h}{\sqrt{h^2 + d^2}}\right)$ (12-13)

Disk source (radius of disk $= d_1$):

$$G = 0.5\left(1 - \frac{h}{\sqrt{h^2 + d^2}}\right) - \frac{3}{16}\left(\frac{dd_1}{h^2}\right)^2 \left(\frac{h}{\sqrt{h^2 + d^2}}\right)^5$$

Scattering

Radiation emitted from a radioactive source in a direction outside the solid angle subtended by a detector may be scattered toward the detector during interactions with the sample container or with shielding

Fig 12-12. – Geometric relationship between a detector and a point or disk source of radioactive material.

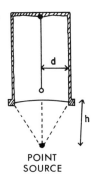

POINT
SOURCE

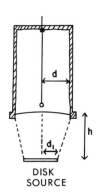

DISK
SOURCE

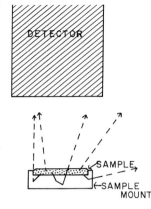

Fig 12-13. — Backscattering of radiation from a radioactive sample.

around the sample and detector. The scattered particles or photons are backscattered if they were emitted originally in a direction away from the detector (Fig 12-13). If the backscattered radiation originates entirely within the mount for the sample, the *percent backscatter %B* and *backscatter factor B* are:

$$\%B = \left[\frac{(\text{Counts with mount present}) - (\text{Counts with mount removed})}{(\text{Counts with mount removed})}\right](100) \tag{12-14}$$

$$B = \frac{(\text{Counts with mount present})}{(\text{Counts with mount removed})} \tag{12-15}$$

The backscatter factor is related to the percent backscatter by

$$\%B = 100(B - 1)$$

For beta particles, the backscatter factor increases with the atomic number of the sample mount and, initially, with the thickness of the mount. *Saturation thickness* is achieved when an increase in thickness does not increase the backscattered radiation. For beta particles, saturation thickness equals about three tenths of the range of the particles in the mount. Backscattering may be reduced by using a sample mount of low atomic number. For beta counting, for example, aluminum planchets often are preferred over copper or steel planchets because the backscatter factor is lower with aluminum. If the sample mount provides saturation thickness, then the backscatter factor for beta particles is almost independent of the energy of the betas.

Sidescatter may be reduced by moving all scattering material (e.g., shielding around the source and detector) far from the path between the source and the detector. Sidescatter may be reduced also with a sleeve of plastic, aluminum or other low-Z material inside the high-Z shield around the source and detector.

Air and Window Absorption

All radiation is attenuated by material between the radioactive source and the sensitive volume of the detector. Usually at least three different attenuators are encountered by radiation moving toward the detector. These attenuators are: (1) the covering over the radioactive source, (2) air between the source and the detector and (3) the entrance window of the detector.

Self-Absorption

This term refers to the attenuation of radiation within the radioactive sample itself. Shown in Figure 12-14 is the increase in count rate for a radioactive sample achieved if the activity of the sample is increased with no change in sample volume. The data describe a straight line, because the fraction of radiation absorbed by the sample remains unchanged. However, if the volume of the sample increases with no change in activity, then the count rate for the sample decreases (Fig 12-15) because an increasing fraction of the radiation is absorbed. In Figure 12-16, the influence upon the count rate is illustrated for a sample with increasing volume and constant specific activity (specific activity = activity of sample/mass of sample). After the sample attains an infinite thickness, the count rate remains constant because the increased absorption of radiation by the sample compensates for the increased activity.

The self-absorption of a sample may be determined by measuring the

Fig 12-14. – Count rate for a sample with constant volume but increasing specific activity.

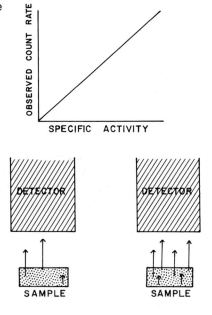

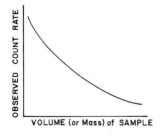

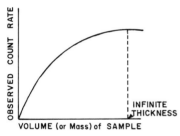

Fig 12-15. — Count rate for a sample with constant activity as the volume of the sample is changed.

Fig 12-16. — Count rate for a sample with constant specific activity as the volume (and, consequently, the total activity) of the sample is increased.

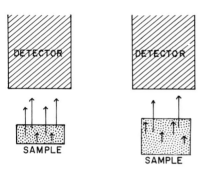

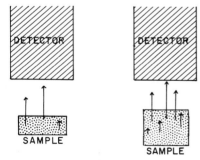

count rate for a series of samples with equal specific activity but different volumes (and, consequently, different total activities). The measured count rate for each sample is divided by the mass or volume of the sample, and the resulting data are plotted as a function of sample mass or volume. By extrapolating the curve to a sample mass or volume of zero, a value for the specific activity of the sample corrected for self-absorption is obtained. The count rate corrected for self-absorption may be determined for any particular sample by multiplying the mass or volume of the sample by the corrected specific activity.

PROBLEMS

*1. Suppose 3,600 counts were accumulated for a sample counted for 10 minutes. Background contributed 784 counts over a counting interval of 6 minutes. What are:

   a. The estimated standard deviation and the percent estimated standard deviation of the sample count rate uncorrected for background?

   b. The estimated standard deviation and the percent estimated standard deviation of the background count rate?

   c. The estimated standard deviation and the percent estimated standard deviation of the sample count rate corrected for background?

*2. A G-M detector that is 60% efficient for counting beta particles subtends a solid angle of 0.2 steradians around a sample of ^{204}Tl ($T_{1/2}$ = 3.8 yr). The counter registers 2 CPS. Assuming that corrections for backscatter, sidescatter, air, window and self-absorption all equal 1.0, compute the number of ^{204}Tl atoms in the sample.

*3. A G-M detector has a resolving time of 300 μsec. What is the count rate corrected for coincidence loss if the measured count rate is 10,000 CPM? What is the maximum count rate if the coincidence loss must not exceed 1%?

*4. The following data were recorded for identical samples:

| "Weightless" Mylar mount | 2,038 CPM |
| Silver backing | 3,258 CPM |

Compute the backscatter factor and the percent backscatter.

5. Explain why there is a saturation or infinite thickness for curves of backscattering (count rate vs thickness of backing material) and self-absorption (count rate vs weight of sample of constant specific activity).

6. The following data were obtained by counting a series of weighed fractions of a radioactive sample:

Mass (mg)	2	4	6	8	10	15	20	25	30	35
CPM (net)	85	160	235	305	335	360	380	398	408	415

Plot a self-absorption curve and determine the specific count rate (CPM/mg) for the sample corrected for self-absorption.

*7. An ^{131}I standard solution was obtained from the National Bureau of Standards. The following information was supplied concerning the solution: as-

---

*For those problems marked with an asterisk, answers are provided on the pages following the appendixes (see pp. 487–488).

say of ^{131}I at 8 A.M., Jan. 1: 2.09 × 10^4 dps/ml ± 2%. On Jan. 15 at 8 A.M., a sample of ^{131}I was counted. This sample had been obtained from a shipment of ^{131}I in the following manner: 20 λ (1 λ = 1 μl) of the shipment was diluted in a volumetric flask to 25 ml; 100 λ of this solution was diluted to 10 ml; 50 λ of this solution was withdrawn, mounted on Mylar, dried, and counted. The dried sample provided a count rate of 4,280 CPM corrected for background. At the same time (8 A.M., Jan. 15) a 50-λ sample of the NBS standard ^{131}I solution was mounted, dried, and counted in the same manner. The count rate for the standard sample was 1,213 CPM corrected for background.

    a. What was the specific activity (mCi/ml) of the ^{131}I shipment at the time the sample from the shipment was counted?

    b. What was the total correction factor between count rate and activity for the system used to count ^{131}I mounted on Mylar?

°8. Compute the equilibrium time for a rate meter with a time constant of 2 seconds, if the equilibrium count rate is 1,800 CPM (30 CPS).

°9. A 2-minute count of 3,310 was measured for a radioactive sample. A second sample furnished 4,709 counts in 3 minutes. Is the difference in count rate between the two samples significant?

°10. Choose the preferred counting system:

	SYSTEM 1	SYSTEM 2
Estimated sample net count rate	51	73
Estimated background count rate	28	37

°11. For time constants of (*a*) 1 second and (*b*) 10 seconds, compare the percent estimated standard deviations for a rate meter reading of 2,000 CPM.

12. A series of radioactive samples of short half-life will be counted one per day over several days. Explain how variations in the observed counts caused by fluctuations in the sensitivity of the counting system can be compensated.

REFERENCES

1. Price, W.: *Nuclear Radiation Detection* (2d ed.; New York: McGraw-Hill Book Co., 1964).
2. Low, F.: Basic Considerations in Nuclear Instrumentation, in Hine, G. (ed.): *Instrumentation in Nuclear Medicine* (New York: Academic Press, 1967), vol. 1, p. 29.
3. England, J., and Miller, R.: Counting times in the measurement of radioactivity, Int. J. Appl. Radiat. Isot. 20:1, 1969.
4. Hendee, W.: *Radioactive Isotopes in Biological Research* (New York: John Wiley & Sons, Inc., 1973).
5. Stearns, R., and Mucci, J.: Using the decay of ^{137}Ba to determine resolving time in G-M counting, J. Chem. Educ. 38:29, 1961.

13 / Gamma-Ray Spectrometry and the Clinical Use of Radioactive Nuclides

ATTENUATION COEFFICIENTS for photoelectric, Compton and pair-production interactions of γ rays in NaI(Tl) are plotted in Figure 13-1 as a function of γ-ray energy. For γ-ray photons with energy less than about 200 keV, photoelectric absorption is the most probable interaction in NaI(Tl). Compton scattering is the dominant interaction between about 200 keV and 7 MeV, and pair production is most important at energies greater than 7 MeV. A γ-ray photon that interacts in a NaI(Tl) crystal may deposit part or all of its energy in the crystal. The size of each voltage pulse from the photomultiplier tube coupled to the crystal is proportional to the energy deposited in the crystal by a particular γ-ray photon. Pulses from the scintillation detector may be sorted with a scintillation spectrometer to yield a pulse height spectrum that reflects the energy distribution of the incident photons.[1, 2]

PULSE HEIGHT SPECTRA

The pulse height spectrum for a particular radioactive source consists of peaks and valleys that reflect the energy of the γ-ray photons from the source, the interactions that occur before the photons reach the scintillation detector, the interactions that occur in the detector and the operating characteristics of the components of the counting system. If the gain of the amplifier or the high voltage across the photomultiplier tube is increased, then the amplification of each pulse is increased proportionally and each pulse is displayed at a position farther along the pulse height scale. Hence, an increase in the high voltage or gain expands the pulse height spectrum over a greater range of pulse heights (Fig 13-2). The height of the spectrum decreases because the voltage pulses encompass a wider range of pulse heights and each pulse height interval contains fewer pulses.

As the window of the pulse height analyzer is widened, more pulses are transmitted to the display device for each position of the window along the pulse height scale. Consequently, the count rate at each window position increases with the window width. With a wider window, however, peaks and valleys in the spectrum are defined less precisely and the resolution of the spectrum is reduced. Pulse height spectra for ^{137}Cs measured with analyzer windows of different widths are shown in Figure 13-3.

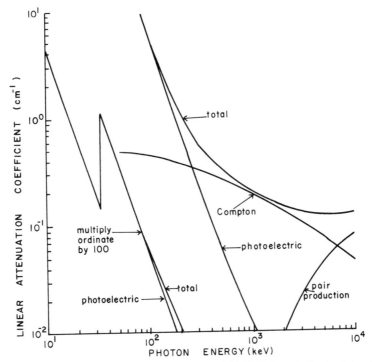

Fig 13-1.—Linear attenuation coefficients of NaI(Tl) for photoelectric absorption, Compton scattering and pair production, plotted as a function of γ-ray energy in kiloelectron volts.

Photopeaks

A *photopeak* on a pulse height spectrum encloses pulses produced by total absorption of γ-ray photons of a particular energy in the scintillation crystal. The energy of the γ-ray photon may have been deposited in the crystal during one interaction or during a series of interactions. The *photofraction* or *peak-to-total ratio* for a photopeak is the quotient of the area enclosed within the photopeak divided by the total area enclosed within the pulse height spectrum. The *intrinsic peak efficiency* is the fraction of the γ rays of a particular energy impinging upon a detector that produces pulses enclosed within the photopeak. The *resolution* of a pulse height spectrum sometimes is described by the *full width at half maximum (FWHM)*, where

$$FWHM = \frac{\text{Width of photopeak at half its maximum height}}{\text{Position of photopeak along pulse height scale}} \quad (13\text{-}1)$$

The full width at half maximum is illustrated in Figure 13-4.

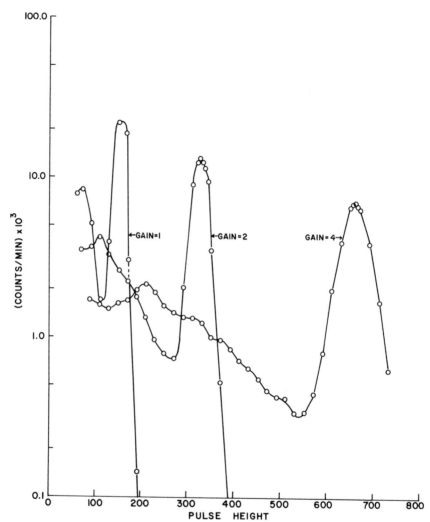

Fig 13-2. — Pulse height spectra for ¹³⁷Cs, measured with different settings of the amplifier gain.

Compton Valley, Edge and Plateau

Compton interactions of incident γ-ray photons in a NaI(Tl) crystal, with escape of the scattered photons from the crystal, result in the formation of voltage pulses smaller than those enclosed within a photopeak. The valley just below a photopeak is referred to as the *Compton valley*. The *Compton edge* is the portion of the pulse height spectrum just below the Compton valley where the height of the spectrum increases rap-

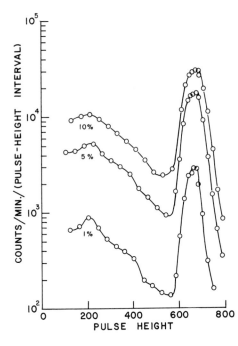

Fig 13-3. — Increased count and decreased resolution are achieved as the width of the window of the pulse height analyzer is increased. Window widths are expressed as a percent of the highest setting of the pulse height scale. Spectra were measured for a ^{137}Cs source in a 2×2 in. NaI(Tl) well detector.

idly. The portion of the pulse height spectrum below the Compton edge is termed the *Compton plateau*.

The relative heights of the photopeak and the Compton edge vary with the size of the NaI(Tl) crystal. In a larger crystal, more scattered photons interact before they escape from the crystal. Hence, the height of the photopeak is increased and the height of the Compton plateau is reduced (Fig 13-5).

X-Ray Escape Peaks

Usually, characteristic x rays are released during photoelectric interactions of γ-ray photons. Gamma rays that interact photoelectrically in a NaI(Tl) crystal usually eject an electron from the K shell of iodine. As the vacancy left by the photoelectron is filled, characteristic x rays are released with an energy equal to the difference in binding energies (28 keV) of L and K electrons in iodine. If a 28-keV characteristic x ray interacts in the scintillation crystal, then the light released during this interaction contributes to the formation of a voltage pulse for the primary γ ray, and this voltage pulse contributes to the photopeak. However, if the x ray escapes from the crystal, then the pulse for the primary γ ray is smaller than those enclosed within the photopeak. If many x rays escape, then a peak occurs on the pulse height spectrum at a location about 28

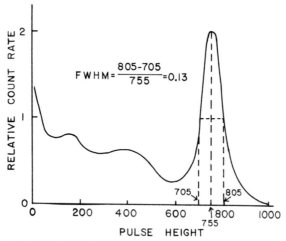

Fig 13-4. — Photopeak resolution, described as the "full width at half maximum" (FWHM).

keV less than the photopeak. This peak is referred to as an *x-ray escape peak* (Fig 13-6). X-ray escape peaks are not observed for γ rays with energy greater than about 200 keV, because the lateral spread of the photopeak for photons of higher energy obscures the presence of the x-ray escape peak. Also, characteristic x rays released during interactions of higher-energy γ rays have a lower probability of escape from the crystal, because most of the higher-energy γ rays penetrate farther into the crystal before interacting.

Fig 13-5. — Pulse height spectra for ^{137}Cs measured with NaI(Tl) crystals of different sizes. The photopeaks are normalized to the same height. (From Heath, R.: *Scintillation Spectrometry Gamma-Ray Spectrum Catalogue* IDO-16408 [Washington, D.C.: Atomic Energy Commission, 1957].)

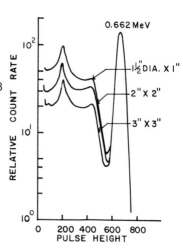

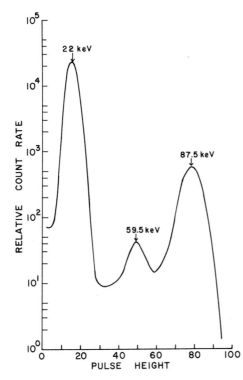

Fig 13-6. — Pulse height spectrum for [109]Cd. An iodine x-ray escape peak is present at a position 28 keV below the photopeak for the 87.5-keV γ rays from [109]Cd. The large photopeak at 22 keV is produced by absorption of characteristic x rays released during decay of [109]Cd by electron capture. (From O'Kelley, G.: *Detection and Measurement of Nuclear Radiation* NAS-NS3105 [Washington, D.C.: Office of Technical Services, Department of Commerce, 1962].)

Characteristic X-Ray Peak

Characteristic x rays released as γ-ray photons from a radioactive source undergo photoelectric interaction in the lead shield around the source and detector. Some of these x rays escape from the shield and strike the NaI(Tl) crystal, producing peaks in the pulse height spectrum. In Figure 13-7, the peak at 0.072 MeV reflects the absorption of characteristic x rays from a lead shield surrounding a scintillation detector and a ^{51}Cr source. The number of characteristic x rays reaching the detector may be reduced by increasing the distance between the detector and the shield or by lining the shield with materials with an atomic number less than the atomic number of lead.

Backscatter Peak

If a photon with energy greater than 200 keV is scattered at a wide angle during a Compton interaction, then the scattered photon has an energy of about 200 keV irrespective of the energy of the primary γ ray. For this reason, photons scattered at a wide angle during Compton interactions in the detector-source shield produce a peak at about 200 keV on the pulse height spectrum (Fig 13-8). This peak is referred to as the

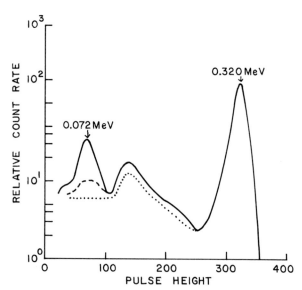

Fig 13-7. — Characteristic x-ray peak at 72 keV produced by x rays from a 6 × 6 in. lead shield surrounding a scintillation detector and a ^{51}Cr source. The x-ray peak may be reduced by increasing the inner dimensions of the shield to 32 × 32 in. *(dotted curve)* or by lining the shield with 0.03 in. of cadmium *(dashed curve)*. The 32 × 32 in. shield was lined with 0.06 in. of cadmium plus 0.005 in. of copper. (Figures 13-7 to 13-11 from Heath, R.: *Scintillation Spectrometry Gamma-Ray Spectrum Catalogue* IDO-16408 [Washington, D.C.: Atomic Energy Commission, 1957].)

backscatter peak. The number of scattered photons received by the detector may be reduced by increasing the distance between the shield and the detector or by choosing a material for the shield in which the number of Compton interactions is reduced.

Annihilation Peak

Pair-production interaction of γ rays with an energy greater than 1.02 MeV is accompanied by the release of 511 keV annihilation photons. If a primary γ ray interacts by pair production in the detector-source shield, then one of the subsequent annihilation photons may escape from the shield and interact in the crystal. This process results in the production of an *annihilation peak* at 511 keV in the pulse height spectrum (Fig 13-9). An annihilation peak at 511 keV also is present in pulse height spectra for positron-emitting nuclides, because annihilation radiation is released as the positron combines with an electron.

Annihilation Escape Peaks

Pair production of high-energy (> 1.02 MeV) photons in the scintillation crystal results in the emission of two 511-keV annihilation photons,

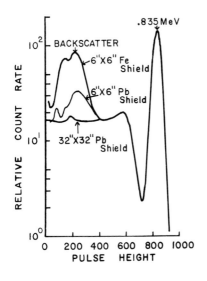
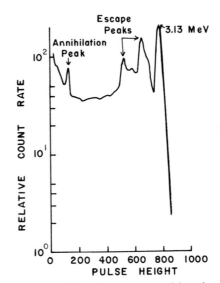

Fig 13-8 (left). — The backscatter peak at about 200 keV is produced by absorption in the detector of photons scattered at a wide angle during Compton interaction of primary γ rays in the detector-source shield. The backscatter peak is greatest for the 6 × 6 in. iron shield, because the relative probability of Compton interaction of the 0.835-MeV γ rays from ⁵⁴Mn is higher for iron than for lead. The backscatter peak is reduced if the distance between the shield and the detector is increased.

Fig 13-9 (right). — Pulse height spectrum for ³⁷S, illustrating single and double escape peaks and an annihilation peak at 0.511 MeV.

one or both of which may escape from the crystal. Pulses that reflect the loss of one annihilation photon contribute to the *single-escape peak* which occurs at a location 0.511 MeV below the photopeak for the primary γ ray. Pulses that reflect the loss of both annihilation photons contribute to the *double-escape peak* which occurs at a location 1.02 MeV below the photopeak. Single- and double-escape peaks, together with an annihilation peak at 0.511 MeV, are present in the pulse height spectrum in Figure 13-9 for ³⁷S, a nuclide that decays by the emission of a β-particle and a γ-ray photon with an energy of 3.13 MeV.

Coincidence Peak

Many radioactive sources decay with the emission of two or more γ rays in cascade. When γ rays from these sources are detected, more than one γ-ray photon released during a disintegration may be absorbed completely in the scintillation crystal. *Coincidence peaks (sum peaks)* on the pulse height spectrum reflect the simultaneous absorption of more than one γ-ray photon in the crystal (Fig 13-10). The relative height of a coincidence peak is reduced if the distance is increased between the

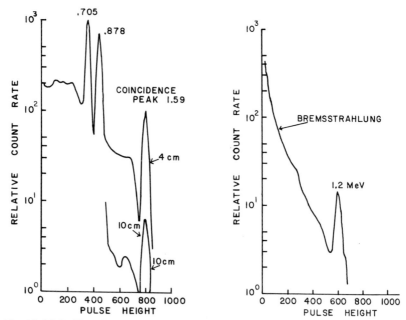

Fig 13-10 (left). — Coincidence peak that reflects the simultaneous absorption of 0.705 MeV and 0.878 MeV γ rays from ⁹⁴Nb. The relative height of the coincidence peak is reduced if the distance between source and detector is increased from 4 cm to 10 cm.

Fig 13-11 (right). — Pulse height spectrum for ⁹¹Y, illustrating the bremsstrahlung contribution characteristic of a radioactive source for which the ratio of γ rays to β-particles is low.

source and the detector because of the reduced probability that two or more photons will strike the crystal simultaneously. For high-activity samples, coincidence peaks may be produced by simultaneous absorption of γ rays released during the decay of different atoms of the sample.

Bremsstrahlung

Bremsstrahlung is released as β-particles from a radioactive source are absorbed in the source or source-detector shield. If the ratio of γ rays to β-particles emitted by the source is low, then the contribution of bremsstrahlung to the pulse height distribution may be noticeable, particularly at the lower end of the pulse height scale (Fig 13-11).

PHOTOPEAK COUNTING

Often, radioactive sources that emit γ rays are counted by sending to the display device only those pulses that are enclosed within a pulse height window centered over the photopeak. Other pulses are rejected because they are larger or smaller than the pulses transmitted by the window. To center the window over the photopeak, the window is positioned at a desired location along the pulse height scale and the amplifier gain or the high voltage is adjusted until a maximum count rate is obtained. For example, if the photopeak for ^{137}Cs is desired at 662 on the pulse height scale, then the window is centered at 662 and the gain or high voltage is increased until a maximum count rate is obtained. If the size of the voltage pulse varies linearly with energy deposited in the crystal, then this procedure furnishes a pulse height scale calibrated from 0 to 1,000 keV, with each division on the pulse height scale representing 1 keV. The pulse height scale may be calibrated from 0 to 2,000 keV by centering the ^{137}Cs photopeak at 331, and from 0 to 500 keV by centering the photopeak for a lower-energy γ-ray photon at an appropriate position on the pulse height scale. A pulse height scale may be calibrated from 0 to 500 keV, for example, by centering the photopeak for ^{99m}Tc (primary γ ray of 140 keV) at 280 on the pulse height scale. The linearity of a scintillation spectrometer may be confirmed by locating photopeaks on the pulse height scale for various sources that emit γ rays of known energy. If the spectrometer is linear, then a plot of the center of the photopeak on the pulse height scale as a function of the γ-ray energy describes a straight line.

The width of the analyzer window most desirable for photopeak counting varies with the relative heights of the photopeak and of the pulse height spectrum for background at the position of the window. For many counting situations, the background spectrum has relatively little structure and is much lower than the photopeak for the sample. For these situations, a relatively narrow (e.g., 2%) window should be centered over the photopeak. If the photopeak is not much higher than background, then the maximum value of (sample net count rate)^2/ (background count rate) may be determined as a function of window width. When the ratio [known as the (signal)^2/background or S^2/B ratio] is maximum, the fractional standard deviation for the net count rate of the sample is minimum. A plot of S^2/B as a function of window width is shown in Figure 13-12 for a ^{137}Cs source and a 2 by 2 in. NaI(Tl) well detector. The optimum window is 70 keV.

Ross and Harris[3] have shown that an acceptable window usually is achieved if lower and upper discriminators are positioned on either side of the photopeak at a location where the count rate is equal to one third of the count rate at the center of the photopeak. About 85% of all pulses enclosed within the photopeak are transmitted by a window defined by discriminators in these positions, and the window is termed an 85% *window*. Ross and Harris suggest an increase in window width if the window or amplifier gain drifts or if the width of the window fluctuates. Under these circumstances the lower and upper discriminators should

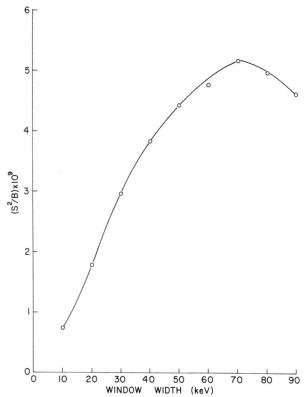

Fig 13-12.—Plot of $S^2 B$ for a ^{137}Cs source and a 2 × 2 in. NaI(Tl) well detector.

intersect the pulse height spectrum at equal heights near the base of the photopeak. If the gain of the amplifier is unstable, then the photopeak should be intercepted by the lower and upper discriminator at relative count rates R_1 and R_2, respectively, where R_1 and R_2 are determined by the expression $R_1/R_2 = V_2/V_1$, and V_1 and V_2 are the positions of the lower and upper discriminators along the pulse height scale.

RADIOACTIVE AGENTS FOR CLINICAL STUDIES

A wide assortment of radioactive nuclides have been administered to patients for the diagnosis and treatment of a variety of conditions. For a nuclide to be acceptable for most applications in nuclear medicine, the half-life for radioactive decay should be between 1 hour and a week or two. Nuclides with half-lives shorter than about 1 hour decay too rapidly for the labeling and sterilizing of radioactive compounds, and nuclides with long half-lives often deliver high radiation doses to patients.

Most radioactive agents administered to patients are injected intravenously and must be sterile. Most agents are sterilized by autoclaving (e.g., heating for 15–20 minutes at a temperature of about 125 C and a pressure of roughly 20 lb/sq in.) or by filtration through fine cellulose-ester membranes. The injected material usually should have a pH near 7 and should either dissolve in an aqueous medium or form a colloidal suspension or a suspension of larger particles. An agent injected intravenously must be free of *pyrogens*, particles that have a diameter of 0.05–1 μ and do not decompose at elevated temperature.[4] The presence of pyrogens in an agent administered intravenously to a patient causes the rapid appearance of characteristic symptoms which have been documented by Miller and Tisdall.[5] Solutions are free from pyrogens only if they are prepared by meticulous chemical techniques. Procedures for testing for the presence of pyrogens are described in the *United States Pharmacopoeia*[6] and other publications.[7]

Other considerations that are important when a radioactive pharmaceutical is used clinically include the following.

1. *Radiochemical purity*, the ratio of the quantity of the desired isotope (or nuclide) present in the desired chemical form to the total quantity of the isotope (or nuclide) in the pharmaceutical.

2. *Radioisotopic purity* (or *radionuclidic purity*), the ratio of the activity of the desired radioactive isotope (or nuclide) to the total activity of radioactive material in the pharmaceutical. Daughter nuclides usually are excluded from the description of radionuclidic purity.

3. Presence of a *carrier* in the pharmaceutical. A solution is *carrier-free* if all isotopes of a particular element in the solution are radioactive.

4. Presence of an *isotope effect*, which is an expression used to describe changes in chemical behavior of the pharmaceutical which are caused by differences in isotopic mass between the radioactive nuclide and its stable counterpart. An isotope effect is observed frequently with compounds labeled with tritium. However, its occurrence decreases rapidly with increasing atomic number of the radioactive nuclide and is rare with compounds labeled with a radioactive nuclide with an atomic number greater than about 15.

5. Presence of *isotope exchange reactions*, during which the radioactive nuclide detaches from the pharmaceutical and adheres to another compound in the body.

6. Radiation dose delivered to critical organs and to the whole body of the patient.

7. Presence of degradation products caused by chemical instability and by self-irradiation of the pharmaceutical.

The localization of a radioactive nuclide administered intravenously, and the rate and mode of excretion of the nuclide from the body, are determined by a number of properties, which include:[8]

1. The oxidation (valence) state of the compound labeled with the nuclide at the pH (7.4) of blood.

2. The solubility of the labeled compound in an aqueous medium. If the compound is insoluble, then the localization and excretion of the compound are determined by the size of the particles formed.

3. The tendency of the nuclide to incorporate into or to bind to organic compounds.

During many clinical applications of radioactive nuclides, radiation emitted by a nuclide distributed within the body is measured with a detector positioned outside the body. For these applications, the nuclide must emit a γ-ray photon (or x-ray photon) with an energy between about 20 and 700 keV. Photons with energy less than about 20 keV are attenuated severely by the patient, and photons with energy greater than about 700 keV are attenuated inadequately by the collimator attached to the detector. Nuclides (e.g., ^{99m}Tc) that decay by isomeric transition are preferred for in vivo studies, because no particulate radiation is emitted from the nucleus during the decay of these nuclides, and the radiation dose delivered to the patient is reduced.

PROBLEMS

1. A pulse height spectrum for ^{113m}In (γ ray of 0.393 MeV) was obtained with a single-channel pulse height analyzer calibrated from 0 to 500 keV. The window width was 2%. Describe the changes in the spectrum if:

   a. A 5% window were used.

   b. The amplifier gain were twice as great.

   c. The amplifier gain were half as great.

   d. The upper discriminator of the window were removed.

°2. ^{24}Na decays to ^{24}Mg by β^- decay with a $T_{1/2}$ of 15 hr. Gamma rays of 4.14 MeV (<1%), 2.76 MeV (100%) and 1.38 MeV (100%) are emitted during the decay process. A pulse height spectrum for this nuclide exhibits peaks at 2.76 MeV, 2.25 MeV, 1.74 MeV, 1.38 MeV, 0.87 MeV, 0.51 MeV and about 0.20 MeV. Explain the origin of each of the peaks.

3. Describe the changes in a pulse height spectrum for ^{51}Cr if:

   a. A larger NaI(Tl) crystal were used.

   b. A 1-in. slab of Lucite were interposed between the ^{51}Cr source and the scintillation detector.

   c. A 1-in. slab of Lucite were placed behind the ^{51}Cr source.

°4. The position of the photopeak for ^{137}Cs γ rays (0.662 MeV) changes with high voltage as shown in the following table when the gain is set at 4.

Position of photopeak on pulse height scale	520	580	650	730	820
High voltage across photomultiplier tube	730	750	770	790	810

°For those problems marked with an asterisk, answers are provided on the pages following the appendixes (see pp. 487–488).

If the gain is reduced to 2 and the high voltage is set at 750, where is the photopeak for the 1.33-MeV γ ray from ^{60}Co on the pulse height scale?

5. Describe the decay characteristics desired for a radioactive nuclide used as a scanning agent.

6. Describe the characteristics desired for a chemical compound used as a scanning agent.

°7. A shipment is labeled "30% ^{14}C-enriched Ba ^{14}CO$_3$ — weight 2,285 mg." This label is interpreted to mean "30% by weight Ba ^{14}CO$_3$, the rest being Ba ^{12}CO$_3$ and Ba ^{13}CO$_3$." What is the activity of ^{14}C in the sample?

°8. Radioactive ^{14}C is produced in the upper atmosphere by neutrons released during cosmic ray bombardment:

$$_0^1n + {}_7^{14}N \rightarrow {}_1^1H + {}_6^{14}C$$

The radioactive carbon is distributed over the earth as ^{14}CO$_2$ in the air and NaH ^{14}CO$_3$ in the sea. Plants and animals incorporate ^{14}C while alive. After a plant or animal dies, the incorporated ^{14}C decays with a half-life of 5,600 yr. The radioactivity in the remains of the plant or animal indicates the time elapsed since the death of the organism. Determination of the age of objects by measurement of their ^{14}C content is termed *carbon dating*. For example, wood from an old mummy case provides a specific count rate of 10.7 CPM/gm. New wood furnishes 16.4 CPM/gm. How old is the mummy case?

°9. What is the specific activity (Ci/gm) of a pure sample of ^{32}P?

REFERENCES

1. Heath, R.: *Scintillation Spectrometry Gamma-Ray Spectrum Catalogue*. 1st ed., AEC report IDO-16408, 1957; 2d ed., AEC report IDO-16880, 1964.

2. O'Kelley, G.: *Detection and Measurement of Nuclear Radiation* NAS-NS3105 (Washington, D.C.: Office of Technical Services, 1962).

3. Ross, D., and Harris, C.: *Measurement of Clinical Radioactivity* ORNL-4153 (Washington, D.C.: Office of Technical Information, Atomic Energy Commission, 1968).

4. Bennett, I., and Beeson, P.: Properties and biological effects of bacterial pyrogens, Medicine 29:365, 1950.

5. Miller, E., and Tisdall, L.: Reactions to 10,000 pooled liquid human plasma transfusions, J.A.M.A. 128:863, 1945.

6. *United States Pharmacopoeia* (17th rev.; Easton, Pa.: Mack Publishing Co., 1965).

7. Moore, J., and Hendee, W.: *Workshop Manual for Quality Assurance of Radiopharmaceuticals and Radionuclide Handling* (Rockville, Md.: Bureau of Radiological Health, 1978).

8. Durbin, D.: Metabolic characteristics within a chemical family, Health Phys. 2:225, 1960.

14 / In Vivo Radionuclide Studies and Radionuclide Imaging

MANY DIAGNOSTIC STUDIES require the use of a detector outside the body to measure the rate of accumulation, release or distribution of radioactivity in a particular region inside the body. The rate of accumulation or release of radioactivity may be measured with one or more detectors, usually NaI(Tl) scintillation crystals, positioned at fixed locations outside the body. Images of the distribution of radioactivity may be obtained with a rectilinear scanner or, more often, with a stationary imaging device.

MEASUREMENT OF RATES OF ACCUMULATION AND EXCRETION

Measurement of the accumulation of radioactive iodine in the thyroid gland was the first routine clinical use of a radioactive nuclide. Since early tests of thyroid function with radioactive iodine, many diagnostic applications of radioactive nuclides have been developed. Many of these applications require measurement of the change in radioactivity in a selected region of the body as a function of time. Some of these applications are discussed briefly in this section.

Thyroid Uptake

The rate of accumulation of iodine in the thyroid gland may be estimated from measurements of the radioactivity in the thyroid at specified times (usually 6 and 24 hr) after a selected amount of radioactive iodine (e.g., 10 μCi of ^{131}I) has been administered orally. The measurement of radioactivity in the thyroid usually is accomplished with a NaI(Tl) scintillation crystal not less than 3 cm in diameter by 3 cm thick, which is positioned 20–30 cm in front of the patient and in line with the isthmus of the thyroid. The *field of view* of the detector is the area perpendicular to the extended axis of the detector at the surface of the patient over which the count rate remains above 90% of the count rate at the center of the field. The detector should be collimated to restrict the field of view to a diameter not greater than 15 cm for adults and proportionately less for children.

To provide a standard sample for determination of thyroid uptake, a vessel resembling the average thyroid (e.g., a 30-ml polyethylene bottle

3 cm in diameter) is filled with an amount of ^{131}I equal to that delivered orally to the patient.* This standard sample is placed at a depth of 0.5 cm behind the surface of a neck phantom composed of a cylinder of Lucite 15 cm in diameter and 15 cm tall. The percent uptake of iodine in the thyroid is the ratio of the net count rate measured in front of the thyroid to that measured under identical conditions with the detector in front of the neck phantom.

$$\text{Uptake } (\%) = (100) \frac{(c)_t}{(c)_s} \tag{14-1}$$

where

$(c)_t$ = count rate for thyroid and $(c)_s$ = count rate for standard.

The contribution of radiation scattered from tissue surrounding the thyroid to the total count rate measured by the detector should be reduced to a minimum during the measurement of thyroid uptake. Radiation scattered from extrathyroidal tissue contributes little to the count rate for a thyroid uptake measured 24 hr after administration of ^{131}I. For an uptake measured at an earlier time or with poor collimation, however, extrathyroidal activity must be considered in the computation of percent uptake. A pulse height analyzer may be used to reject pulses produced by γ rays scattered into the detector from extrathyroidal tissue (Fig 14-1). Alternately, a lead absorber (A-block) 1.5 mm thick may be used to provide an energy distribution for the γ rays striking the crystal which does not vary greatly with different thicknesses of tissue around the patient's thyroid. With another method for correction for extrathyroid activity, the count rates for the patient and the phantom are measured before and after a lead block (B-block) about ½ in. thick has been placed over the thyroid and the radioactive source in the phantom. The percent uptake is

$$\text{Uptake } (\%) = (100) \frac{(c)_t - (c)_{tL}}{(c)_s - (c)_{sL}} \tag{14-1}$$

where

$(c)_t$ = Count rate for thyroid.
$(c)_{tL}$ = Count rate for thyroid shielded by lead block.
$(c)_s$ = Count rate for standard.
$(c)_{sL}$ = Count rate for standard shielded by lead block.

Example 14-1

The following count rates were obtained 24 hr after administration of 10 μCi of ^{131}I to a patient:

*Sometimes a standard count rate is obtained by counting the capsule of ^{131}I before it is administered to the patient.

For patient's thyroid	537 CPM
For patient's thyroid shielded by lead block	193 CPM
For standard	3,215 CPM
For standard shielded by lead block	182 CPM

What is the percent uptake?

$$\text{Uptake } (\%) = (100)\ \frac{(c)_t - (c)_{tL}}{(c)_s - (c)_{sL}}$$
$$= (100)\ \frac{537 - 193}{3,215 - 182}$$
$$= 11$$

The percent uptake that indicates normal or abnormal function of the thyroid varies widely from one laboratory to another. Hence, an uptake of 11% may indicate hypothyroidism in one laboratory and a normal thyroid in another.

Dilution Studies

Dilution measurements with radioactive nuclides are used for a variety of diagnostic tests in clinical medicine. If a solution of volume v_i

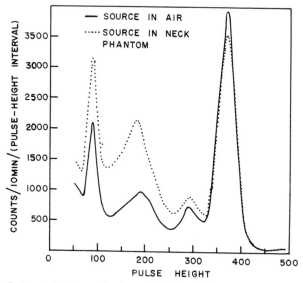

Fig 14-1. — Pulse height spectra for a 1 ml, 5 μCi ^{131}I source in air and in a neck phantom at a distance of 30 cm from a 1.5 in. diameter, 1 in. thick NaI(Tl) crystal. Radiation scattered by material around the radioactive source increases the height of the Compton plateau. (From Hine, G., and Williams, J.: Thyroid Radioiodine Uptake Measurements, in Hine, G. [ed.]: *Instrumentation in Nuclear Medicine* [New York: Academic Press, 1967], vol. 1.)

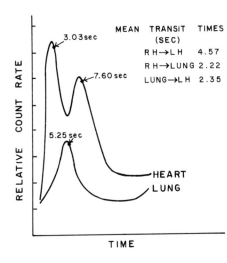

MEAN TRANSIT TIMES
(SEC)

RH→LH 4.57
RH→LUNG 2.22
LUNG→LH 2.35

3.03 sec

7.60 sec

5.25 sec

HEART
LUNG

RELATIVE COUNT RATE

TIME

Fig 14-2. — Time-concentration curve obtained by recording signals from scintillation detectors over the precordium *(upper curve)* and over the lung *(lower curve)* after intravenous injection of a mixture of ^{125}I and ^{131}I. (From Johnson, D., et al.: Radiopulmonary Cardiography for Measurement of Central Mean Transit Time and Its Arterial and Venous Subdivisions, in Kniseley, R., Tauxe, W., and Anderson, E. [eds.]: *Dynamic Clinical Studies with Radioisotopes* TID 7678 [Springfield, Va.: Clearinghouse for Federal Scientific and Technical Information, 1964].)

which contains a known concentration $(CPM/ml)_i$ of radioactive material is mixed thoroughly with a large volume of nonradioactive solution, then the volume v_f of the final solution may be estimated by measuring the specific count rate $(CPM/ml)_f$ of the final solution:

$$v_f = \frac{(CPM/ml)_i}{(CPM/ml)_f} v_i \qquad (14\text{-}2)$$

Since $(CPM/ml)_i \, v_i$ = total CPM $[(CPM)_i]$ of the injection solution, equation (14-2) may be written as:

$$v_f = \frac{(CPM)_i}{(CPM/ml)_f}$$

The specific count rates $(CPM/ml)_i$ and $(CPM/ml)_f$ must be corrected for background. The difference $v_f - v_i$ is the volume of the nonradioactive solution with which the solution of volume v_i is mixed.

During some applications of the dilution technique, the specific count rate $(CPM/ml)_f$ of the final solution must be corrected for activity that escapes from the volume to be measured. For example, estimates of blood volume with serum albumin labeled with ^{131}I sometimes are made at intervals over the first hour after intravenous injection of the labeled compound. To correct for the escape of serum albumin from the circulation, the specific count rate may be plotted as a function of time and extrapolated back to the moment of injection. Alternately, the blood volume may be measured at a specific time (e.g., 10 minutes) after injection of the labeled albumin, and a predetermined correction factor may be applied to the measured volume.

Example 14-2

Ten microcuries of serum albumin tagged with ^{131}I (radioiodinated human serum albumin or RISA) were injected intravenously into a patient. After the labeled albumin had mixed thoroughly in the patient's circulatory system, 5 ml of the patient's blood was withdrawn. The 5-ml sample yielded a count rate of 2,675 CPM. Another 10-μCi sample of RISA was diluted to 2,000 ml. A 5-ml aliquot from this standard solution yielded a count rate of 6,343 CPM. The background count rate was 193 CPM. What was the total blood volume?

$$\text{Sample net specific count rate} = (2,675 - 193) \text{ CPM/5 ml}$$
$$= 495 \text{ CPM/ml}$$
$$\text{Standard net specific count rate} = (6,343 - 193) \text{ CPM/5 ml}$$
$$= 1,230 \text{ CPM/ml}$$
$$\text{Count rate for 10-}\mu\text{Ci sample} = (1,230 \text{ CPM/ml})(2,000 \text{ ml})$$
$$= 246 \times 10^4 \text{ CPM}$$

If the volume of the injected RISA is ignored, the blood volume v_f is

$$v_f = \frac{(\text{CPM})_i}{(\text{CPM/ml})_f}$$
$$= \frac{246 \times 10^4 \text{ CPM}}{495 \text{ CPM/ml}}$$
$$\approx 5,000 \text{ ml}$$

Time-Concentration Studies

A number of diagnostic tests have been devised in which an external detector is used to measure the radioactivity in an organ or in the blood flow to an organ as a function of time after the administration of a radioactive compound. For example, the *mean transit time* of blood between the right side of the heart, lungs and the left side of the heart may be estimated by recording the signals from detectors over the precordium and over the lung after intravenous injection of ^{131}I and ^{125}I.[1] The counting system for the detector over the precordium records the ^{131}I activity, and the counting system for the detector over the lung records the ^{125}I activity. The first peak in the upper curve in Figure 14-2 reflects the accumulation of activity in the right chamber of the heart, prior to its release into the lungs. The second peak reflects the return of activity from the lungs to the left chamber of the heart. The valley between the peaks corresponds to the time when the activity is greatest in the lungs. Data such as those in Figure 14-2 may be used for the detection of pulmonary hypertension and abnormal cardiac output.

Time-concentration curves may be used also to estimate the rate of blood flow to the liver and to the kidneys. The functional capability of the liver may be estimated by measuring the rate at which rose bengal dye labeled with ^{131}I is accumulated and released by the liver.[2] Hippuran tagged with ^{131}I has been used for the study of kidney function. For

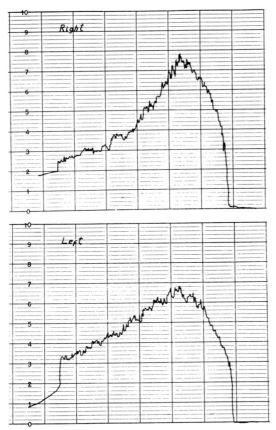

Fig 14-3.—Renogram measured with ^{131}I-Hippuran for a normal right kidney and a left kidney with increased retention of activity.

this study, two scintillation detectors are used to measure the activity in both kidneys simultaneously as a function of time. The renogram in Figure 14-3 depicts the accumulation of ^{131}I-Hippuran by each kidney and its subsequent release into the urine. The greater activity retained by the left kidney suggests that an obstruction in the kidney or ureter interferes with the release of urine into the bladder.

RECTILINEAR SCANNERS

Rectilinear scanners consist of a radiation detector which moves in a plane above or below the patient, and a recording device which moves in synchrony with the detector (Fig 14-4). In earlier scanners, the motion of the detector was synchronized with the recording device by a mechanical linkage. In later versions, electronic rather than mechanical

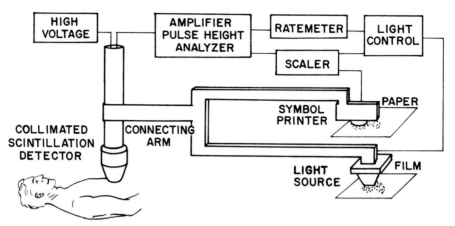

Fig 14-4. — Diagram of a rectilinear scanner with mechanical linkage.

linkage has been used, and the recording device usually is separated physically from the detector.

The first practical rectilinear scanner was developed in 1951 by Cassen and colleagues.[3] In this scanner, a small crystal of calcium tungstate was used as the radiation detector. However, the superior properties of sodium iodide (NaI) for detecting γ rays were quickly recognized, and essentially all scanners now in use employ this type of detector. In earlier scanners, the NaI crystal was typically 3 in. in diameter and 2 in. thick. In more recent scanners, the crystal diameter has increased to 5 or 8 in. to improve the efficiency of γ-ray detection. With a larger crystal, images may be obtained more quickly or, alternately, less "noisy" images may be obtained in comparable imaging times. Although the larger crystals collect more γ rays because of their larger field of view, they exhibit a more limited depth of focus, and radioactivity above and below the focal plane of the collimator is imaged less sharply.

Collimation

As the NaI detector moves across a patient, γ rays from the patient's body impinge upon the detector to produce electric pulses which are processed to yield an image. At each location along the path of the detector, the small region of the patient's body from which γ rays are detected

Fig 14-5. — Typical configurations of channels in collimators for rectilinear scanners.

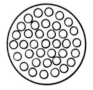

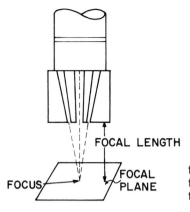

Fig 14-6. — Simplified multihole focused collimator illustrating the focal length, focal plane and focus of the collimator.

is identified by a collimator attached to the detector. In almost all applications, the collimator is a focused collimator consisting of small circular or hexagonal channels in a block of lead or tungsten (Fig 14-5). A collimator with hexagonal channels provides a slightly higher efficiency of γ-ray collection. Imaginary lines through the channels converge to a point a few inches in front of the face of the collimator. This point is referred to as the *collimator focus.* The plane parallel to the collimator face and containing the focus is termed the *focal plane* of the collimator, and the distance from this plane to the collimator face is the *collimator focal length* (Fig 14-6). In most applications of the rectilinear scanner, the patient is positioned with the focal plane of the collimator centered in the region of interest for the patient.

To localize the region from which γ rays emerging from the patient may strike the crystal, the collimator channels must be separated by intervening lead or tungsten leaves, termed *septa*, which are thick enough to attenuate most of the γ rays originating outside the region of interest. Rather thick septa are required for high-energy photons, whereas the septa may be much thinner for γ rays of lower energy. Hence, collimators may be termed *high* energy, *medium* energy or *low* energy, depend-

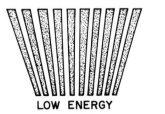

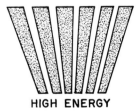

LOW ENERGY   HIGH ENERGY

Fig 14-7. — Multihole focused collimators. Thicker lead septa are required to attenuate high-energy photons.

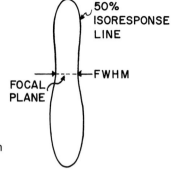

Fig 14-8.—Spatial resolution of collimator described as the "full width at half maximum" (FWHM).

ing on the thickness of the septa and, consequently, on the energy of the γ rays for which they are to be used (Fig 14-7). Collimators also may be characterized as *high resolution* or *high sensitivity*. High-resolution collimators have many holes of small diameter, and high-sensitivity collimators have fewer holes of larger diameter so that more of the crystal is

Fig 14-9.—Relative resolution of two collimators: a high-resolution collimator *(left)* and a high-sensitivity collimator *(right)*.

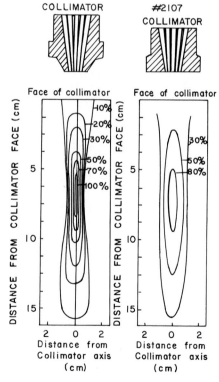

exposed to radiation. Alternately, the resolution of a collimator may be improved by increasing the height of the collimator rather than the number of holes. In general, a high-resolution collimator has relatively low sensitivity, and vice versa.

To determine the spatial resolution of a collimator, a point source is moved to a variety of positions in a series of planes parallel to the face of the collimator, and the detector response is determined as a percent of the response with the source at the focus. Curves connecting points of equal percent response are termed *isoresponse curves*. The distance between the 50% isoresponse curves in the focal plane often is called the *collimator resolution width*. Sometimes this width is termed the *full width at half maximum* (FWHM) for the collimator (Fig 14-8). A high-resolution collimator has a relatively small resolution width or FWHM, whereas a high-sensitivity collimator has a wider resolution width (Fig 14-9).

Scintillation Crystal and Electronics

When a γ ray traverses the collimator and interacts in the crystal, a flash of light is produced which varies in brightness with the amount of energy deposited in the crystal by the γ ray. This light is directed onto the photocathode of the photomultiplier (PM) tube and electrons are ejected from the photocathode. The number of electrons ejected is proportional to the incident light and, hence, to the energy deposited in the crystal by the incoming γ ray. The number of electrons is amplified in the PM tube, and the resulting electron pulse is collected at the PM-tube anode and converted to a voltage pulse. The voltage pulse is transmitted through the preamplifier and amplifier to a pulse height analyzer in the manner described in Chapter 12.

In the pulse height analyzer, a window is available to select only the voltage pulses that correspond to total absorption of the γ rays of interest in the crystal. The position and width of this window are critically important to the production of high-quality images. Even with careful selection of the window, certain problems are very difficult to solve. With high patient activities, for example, 72-keV fluorescence x rays from the lead collimator may sum in the detector to yield voltage pulses corresponding to 144 keV. Even the most carefully chosen window for imaging ^{99m}Tc (140 keV) cannot reject these pulses.

Rate Meter

In a rectilinear scanner, pulses accepted by the window of the pulse height analyzer are transmitted to a rate meter where the rate of receipt of pulses is registered on a meter or digital display. In the rate meter, the time over which counts are averaged to yield an estimate of count rate is related to the time constant of the rate meter. Usually, the time constant

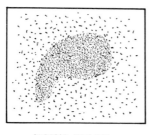
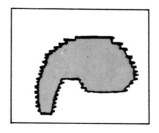

NOISY IMAGE   **IMAGE SCALLOPING**

Fig 14-10. — Effect of rate meter response on images obtained with the rectilinear scanner. A short time constant may yield a noisy image, whereas a long time constant leads to image scalloping.

can be varied with a control on the front of the rate meter. A short time constant provides a rapid response to changes in activity as the detector scans over the patient. However, the indicated count rate is susceptible to statistical fluctuations, and the resulting image may be rather "noisy." This susceptibility can be reduced (i.e., the count rate can be smoothed) by increasing the time constant of the rate meter. However, a longer time constant reduces the responsiveness of the scanner to abrupt changes in activity as the detector scans across the patient (Fig 12-8). This decrease in responsiveness leads to distortion of the image, which is referred to as *scalloping* (Fig 14-10).

Photorecording Display Device

From the rate meter, the count rate signal is transmitted to the display section where an image is made of the distribution of radioactivity in the patient. In the display section, a collimated light source (usually a small cathode-ray tube) moves across a photographic film in synchrony with the motion of the detector across the patient. The light source turns on and off in response to the count rate, with higher count rates causing the light source to remain on for longer periods of time. Hence, the film is darker in regions corresponding to higher count rates. The brightness of the light source, and hence the overall average density of the image, is determined by the density setting on the panel of the photorecording display device, as well as by the size of the collimator selected for the light source.

Contrast Enhancement Control

In scanning across a particular region of a patient, the count rate may vary from background to some maximum value depending upon the activity present at each location within the region. Since the background count rate provides no information about the patient, many scanners provide a control to subtract background from the count rate furnished to

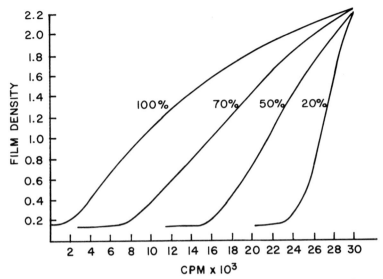

Fig 14-11.—Film density as a function of count rate at different settings of the contrast enhancement control.

the display device. With this control set so that count rates slightly higher than background correspond to white in the image, and maximum count rates correspond to black, the entire distribution of radioactivity in the region of interest can be displayed as shades of gray in the image. In this case, however, slight differences in activity, which may represent pathologic conditions in the patient, may not be displayed as gray levels sufficiently different to be appreciated visually. To accentuate subtle differences in count rate, the photorecording device provides a control with which the available shades of gray can be applied over the count rate range of interest. This control may be labeled *contrast enhancement, count rate differential,* or *range differential.* To utilize the contrast enhancement capability of the scanner, the density control is adjusted so that the maximum count rate of interest is displayed as black in the image. Then the contrast enhancement control is adjusted so that the minimum count rate of interest is displayed as white in the image. For example, setting the contrast enhancement control at 40% on one type of scanner insures that count rates less than 60% of maximum are displayed as white areas in the image, and the available gray scale of the image is superimposed over the upper 40% of the measured count rates (Fig 14-11). Although contrast enhancement is very useful in revealing subtle differences in the distribution of radioactivity in the patient, the control must be used with care since it can also delete information from the image which may be necessary for diagnosis of the patient's condition.

The rectilinear scanner may provide a second type of display referred to as a *dot scan*. To produce this type of image, a mechanical device moves across a sheet of paper in synchrony with the moving detector, and imprints a symbol on the paper each time some preset number of counts has been accumulated. The number of counts per imprint is determined by the *dot factor* or *scale factor* set on the console of the display device. With a dot scan, the operator can monitor the production of an image of the distribution of radioactivity in the patient. Monitoring the image is not possible with the photographic image, because the image is not available until after the scan has been completed and the film has been processed. Although dot scans are useful to monitor image production, they seldom are used for image interpretation because the photographic display is more useful for clinical diagnosis.

Minified Images

Sometimes scan images are made life size by a one-to-one relationship between the motion of the detector across the patient and the motion of the light source across the film. However, it also is possible to change this ratio to provide a minified image of a region of interest in the patient. Minified images are particularly useful when large areas of the patient are scanned, such as whole body images of the distribution of radioactivity in soft tissues or the skeleton of the patient.

Information Density

To obtain an image with a rectilinear scanner, two control settings must be selected that are related to the mechanical motion of the scanning detector. These controls are the scan speed and line spacing. Usually, the line spacing is $\frac{1}{8}$ or $\frac{1}{16}$ in., and the light collimator in the photorecording device is chosen to correspond to this spacing. Then the scan speed is selected from the relationship:

$$\text{Information density} \left(\frac{\text{counts}}{\text{sq cm}}\right) = \frac{\text{Count rate (CPM)}}{[\text{Scan speed (cm/min)}][\text{Line spacing (cm)}]}$$

From an estimate of the average count rate over the region of interest, the scan speed may be selected to yield a desired information density in the image. Usually, information densities of 1,000–1,200 counts/sq cm are desired. However, lower densities are tolerated in some examinations in which long scan times or low patient activities are encountered.

High-Speed Rectilinear Scanner

The high-speed rectilinear scanner utilizes a linear array of 10 crystals, each associated with its own focused collimator, photomultiplier tube, amplifier and pulse height analyzer. In one high-speed rectilinear scanner, the collimators, a 24 by 4.9 in. array of crystals, and associated electronics are contained in a scanning head which is positioned perpendic-

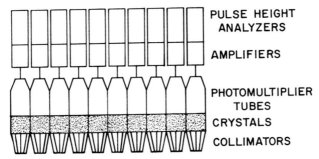

PULSE HEIGHT
ANALYZERS

AMPLIFIERS

PHOTOMULTIPLIER
TUBES

CRYSTALS

COLLIMATORS

Fig 14-12. — Scanner head of a high-speed rectilinear scanner.

ular to the scanning table (Fig 14-12). Scanning is accomplished by movement of the detector back and forth across a distance of approximately 2.5 in. perpendicular to the table axis, together with a continuous sweep of the scanning head parallel to the table axis. Counts from each photomultiplier tube are analyzed separately and stored on a magnetic disk. These data may be played back to a cathode-ray tube (CRT) for storage on Polaroid or photographic film. Storage on the disk also allows the data to be manipulated in a nondestructive manner. For example, background may be subtracted or contrast enhanced as the data are played back to the CRT. The high-speed rectilinear scanner allows studies such as bone scans to be performed quickly as compared with the time required for a traditional rectilinear scanner.

STATIONARY IMAGING DEVICES

With a stationary imaging device, areas of activity within a regional distribution of radioactivity may be visualized simultaneously without moving either the patient or the detector. Since mechanical motion of the detector is not required, images can be obtained much more rapidly with this device than with a rectilinear scanner. Also, studies can be made of rapidly occurring changes in the distribution of radioactivity within a region of interest. Because of these advantages, stationary imaging devices, primarily the scintillation camera, have become the principal instruments in most nuclear medicine laboratories for studying almost all body parts, with the possible exception of the thyroid and skeleton.

The Single-Crystal Scintillation Camera

The first single-crystal scintillation camera was assembled in 1956 by Anger at the University of California.[4] This camera contained a 1/4 in. thick sodium iodide [NaI(Tl)] crystal only 5 in. in diameter. It was viewed by seven photomultiplier (PM) tubes, each 1.5 in. in diameter. Six

PM tubes were hexagonally arranged about the seventh tube at the center. In 1960, an improved version of the Anger camera was made available commercially. In 1963, a larger scintillation camera was built with an 11.5-in. crystal and 19 PM tubes arranged in hexagonal fashion. In this camera, as in earlier versions, the PM tubes were optically coupled to the scintillation crystal with mineral oil, a technique that furnished efficient transmission of light from the crystal but restricted the position of the detector to an overhead view of the patient. A major improvement in camera design was achieved when the mineral oil was replaced by a solid plastic light guide and optical coupling grease, eliminating the oil seals required for earlier cameras and permitting rotation of the detector head to any desired position.

Although the basic design of the scintillation camera has not changed much since 1963, many improvements have been added that have increased the speed and versatility of this instrument and enhanced its usefulness in clinical nuclear medicine. Among these improvements are electronic changes such as replacement of vacuum tubes by integrated circuits, and precision electronic components to obtain a more rapid and reliable signal which is less sensitive to environment and power fluctuations. Currently, scintillation cameras are available with crystals up to 20 in. in diameter coupled to as many as 91 PM tubes to improve the quality of scintillation camera images. Another development that has enhanced the usefulness of the scintillation camera for certain nuclear medicine procedures has been the interfacing of the camera to data storage and processing systems. Other modifications in present-day cameras include the use of more efficient bialkali photomultiplier tubes in place of the conventional tubes used earlier, the use of multichannel analyzers for window selection and adjustment, and the incorporation of region of interest and count summation circuits into the image display network.

One factor that has contributed greatly to the popularity of the scintillation camera has been the widespread utilization of ^{99m}Tc. This radionuclide emits a γ ray of 140 keV, an ideal energy for scintillation camera imaging, with only slight contamination by particles and photons of undesired energies. In addition, ^{99m}Tc has a short half-life (6 hr) and can be incorporated into a variety of compounds and drugs. Compared to many other radionuclides, the short half-life of ^{99m}Tc permits administration of large amounts of radioactive material without excessive radiation dose to the patient. This increased administration of radioactivity means that more γ rays are emitted over a shorter period of time, permitting the scintillation camera to be used to its full advantage.

Principles of Scintillation Camera Operation

A single-crystal scintillation camera can be separated into four sections: the collimator, the detector, the data processing section, and the display unit.

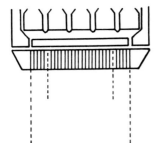

Fig 14-13.—Parallel multihole collimator.

COLLIMATORS.—To produce an image of the distribution of radioactivity in a patient, the sites of absorption of γ rays in the scintillation camera crystal must be related clearly to the origin of the γ rays within the patient. This relationship can be achieved by placing a collimator between the crystal and the patient. The most commonly used collimator is the parallel multihole collimator, comprised of small straight cylinders separated by lead or tungsten septa (Fig 14-13). Relatively thin septa are used

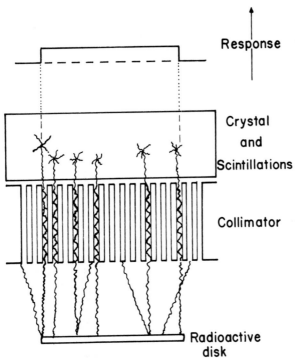

Fig 14-14.—With a multihole collimator, γ rays emitted in line with the collimator holes are transmitted to the crystal, whereas γ rays emitted obliquely are absorbed by the collimator septa.

in low-energy collimators designed for use with radionuclides emitting low-energy photons. Thicker septa are required for collimators used with nuclides emitting higher-energy photons. The ability of high-energy photons to traverse even relatively thick septa establishes an upper limit of about 600 keV on the photon energy range amenable to scintillation camera imaging. As a general rule, the minimum path length through septa of the collimator should be at least 5 mean free paths (< 1% transmission) for the photons with which the collimator is to be used.

A γ ray moving from the patient toward the crystal in a direction in line with one of the collimator cylinders can pass through the cylinder and interact in the crystal, whereas a γ ray emerging obliquely from the patient would have to traverse one or more of the lead septa in the collimator before reaching the crystal (Fig 14-14). Hence, γ rays emitted obliquely have a much lower probability of reaching the detector. By this mechanism, γ rays interacting in the crystal can be related reasonably well to their origin in small discrete volumes of tissue directly below the collimator.

A collimator with many cylinders of small diameter is termed a *high-resolution collimator*; a collimator with fewer cylinders of larger diameter or with shorter cylinders of the same diameter allows more photons to reach the crystal and is termed a *high-sensitivity collimator*. In the selection of parallel multihole collimators, a gain in sensitivity is accompanied by a loss of resolution, and vice versa.

As the diameter of the collimator cylinders is reduced, fewer photons are admitted through each cylinder into the scintillation crystal, and the statistical influence of variations in photon emission (i.e., quantum noise or mottle) is increased. The only way to prevent an increase in image noise is to increase either the imaging time or the emission from the source, so that the number of photons passing through each cylinder of the collimator remains constant. As an example, suppose the intrinsic resolution of a nuclear medicine imaging system is improved by a factor of two by decreasing the diameter of the collimator cylinders, and suppose that this improvement is accompanied by a twofold reduction in the number of photons reaching the crystal. To keep the quantum noise of the image at the original level, the number of photons incident upon the collimator must be increased by a factor of two. To reduce the quantum noise to a level corresponding to the finer resolution of the new collimator, however, an additional fourfold increase is required in the number of photons incident upon the collimator. That is, a twofold improvement in the resolution of an imaging system achieved by reducing the diameter of the collimator cylinders should be accompanied by an eightfold increase in photon emission or imaging time to obtain a parallel improvement in image noise.

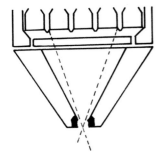

Fig 14-15.—Pinhole collimator.

As the distance is increased between the face of a parallel multihole collimator and a radioactive object (e.g., a patient), the resolution decreases because each open cylinder in the collimator views a larger cross-sectional area of the object. For the same reason, the sensitivity does not change significantly with the distance between a multihole collimator and the object. Although the number of photons collected by each collimator cylinder from a unit area of the object decreases with the square of the collimator–object distance, the area viewed by each cylinder increases as the square of the distance. These two influences counteract each other so that the sensitivity does not change appreciably as the collimator–object distance is changed.

Other types of collimators used occasionally with scintillation cameras include the pinhole collimator, the diverging collimator and the converging collimator.

The pinhole collimator (Fig 14-15) is used primarily to obtain high-resolution images of small organs (e.g., the thyroid) that can be positioned near the pinhole. The major disadvantage of the pinhole collimator is its low sensitivity, since only a few of the photons emitted by the object are collected to form an image. Occasionally, a pinhole collimator with three apertures is used to provide three different views of a small organ simultaneously.

The diverging collimator (Fig 14-16) permits the scintillation camera

Fig 14-16.—Diverging collimator.

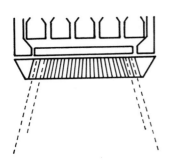

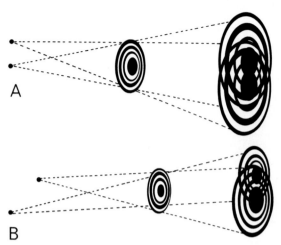

Fig 14-17.—In zone plate imaging, each point of radioactivity casts a unique shadow onto the detector. (From Farmelant, M., DeMeester, G., Wilson, D., and Barrett, H.: Initial clinical experiences with a Fresnel zone-plate imager, J. Nucl. Med. 16:183, 1975. Reprinted with permission.)

to image anatomical regions larger than the dimensions of the crystal. Compared to a parallel multihole collimator, there is some reduction in resolution with a diverging collimator. With the converging collimator, images with improved resolution can be obtained for organs smaller than the dimensions of the crystal. The resolution is improved because the object is projected over the entire crystal face, rather than onto a limited region of the crystal. Also, the photon collection efficiency is greater for a converging collimator than for a parallel multihole collimator used to image a small object. Hence, the influence of quantum noise is often less noticeable in images obtained with a converging collimator. Collimators that can be used in both the converging and diverging modes often are referred to as *div/con* collimators.

CODED APERTURE SUBSTITUTES FOR COLLIMATORS.—Conventional collimators provide the necessary positional relationship between the interaction of a γ ray in the crystal and the origin of the γ ray in the patient. However, they are inefficient collectors of γ rays because they reject all γ rays except those arising within a relatively small solid angle. Also, conventional collimators often are the major factor influencing the resolution of a scintillation camera image. As substitutes for conventional collimators, various coded apertures have been proposed. One of the simplest of these devices is the Fresnel zone plate, in which each point of radioactivity in front of the plate casts a unique shadow of the zone plate onto the detector (Fig 14-17). That is, points of radioactivity at the same

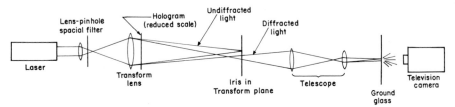

Fig 14-18.—Optical reconstruction system for coded aperture imaging. (From Farmelant, M., DeMeester, G., Wilson, D., and Barrett, H.: Initial clinical experiences with a Fresnel zone-plate imager, J. Nucl. Med. 16:183, 1975. Reprinted with permission.)

distance from the zone plate cast shadows on the detector that are laterally displaced from each other, and points at different distances from the zone plate cast shadows of different sizes. Because of the latter effect, information is projected onto the detector about the three-dimensional distribution of radioactivity in the patient.

To retrieve this information, the transmission data projected onto the detector may be recorded in coded form on film. When this coded image is placed in a coherent light beam, diffraction of the light produces an interpretable image that can be viewed telescopically (Fig 14-18). This image is tomographic, and movement of the eyepiece of the telescope allows one to visualize the distribution of radioactivity at different depths in the patient.

Many other coded apertures have been studied, including some that change continuously over the time in which radiation from the object is detected. All coded apertures developed so far have one major limitation, however; they exhibit very low sensitivity to large areas of radioactivity such as those usually encountered in nuclear medicine.

SCINTILLATION CRYSTAL.—Although NaI(Tl) crystals up to 20 in. in diameter are used in single-crystal scintillation cameras, the periphery of the crystal is always masked and does not contribute to image formation. With an 11.5-in. diameter crystal, for example, only the center 10 in. is used to create an image. Masking is necessary to prevent distortion in the image caused by inefficient collection of light at the periphery of the crystal. To prevent physical damage to the crystal and to keep it free of moisture, the crystal is sealed between a thin ($<$ 1 mm) aluminum canister on the exterior surface and a glass or plastic plate on the interior surface.

The photopeak detection efficiency of a 0.5 in. thick NaI(Tl) detector varies from about 80% for ^{99m}Tc (140 keV) to about 10% at 511 keV. Although increased detection efficiency could be achieved with thicker crystals, multiple scattering within the crystal also would increase, causing a reduction in the photon positioning accuracy of the camera. To facilitate the escape of scattered photons from the crystal without multiple interactions, the thickness of the crystal is maintained purposefully at 0.5 in.

When a γ ray traverses the collimator and interacts in the crystal, it produces a flash of light that varies in brightness with the amount of energy deposited in the crystal by the γ ray. This light radiates from the interaction site and impinges upon the light guide between the NaI(Tl) crystal and the PM tubes.

LIGHT GUIDE.—In addition to the protective glass plate, most camera detectors have a light guide, usually composed of Plexiglas, which transmits and distributes the light from the primary interaction site in the crystal to the surrounding PM tubes (Fig 14-19). The distribution of light within a light guide of properly chosen thickness (usually about 4 cm from the central plane of the crystal to the face of the PM tubes) results in increased counting efficiency and positioning accuracy. The light is transmitted with almost no loss because the sides of the light guide are coated with a reflective covering. Because the light guide is solid, the detector assembly can be positioned in different orientations without difficulty.

PHOTOMULTIPLIER TUBES.—The light transmitted to a particular PM tube strikes the photocathode element of the tube. In response, electrons are ejected from the photocathode and focused upon the first of $8-14$ positively charged electrodes referred to as *dynodes*. The number of electrons ejected from the photocathode depends upon the amount of incident light. This number of electrons is multiplied in the remaining dynodes to yield 10^6-10^8 electrons collected as a negative current pulse at the final electrode or anode for each electron released at the photocathode. The actual number of electrons finally collected at the anode

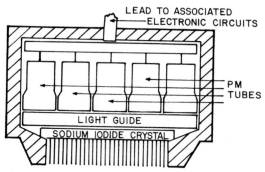

Fig 14-19.—Detector assembly of a single-crystal scintillation camera.

(i.e., the size of the output signal) varies in direct proportion to the amount of light striking the photocathode.

One of the restrictions on image quality with a single-crystal scintillation camera is the statistical fluctuation in the number of electrons ejected from the photocathode for a given amount of energy arriving at the photocathode in the form of visible light. This statistical fluctuation is determined primarily by the average number of electrons ejected per unit incident energy, and has been improved markedly by replacement of older S11-type PM tubes with tubes having photocathodes that release more electrons per unit of incident energy. Another improvement in noise reduction is the use of threshold preamplifiers that reject small signals from PM tubes distant from the interaction site in the crystal. These signals are rejected because they add significant noise without contributing substantially to image formation. Even with the newer tubes, however, statistical fluctuations in electron ejection from PM tube photocathodes establish a lower limit of about 70 keV for the energy range of γ rays amenable to single-crystal scintillation camera imaging. Also contributing to this lower energy limit is the difficulty in using pulse height analysis to distinguish primary from scattered photons when the primary photon energies are low. For example, a 140-keV photon from ^{99m}Tc that is scattered at 45 degrees has an energy of 131 keV. This photon would be accepted by a 15% pulse height analyzer window centered on the photopeak and transmitting pulses corresponding to energies between 129.5 and 150.5 keV.

PHOTOMULTIPLIER TUBE PREAMPLIFIERS.—Each PM tube transmits its output electric signal to its own preamplifier (Fig 14-20). This circuit is used primarily to match the PM tube to the succeeding electric circuits; that is, the actual amplification of the signal usually is insignificant in the preamplifier. Preamplifiers offer the opportunity to tune the detector so that signals from the PM tubes are identical for a given amount of energy

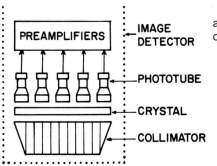

Fig 14-20.—Detector assembly and preamplifiers of a scintillation camera.

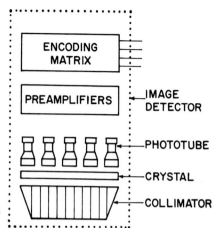

Fig 14-21.—Preamplifiers and position encoding matrix circuits of the scintillation camera.

absorbed in corresponding regions of the detector. Many scintillation cameras use this approach to tuning the PM tube array.

POSITION ENCODING MATRIX.—The PM tubes are positioned in a hexagonal array above the scintillation crystal, with the spacing and separation from the crystal carefully controlled to provide an optimum combination of spatial uniformity and resolution. For the distribution of electric signals emerging from the preamplifiers of these PM tubes, some operation must be performed to determine the site of energy absorption in the crystal. This operation is the function of the position encoding matrix (Fig 14-21). The signal from each preamplifier enters the matrix and is applied across four precision resistors to produce four separate electric signals for each PM tube. These signals are labeled: +x, −x, +y and −y.

For the PM tube in the center of the array, all four resistors are equal and all four signals are identical. On the other hand, a PM tube in the lower left quadrant in the array is represented in the matrix by +x and

Fig 14-22.—In the position encoding matrix for each photomultiplier tube, the PM signal is separated into four signals of relative sizes which reflect the position of the particular PM tube within the PM tube array.

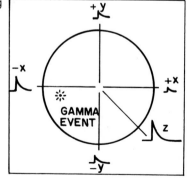

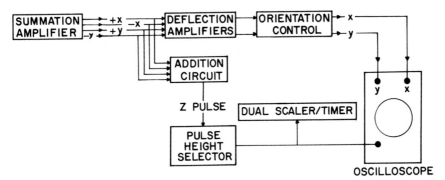

Fig 14-23.—Position and pulse height control circuitry of a scintillation camera.

+y resistors that are significantly different from the −x and −y resistors. A signal from the preamplifier of this PM tube furnishes −x and −y signals that are larger than the +x and +y signals (Fig 14-22). The actual magnitude of the signals from each four-resistor component of the encoding matrix reflects the proximity of the corresponding PM tube to the origin of the light flash within the crystal.

SUMMATION AMPLIFIERS.—From the encoding matrix, the position signals for each PM tube are transmitted to four summation amplifiers. The +x signals for all of the PM tubes are added in one amplifier; the −x signals for all of the tubes are added in a second summation amplifier; and so forth. The product of the summation operation is four electric signals, one for each of the four deflection plates in the cathode-ray tube.

DEFLECTION AMPLIFIERS.—Before the signals are applied to the plates, however, they are transmitted to four deflection amplifiers where they are amplified, differentiated and shaped (Fig 14-23). Here the signals also are divided by the Z pulse (see below) to normalize the positioning signals to the summation signal representing the particular interaction. This normalization process permits the use of a relatively wide pulse-size acceptance range (i.e., a relatively wide window) without an unacceptable reduction in position accuracy. Among other adjustments in the deflection amplifiers, the signals are modified to furnish the exact size of image desired on the cathode-ray tube. Malfunctions of the deflection amplifiers often are responsible for distortions of the image, such as the production of elliptical images for circular distributions of radioactivity. Following the deflection amplifiers, the positioning signals are fed to the orientation control, where rotation switches on the camera console can be manipulated to alter the left–right and top–bottom presentation of the image on the camera console.

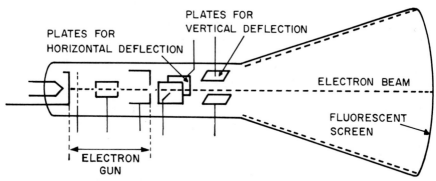

Fig 14-24. — Cathode-ray image display device.

PULSE SUMMATION (ADDITION) CIRCUIT. — In a circuit parallel to the deflection amplifiers, the four position signals are added to form the Z pulse, which is transmitted to the Z-pulse-forming circuit where it is differentiated and shaped. Next, the Z pulse is sent to the pulse height analyzer (PHA). In many cameras the PHA is a fixed bias circuit and the pulse height selection window is nonvariable. With a fixed bias PHA, pulses must be attenuated with an isotope range switch so that pulses representing total absorption of photons of a desired energy will be of the proper size to be accepted by the analyzer. Usually, the isotope range switch, with different attenuation settings for different photon energy ranges, is positioned in the camera circuitry before the positioning signals branch to the addition circuit and deflection amplifiers.

If a particular pulse triggers the lower, not the upper, discriminator of the PHA, a microsecond negative pulse is transmitted to one input of an AND gate. The second input to the AND gate is furnished as soon as any previous pulse has dissipated. When the AND gate is activated, a microsecond unblanking pulse is furnished to the display cathode-ray tube, where it activates the CRT electron beam to produce a short burst of electrons. This burst of electrons produces a tiny light flash on the cathode-ray screen. The number of electrons in the burst, and hence the brightness of the light flash on the cathode-ray screen, is adjusted with the intensity control on the console of the scintillation camera. The unblanking pulse also is transmitted to a scaler, which records the counts forming the image.

CATHODE-RAY TUBE (CRT). — The cathode-ray tube consists essentially of an electron gun, four deflection plates and a fluorescent screen that furnishes a flash of light when struck by the electron beam from the electron gun (Fig 14–24). Normally, the electron beam is prevented from flowing across the cathode-ray tube; only during the brief interval when the signal from the PHA is received at the cathode-ray tube is the electron beam permitted to flow and produce a light flash on the screen. During this brief interval, the position signals are applied to the deflection plates so that the light flashes on the screen at a position corresponding to the site of γ-ray absorption in the crystal.

Resolving Time Characteristics of Scintillation Cameras

At relatively low sample activities, the count rate from a single-crystal scintillation camera varies linearly with the sample activity. At higher sample activities, however, this relationship is not maintained, and the count rate increases less rapidly than expected as the activity of the sample is increased. The resulting loss of counts is termed the *coincidence loss*, and its magnitude depends on the resolving time of the camera. The resolving time is the minimum time required between successive interactions in the scintillation camera crystal for the interactions to be recorded as independent events.

When scintillation cameras are used for dynamic function studies, the loss of counts at high count rates may be a significant problem. In studies of the heart, for example, a 15–20 mCi bolus of activity may be present in the camera's field of view. This high activity may yield as many as 80,000 scintillations per second in the detector, and possibly even more if a converging collimator is used. At count rates this high, significant count rate losses occur, and quantitative interpretation of count rate data can be severely misleading.

For purposes of resolving time considerations, a scintillation camera may be considered as a two-component system, with a paralyzable component followed by a nonparalyzable component.[5] In a paralyzable counting system, the minimum time required for the independent detection of two separate interactions is extended if an interaction occurs within the recovery interval. With such a system, the count rate may de-

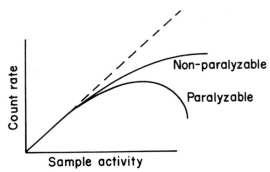

Fig 14-25.—Count rate characteristics of a paralyzable and a nonparalyzable counting system.

crease dramatically (i.e., the system may be paralyzed) for samples of exceptionally high activity (Fig 14-25). In a nonparalyzable system, a certain minimum time is required to process each interaction, but this time is not extended by an interaction occurring within the processing interval. With a nonparalyzable system and high sample activity, the count rate may reach a maximum plateau but will not decrease as the activity is increased. Many scintillation cameras exhibit a behavior intermediate between paralyzable and nonparalyzable systems. In general, the paralyzable component is the part of the camera that precedes the pulse height analyzer, and is a reflection primarily of the fluorescence decay time of the scintillation crystal. The fluorescence decay time of a NaI(Tl) crystal is characterized by a 0.25-μsec decay constant, with 0.8 μsec required for 98% of all light to be released. The nonparalyzable component is the part of the camera, including scalers and data processing equipment, that follows the pulse height analyzer.

A number of methods have been proposed for correcting scintillation camera data for coincidence count rate loss. If the resolving time were known for a particular camera, for example, one could estimate true counts from observed counts, provided that the resolving time is independent of factors such as activity position across the detector face, and

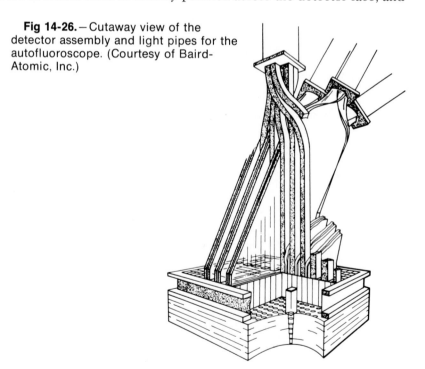

Fig 14-26.—Cutaway view of the detector assembly and light pipes for the autofluoroscope. (Courtesy of Baird-Atomic, Inc.)

that the summation of small coincident pulses to produce pulses transmitted by the PHA could be estimated. One rather widely used method to correct for coincidence count rate loss utilizes the count rate from a small radioactive marker source positioned near the periphery of the camera's field of view. In place of the radioactive marker source, an electronic marker such as a pulse generator may be used.

The Multiple-Crystal Scintillation Camera

The multiple-crystal approach to scintillation camera design was pioneered by Bender and Blau, who introduced the concept of the autofluoroscope in 1963.[6] In this device, 294 discrete NaI(Tl) crystals are arranged in a matrix of 21 columns and 14 rows, with each crystal $5/16$ by $5/16$ in. in cross section and 1.5 in. thick (Fig 14-26). The center-to-center spacing of the crystals is $7/16$ in., yielding dimensions of 6 by 9 in. for the entire crystal array. For most applications, each crystal is equipped with its own collimator and contributes one resolution element to the image. Each crystal in the array is viewed by two Plexiglas light guides, with each guide receiving half the light released during an interaction in the crystal. One of the light guides is coupled to one of 21 "column" PM tubes, and the other is coupled to one of 14 "row" PM tubes. With this coupling arrangement, each of the 294 crystals is identified uniquely by the combination of column and row PM tubes to which it is connected. Pulses arising simultaneously from light flashes in more than one crystal are rejected by anticoincidence circuitry, so that interactions caused by scattering of photons between crystals in the detector matrix are not registered. From each PM tube, the signal is fed through a preamplifier and linear amplifier to a specific location in computer memory. When a signal is received, the number stored at this location is increased by 1, provided that the signal represents the total absorption of a photon of interest in the crystal. This requirement is satisfied if the summed signal from all 35 PM tubes passes the pulse height analyzer, and if only one signal is received from all 21 column PM tubes and only one signal is received from all 14 row PM tubes.

In a single-crystal scintillation camera, the detection of γ-ray interactions includes determination of the spatial coordinates of the interaction. In a multiple-crystal camera, the detection of an interaction does not include the collection of position information, and much higher count rates can be processed without significant count rate loss or positioning errors. In the multiple-crystal camera, the resolving time is determined essentially by the speed with which an event can be processed electronically, rather than by the fluorescence decay time of the crystal.

The resolution of the multiple-crystal camera is limited intrinsically by the size of each detector element. However, the resolution can be

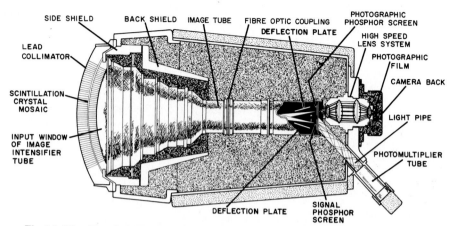

Fig 14-27.—The CsI (Tl) mosaic multiple-crystal scintillation camera (Quanta-scope). (Courtesy of Harshaw Chemical.)

improved markedly by moving the patient incrementally in the x and y directions so that each resolution element is divided into 16 subelements. With this motion of the scanning bed supporting the patient, the 294 resolution elements are subdivided essentially into 294 × 16 = 4,704 subelements, with the final image reassembled by computer. For anatomical regions larger than the 9.3 by 6.3 in. viewing area of the detector, two successive adjacent 16-position images can be reassembled by computer to furnish a single image containing 9,408 picture elements.

A second approach to the design of a multiple-crystal scintillation camera utilizes a mosaic of 2,515 CsI(Tl) crystals, each ⅛ in. wide and ⅝ in. long (Fig 14-27). The crystal mosaic is positioned on the face of an image intensifier tube with a 10 in. diameter photocathode. This instrument provides pulse height discrimination with a light deflection plate mounted behind the output phosphor. The plate guides the light from a single interaction onto a photomultiplier tube connected to an amplifier and pulse height analyzer. If the amount of light corresponds to the total interaction of a γ ray of interest, a returning pulse from the PHA circuit moves the deflection plate so that the remaining light pulse is recorded on photographic film. This approach to pulse height discrimination is somewhat marginal, because only the first part of the light pulse is available for analysis, as the remainder of the pulse must either be recorded or not recorded. However, pulse height analysis is not required in applications such as radionuclide angiocardiography. The major advantage of the CsI(Tl) mosaic scintillation camera is its high count rate capacity, limited only by the fluorescence decay time of the CsI(Tl) mosaic and the output phosphor of the image intensifier tube. The capacity of the

CsI(Tl) mosaic camera to function at high count rates has facilitated applications of this device to radionuclide angiocardiographic studies in which rapid sequential images are obtained of the passage of high-activity boluses through the heart.[7]

MULTIPLANE TOMOGRAPHY

The multiplane tomographic scanner provides multiple tomographic images at different depths following a single rectilinear scan of the patient. With a single-detector scanner, six tomographic images are provided; this number of images is doubled with a dual-head scanner that has detectors on opposite sides of the patient. In each image, point sources are imaged faithfully if they are in the corresponding tomographic plane. They are imaged as blurred disk sources if they are above or below the tomographic plane. In the commercial version of the multiplane tomograph, an 8.5 in. diameter by 1 in. NaI(Tl) crystal is viewed by seven 3 in. diameter PM tubes. The crystal is equipped with a collimator that is focused about 3.5 in. below the collimator face. The circuitry for the PM tubes and successive electronics is similar to that described for the scin-

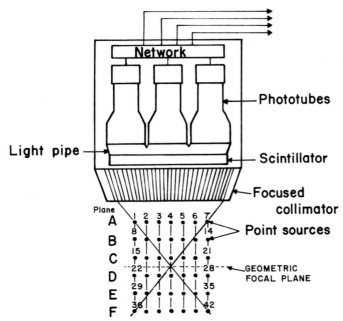

Fig 14-28. — Detector assembly for the multiplane tomographic scanner. (From Anger, H. O.: Tomography and Other Depth-Discrimination Techniques, in Hine, G. [ed.]: *Instrumentation in Nuclear Medicine* [New York: Academic Press, 1974], vol. 2, p. 71. Reprinted with permission.)

tillation camera, including a cathode-ray tube that provides light flashes on a fluorescent screen at locations corresponding to the sites of interactions of γ rays in the crystal.

To understand the operation of a multiplane tomographic scanner, consider a detector moving from right to left across a point source in plane A (Fig 14-28). On the cathode-ray tube, the image of the point source moves from left to right across the screen. Next consider the detector moving from right to left across a similar source in plane B. At the periphery of plane B, the source is outside the field of view of the detector and no image of the source is produced. As the source enters the field of view, an image is produced and moves left to right across the screen at a faster rate than the source in plane A. This situation is accentuated for a source in plane C, since the source appears for only a moment in the field of view and moves very rapidly across the screen. A source in plane D behaves as one in plane C, except that the image is inverted and the source appears to move from right to left. Similarly, plane E is like plane B, and plane F is like plane A, except that the source moves in the opposite direction.

In the photographic display unit, the apparent relative motion of the cathode-ray tube and film is synchronized with the motion of the detector across the patient. During this motion, the image of the cathode-ray tube is projected sequentially and repeatedly to 6 (or 12 with the dual-head scanner) different regions of the film, with each region furnishing an image of a separate tomographic plane in the patient. For each image, the sweep frequency of the cathode-ray tube is adjusted so that the electron beam of the CRT sweeps across the fluorescent screen at the same velocity but in the opposite direction to the movement across the screen of the image of a point source in the corresponding tomographic plane. In this manner, the image of a point source remains stationary on the fluorescent screen, provided that the point source is in the tomographic plane. That is, an in-focus image of the point source is produced on the screen. For a point source above or below the tomographic plane, the movement of the image of the source across the screen is not balanced by the sweep velocity of the electron beam, and the image is blurred across the fluorescent screen. Hence, only point sources in the tomographic plane are maintained in focus in the corresponding image. By changing the sweep velocity of the electron beam from one of the six images to the next, six tomographic images at different depths in the patient can be obtained.

The first multiplane tomographic scanner was developed by Anger in 1969. Although in-depth resolution is available with this scanner, it is important to note that the blurring of activity outside a particular tomographic plane may not be complete if the activity is well localized and considerably different from the activity in the tomographic plane.

PROBLEMS

°1. The uptake of ^{131}I was measured for a patient treated for hyperthyroidism with the same radioactive nuclide 2 months previously. The count rates were:

For ^{131}I standard on day 0	13,260 CPM
For ^{131}I standard 24 hr later	12,150 CPM
For patient on day 0 before ^{131}I administered	6,140 CPM
For patient 24 hr later	12,840 CPM

Compute the percent uptake of ^{131}I in the thyroid gland. Ignore the contribution of background radiation to the count rates, but include the contribution from residual ^{131}I.

°2. A patient was given 3 μCi of ^{131}I-RISA. A second 3-μCi sample was diluted to 3,000 ml. A 5-ml aliquot of this solution provided a count rate of 3,050 CPM. A 5-ml sample of the patient's blood provided a count rate of 1,660 CPM. What is the patient's blood volume?

3. Describe a method with a radioactive nuclide to determine the volume of a large container.

°4. The following count rates were recorded 24 hr after administration of 10 μCi ^{131}I to a patient:

For patient's thyroid	1,831 CPM
For patient's thyroid shielded by lead block	246 CPM
For standard source in thyroid phantom	3,942 CPM
For standard shielded by lead block	214 CPM

What is the percent uptake?

°5. Line-source response functions were measured for a NaI(Tl) scintillation detector and a multihole focused collimator. Which functions resemble a normal probability curve more closely:

a. A response function measured with a ^{198}Au source (γ ray of 412 keV) or a response function measured with an ^{241}Am source (γ ray of 60 keV)?

b. A response function measured with a ^{51}Cr source (γ ray of 320 keV) or a response function measured with a ^{197}Hg source (γ and x rays of about 70 keV)?

6. Explain the use with a gamma camera of: (a) a pinhole collimator, (b) a parallel multihole collimator, (c) a diverging collimator and (d) a converging collimator. Explain why the sensitivity does not change greatly as the distance varies between the patient and the face of a parallel multihole collimator.

7. Explain why the minimum resolution distance of an autofluoroscope is about equal to the width of a crystal in the detector mosaic.

8. *Scalloping* refers to the uneven borders of the image produced by a single-crystal rectilinear scanner. Explain why scalloping occurs. Why is scalloping enhanced if a longer time constant is used and reduced if a shorter time constant is used?

9. Explain the operation and usefulness of the contrast enhancement control of a rectilinear scanner.

°10. For an information density of 1,200 counts/sq cm, what scan speed is necessary if the line spacing is $\frac{1}{16}$ in. and the average count rate is 7,500 CPM?

11. Describe the reasons for limiting the useful range of a scintillation camera from about 70 keV to about 600 keV.

°For those problems marked with an asterisk, answers are provided on the pages following the appendixes (see pp. 487–488).

12. Explain why, compared to a parallel multihole collimator, a converging collimator yields superior images for small distributions of radioactivity.

REFERENCES
1. Johnson, D., et al.: Radiopulmonary Cardiography for Measurement of Central Mean Transit Time and Its Arterial and Venous Subdivisions, in Kniseley, R., Tauxe, W., and Anderson, E. (eds.): *Dynamic Clinical Studies with Radioisotopes* TID 7678 (Springfield, Va.: Clearinghouse for Federal Scientific and Technical Information, 1964), p. 249.
2. Taplin, G., Dore, E., and Johnson, D.: Hepatic Blood-Flow and Reticuloendothelial System Studies with Radiocolloids, in Kniseley, R., Tauxe, W., and Anderson, E. (eds.): *Dynamic Clinical Studies with Radioisotopes* TID 7678 (Springfield, Va.: Clearinghouse for Federal Scientific and Technical Information, 1964), p. 285.
3. Cassen, B., et al.: Instrumentation for ^{131}I use in medical studies, Nucleonics 9(2):46, 1951.
4. Anger, H.: Scintillation camera, Rev. Sci. Instrum. 29:27, 1958.
5. Sorenson, J.: Deadtime characteristics of Anger cameras, J. Nucl. Med. 16:284, 1975.
6. Bender, M., and Blau, M.: The autofluoroscope, Nucleonics 21:52, 1963.
7. Kirch, D., et al.: Application of a computerized image intensifier radionuclide imaging system to the study of regional left ventricular dysfunction, IEEE Trans. Nucl. Sci. NS-23:507, 1976.

15 / Roentgenography

THE EXPRESSION *roentgenography* refers to procedures for recording, displaying and using information carried to a film by an x-ray beam. Satisfactory images are recorded only if enough information is transmitted to the film by x rays emerging from the patient. Also, unnecessary information and background "noise" must not interfere with extraction of the information desired. Procedures for recording the information desired and for reducing extraneous information and noise are described in this chapter.

X-RAY FILM

X-ray film is available with an emulsion on one side (single-emulsion film) or both sides (double-emulsion film) of a transparent film base which is about 0.2 mm thick (Fig 15-1). The base is either cellulose acetate or a polyester resin. Single-emulsion film is less sensitive to radiation and is used primarily when exceptionally fine detail is required in the image. The emulsion is composed of silver halide granules, usually silver bromide, which are suspended in a gelatin matrix. The emulsion is covered with a protective coating (T coat) and is sensitive to visible and ultraviolet light and to ionizing radiation. Film used with intensifying screens is most sensitive to the wavelengths of light emitted by the screens. Nonscreen film is designed for direct exposure to x rays and is less sensitive to visible light.

The Photographic Process

The granules of silver bromide in the emulsion of an x-ray film are affected when the film is exposed to ionizing radiation or to visible light. Electrons are released as energy is absorbed from the incident radiation. These electrons are trapped at "sensitivity centers" in the crystal lattice of the silver bromide granules. The trapped electrons attract and neutralize mobile silver ions (Ag^+) in the lattice. Hence, small quantities of metallic silver are deposited in the emulsion, primarily along the surface of the silver bromide granules. Although these changes in the granules are not visible, the deposition of metallic silver across a film exposed to an x-ray beam is a reflection of the information transmitted to the film by the x radiation. This information has been captured and stored as a *latent image* in the photographic emulsion.

When the film is placed in a developing solution, additional silver is

Fig 15-1.—Cross section of an x-ray film. The base is cellulose acetate or a polyester resin, and the emulsion usually is silver bromide suspended in a gelatin matrix.

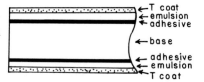

deposited at the sensitivity centers. Hence, the latent image induced by the radiation serves as a catalyst for the deposition of metallic silver upon the film base. No silver is deposited along granules that are unaffected during exposure of the film to radiation, and these granules are removed by sodium thiosulfate or ammonium thiosulfate present in the fixing solution. The fixing solution also contains potassium alum to harden the emulsion and acetic acid to neutralize residual developer present on the film. The degree of blackening of a region of the processed film depends on the amount of free silver deposited in the region and, consequently, on the number of x rays absorbed in the region.

Optical Density and Film Gamma

The amount of light transmitted by a region of processed film is described by the *transmittance T*, where

$$T = \frac{\text{Amount light transmitted by a region of film}}{\text{Amount light received at same location with film removed}}$$

(15-1)

The degree of blackening of a region of film is described as the *optical density (OD)* of the region. The optical density is

$$OD = \log\left(\frac{1}{T}\right) \tag{15-2}$$

Often, the optical density is referred to as the "density" of the film.

Example 15-1

A region of processed film transmits 10% ($T = 0.1$) of the incident light. What is the optical density of the region?

$$T = 0.1$$
$$OD = \log\left(\frac{1}{T}\right)$$
$$= \log\left(\frac{1}{0.1}\right)$$
$$= \log(10)$$
$$= 1$$

Example 15-2

A second film with a transmittance of 0.1 is superimposed over the film described in Example 15-1. What is the optical density of the combination?

The transmittance of the combination is

$$T = (0.1)(0.1) = 0.01$$

The optical density is

$$OD = \log\left(\frac{1}{T}\right)$$
$$= \log\left(\frac{1}{0.01}\right)$$
$$= \log(100)$$
$$= 2$$

The relationship between transmittance and optical density is depicted graphically in Figure 15-2. The optical density across most roentgenograms* varies from 0.3 to 2, corresponding to a range of trans-

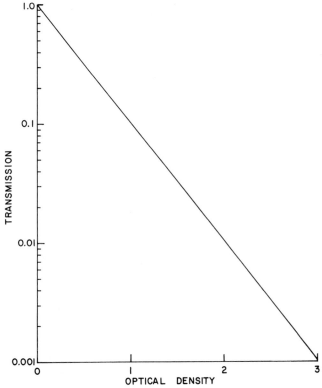

Fig 15-2.—The relationship between optical density and transmittance of x-ray film.

*A *roentgenogram* is a processed film that has been exposed to x radiation or to light from intensifying screens. A *roentgenographic image* is an image present on a roentgenogram.

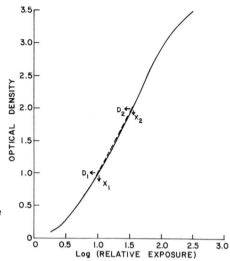

Fig 15-3.—Characteristic curve for an x-ray film. The average gradient for the film is 1.9 over the density range 1.0–2.0.

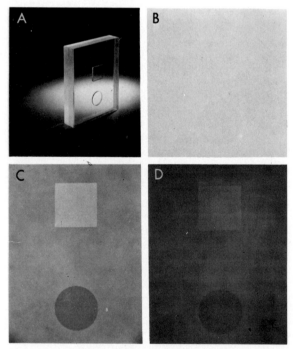

Fig 15-4.—Photograph **(A)** of a plastic test object and roentgenograms of the object obtained with screen-type films, and an exposure on the toe **(B)**, middle **(C)** and shoulder **(D)** of the characteristic curve. The contrast of the image is highest for the exposure on the straight-line portion of the curve. (Figures 15-4 to 15-10 from *Sensitometric Properties of X-ray Films* [Rochester, N.Y.: Radiography Markets Division, Eastman Kodak Company].)

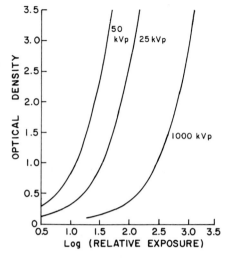

Fig 15-5. — Characteristic curves for a nonscreen x-ray film exposed to heavily filtered x-ray beams generated at different tube voltages. Developing conditions were constant for all curves.

mittance from 50% to 1%. Roentgenograms with an optical density greater than 2 usually must be viewed with a light source (a "hot light") more intense that the ordinary viewbox.

The optical density of a particular film or combination of film and intensifying screens may be plotted as a function of the exposure or [log (exposure)] to the film. The resulting curve is termed the *characteristic curve, sensitometric curve* or *H-D curve* for the particular film or film-screen combination (Fig 15-3). The expression "H-D curve" is derived from the names of Hurter and Driffield, who in 1890 first used characteristic curves to describe the response of photographic film to light. The

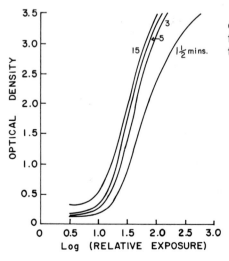

Fig 15-6. — Characteristic curves for a screen-type x-ray film developed for a series of times at 68 F.

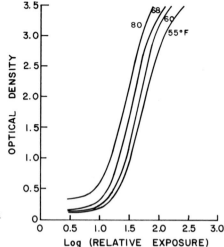

Fig 15-7.–Characteristic curves for a screen-type x-ray film developed for 5 minutes at a series of developing temperatures.

region below the essentially straight-line portion of the characteristic curve is referred to as the *toe* of the curve. The *shoulder* is the region of the curve above the straight-line portion. A roentgenogram with optical densities in the region of the toe or the shoulder furnishes an image with inferior contrast (Fig 15-4). The exposure range over which acceptable optical densities are produced is known as the *latitude* of the film. The shape of the characteristic curve for a particular film is affected by the quality of the x-ray beam used for the exposure (Fig 15-5) and by the conditions encountered during development (Figs 15-6 and 15-7). Consequently, the tube voltage used to generate the x-ray beam and the temperature, time and solutions used for processing the film should be stated when a characteristic curve for a particular film or film-screen combination is displayed.

The radiation exposure to an x-ray film should be sufficient to place the range of optical densities exhibited by the processed film along the essentially straight-line portion of the characteristic curve. The average slope of this portion of the curve is referred to as the *average gradient* of the film. The *average gradient* for a film is

$$\text{Average gradient} = \frac{D_2 - D_1}{\log X_2 - \log X_1} \tag{15-3}$$

where D_2 is the optical density resulting from an exposure X_2, and D_1 is the optical density produced by an exposure X_1 (Fig 15-3). Often, D_1 and D_2 are taken as optical densities of 0.3 and 2.0, respectively. Films with higher average gradients tend to furnish images with higher contrast

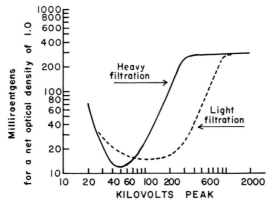

Fig 15-8.—Exposure for an optical density of 1.0 above base density, expressed as a function of the quality of the x-ray beam used to expose the film. The speed of the film is the reciprocal of the exposure in roentgens required for a density of 1.0 above base density.

(more blacks and whites and fewer shades of gray) than do films with lower values of the average gradient. Since contrast and latitude are reciprocally related, films with high average gradients also provide relatively short latitudes, and vice versa. The maximum value of the slope of the characteristic curve is termed the *gamma* (γ) of the film. The gamma for a film may be defined explicitly as the slope at the inflection point of the characteristic curve.

Example 15-3

In Figure 15-3, $D_2 = 2.0$, $\log X_2 = 1.52$, $D_1 = 1.0$ and $\log X_1 = 1.00$. What is the average gradient for the film in this region of optical density?

$$\text{Average gradient} = \frac{D_2 - D_1}{\log X_2 - \log X_1} \qquad (15\text{-}3)$$
$$= \frac{2.0 - 1.0}{1.52 - 1.00}$$
$$= 1.9$$

Film Speed

The length of the toe of a characteristic curve and the position of the characteristic curve along the exposure axis are described by the *film speed* or *film sensitivity*. The film speed is

$$\text{Film speed} = \frac{1}{\text{Exposure in R required for an } OD \text{ of 1.0 above base density}}$$
$$(15\text{-}4)$$

Example 15-4

What is the speed of the x-ray film in Figure 15-3, if 20 milliroentgens (mR) are required to produce an optical density of 1.0 above base density?

$$\text{Film speed} = \frac{1}{\text{Exposure in R required for an } OD \text{ of 1.0 above base density}}$$

$$= \frac{1}{0.02} \qquad (15\text{-}4)$$

$$= 50$$

The toe is short for high-speed film or film-screen combinations, and longer for film with lower speed. High-speed film is referred to as "fast" film and film with lower speed is said to be "slow." The speed of a film depends primarily on the size of the silver bromide granules in the emulsion. A film with large granules is faster than a film with smaller granules. Speed is gained by requiring fewer x-ray or light photons to form an image. Hence, a fast film furnishes a "noisier" roentgenographic image in which fine detail in the object may be less visible (see chap. 18).

Film speed varies with the energy of the x rays used to expose the film (Fig 15-8). For nonscreen film, the film speed is greatest when the spectral distribution of the x-ray beam is centered over the K-absorption edge (25 keV) of silver.

Film Reciprocity

For most exposure rates encountered in roentgenography, the shape of the characteristic curve is unaffected by changes in the rate of exposure of the film to x radiation. The independence of optical density and exposure rate is referred to as the *reciprocity law*. The reciprocity law sometimes fails if a film is exposed at either a very high or a very low exposure rate. In these situations, a particular exposure delivered at a very high or very low rate provides an optical density less than that furnished by an exposure delivered at a rate nearer optimum. However, a decrease in optical density usually is not noticeable unless the film is exposed with intensifying screens and unless the exposure rate differs from the optimum by a factor of at least eight.[1] For film exposed with rare earth intensifying screens, failure of the reciprocity law has been observed over a more restricted range of exposure rates.[2]

Inherent Optical Density and Film Fogging

The optical density of film processed without exposure to radiation is referred to as the *inherent optical density (base density)* of the film. The inherent optical density is a reflection primarily of the absorption of light in the film base, which may be tinted slightly. Most x-ray film has an inherent optical density of about 0.07.

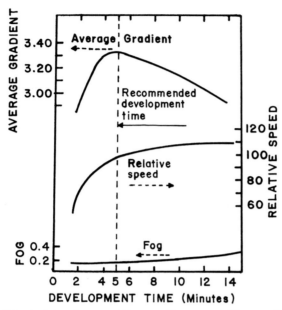

Fig 15-9. — Effect of development time on film speed, film gradient and fog.

Fogging of an x-ray film is caused by the deposition of metallic silver without exposure to radiation and by the undesired exposure of a film to radiation (usually background radiation). For example, an exposure as small as 1 mR to a high-speed film may produce a significant amount of fogging. The optical density attributable to fog may be as low as 0.05 for fresh film but increases with the storage time of the film, particularly if the temperature of the storage facility is not below room temperature. An inherent-plus-fog optical density greater than 0.2 is considered excessive.[3]

Processing X-Ray Film

Properties of x-ray film that affect the quality of a roentgenographic image include contrast, speed and the ability of the film to record fine detail. Any two of these properties may be improved at the expense of the third, and a particular type of film is chosen only after a compromise has been reached among the various properties.

The properties of x-ray film are affected to some extent by the conditions encountered during processing. The speed of an x-ray film increases initially with development time. With a long development time, however, film speed reaches a plateau and even may decrease (Fig 15-9). Fogging of an x-ray film increases with time spent in the developing solution. The average gradient of a film increases initially with develop-

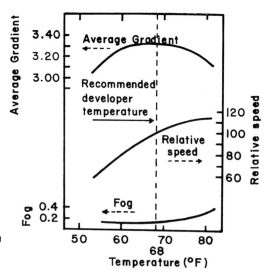

Fig 15-10. — Effect of temperature of the developing solution on film speed, fog and inherent contrast.

ment time and then decreases. The development time recommended by the supplier of a particular type of x-ray film is selected to provide acceptable film contrast and speed with minimum fogging of the film.

The temperature of the developing solution also affects film speed, fog and contrast (Fig 15-10). For films processed manually, a temperature of 68 F usually is recommended for the developing solution, and the development time is chosen to furnish satisfactory contrast and speed with minimum fogging. With automatic, high-speed processors, the temperature of the developing solution is elevated greatly (85–95 F), and the development time is reduced. The relationship between development time and temperature of the developing solution is illustrated in Table 15-1.

TABLE 15-1. — RELATIONSHIP BETWEEN
DEVELOPMENT TIME AND
TEMPERATURE OF DEVELOPING
SOLUTION FOR PARTICULAR
X-RAY FILM*

DEVELOPER TEMPERATURE (°F)	DEVELOPMENT TIME (min)
60	9
65	6
68	5
70	4¼
75	3

* From Seemann.[3]

Contrast, speed and fog are not affected greatly by changes in the fixation time or the temperature of the fixing solution. However, a decrease in film speed and contrast and an increase in film fog may be noticeable if the fixation time is prolonged greatly.

Film Resolution

The *resolution* (detail, definition, sharpness) of roentgenographic and fluoroscopic images is discussed in detail in Chapter 18. In general, resolution describes the ability of an x-ray film or a fluoroscopic screen to furnish an image that depicts differences in the transmission of radiation by adjacent small regions of a patient. A detector with "good" or "high" resolution provides an image with a good rendition of fine structures in the patient. A detector with "poor" or "coarse" resolution furnishes an image that depicts only relatively large anatomical structures in the patient.

Xeroradiography and Ionic Radiography

X-ray film is expensive and is not reusable, although unused silver can be retrieved from processing solutions. Hence, alternate methods for recording the roentgenographic image are of considerable interest. One alternate method is xeroradiography, in which a positively charged selenium plate replaces the x-ray film. When the selenium plate is exposed to radiation, the positive charge is reduced in different regions across the plate, depending upon the exposure delivered to each region. The resulting distribution in residual positive charge constitutes a latent image on the plate. The latent image is developed by dusting a plastic sheet over the plate with a blue developing powder called *toner*. The amount of toner collected in each region depends on the residual positive charge of the region. After the toner has settled, it is fixed into position and the

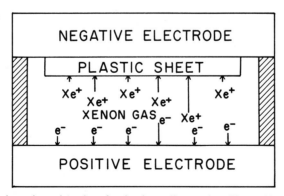

Fig 15-11.—Imaging chamber for ionic radiography. (From Hendee, W., Chaney, E., and Rossi, R.: *Radiologic Physics, Equipment and Quality Control* [Chicago: Year Book Medical Publishers, Inc., 1977].)

sheet is removed and viewed by reflected light. Because the toner tends to accumulate at boundaries where the distribution of positive charge is changing, the xeroradiographic process enhances the image of edges between different structures in the patient.[4] Xeroradiography is considered by many clinicians to be the preferred imaging technique for mammography. Other applications such as identification of hairline fractures in the extremities are being developed for this technique.

A related substitute for x-ray film is electronic or ionic radiography. In this approach, an uncharged plastic sheet is placed on the negative electrode of an exposure chamber containing xenon gas under pressure (Fig 15-11). During exposure of the chamber, the xenon gas is ionized and the positive ions are collected by the plastic sheet. In each region of the sheet, the positive charge collected depends on the amount of ionization occurring in the chamber immediately below the region. This distribution of positive charge contributes a latent image. As in xeroradiography, the latent image may be developed with a dry powder, although processing with wet chemicals has been more successful with ionography. Since the plastic sheet is transparent, it may be viewed with transmitted light from a conventional viewbox. Although ionic radiography is a relatively recent development, it is a promising replacement for x-ray film.

INTENSIFYING SCREENS

For an x-ray beam of diagnostic quality, only about 2–6% of the total energy in the beam is absorbed in the emulsion of an x-ray film exposed directly to the beam. The amount of energy absorbed is even smaller for x rays of greater energy. Consequently, direct exposure of film to x rays is a very inefficient utilization of energy available in the x-ray beam. This procedure is used only when images with very fine detail are required. For most roentgenographic examinations, the x-ray film is sandwiched between *intensifying screens*. The intensifying screens furnish a light image that reflects the variation in exposure across the x-ray beam. This light image is recorded by film that is sensitive to the wavelengths of

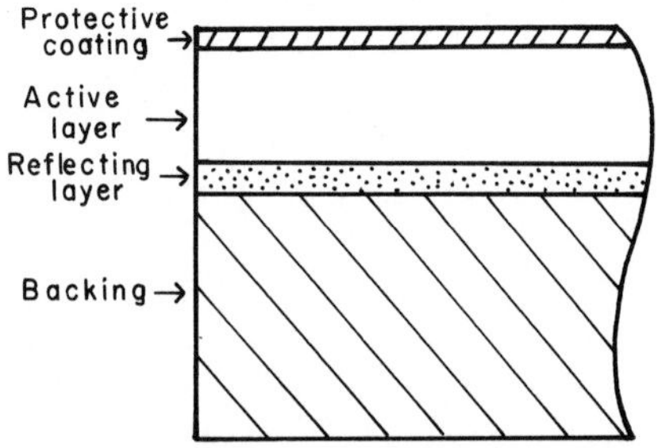

Fig 15-12. — Construction of a typical intensifying screen.

Protective coating →
Active layer →
Reflecting layer →
Backing →

light emitted by the screen. The mechanism for the radiation-induced fluorescence of an x-ray intensifying screen is similar to that discussed in Chapter 11 for a NaI(Tl) scintillation crystal.

Composition and Properties

The construction of an intensifying screen is diagramed in Figure 15-12. The backing is cardboard, plastic or, less frequently, metal. The backing is coated with a white pigment which reflects light. The reflecting layer is covered by an active layer, which is composed of small granules of fluorescent material embedded in a plastic matrix. The granule diameters range from about 4 to about 8 microns. The thickness of the active layer ranges from perhaps 50 μ for a detail screen to about 300 μ for a fast screen. The active layer is protected by a coating about 0.001 in. thick, which is transparent to the light produced in the active layer.

Desirable properties of an x-ray intensifying screen include:

1. A high attenuation coefficient for x rays of diagnostic quality.

2. A high efficiency for the conversion of energy in the x-ray beam to light.

3. A high transparency to light released by the fluorescent granules.

4. A low refractive index so that light from the granules will be released from the screen and will not be reflected internally.

5. An insensitivity to handling.

6. An emission spectrum for the radiation-induced fluorescence which matches the spectral sensitivity of the film used.

For use with conventional x-ray film, the light should fall in the blue-violet or near-ultraviolet range of wavelengths.

7. A reasonably short time for fluorescence decay.

8. A minimum loss of light by lateral diffusion through the fluorescent layer. To reduce this loss of light, the fluorescent layer is composed of granules and is not constructed as a single sheet of fluorescent material.

9. Low cost.

Crystalline calcium tungstate, with an emission spectrum peaked at 4,200 Å, is the fluor used in most x-ray intensifying screens. For most calcium tungstate screens, the efficiency is about 20–50% for the conversion of energy in the x-ray beam to light.[5, 6] Barium lead sulfate, with an emission spectrum peaked in the ultraviolet region (3,600 Å), is used also as a fluorescent material in intensifying screens. This material is useful particularly for roentgenography at higher tube voltages. Zinc sulfide (4,400 Å) is used occasionally in intensifying screens, particularly for radiography at lower tube voltages. Ter-Pogossian[7] has shown that screens with fluorescent layers of potassium iodide activated with thallium (4,300 Å) are five times faster than medium-speed calcium tungstate screens and provide almost the same resolution.

The K-absorption edge (69.5 keV) of tungsten, the principal absorbing element in calcium tungstate screens, is above the energy of most photons in a diagnostic x-ray beam. Increased absorption of diagnostic x rays would occur if tungsten were replaced by an absorbing element of reduced Z with a K-absorption edge in the range of 35 to 50 keV. Elements with K-absorption edges in this energy range include rare earth elements such as gadolinium, lanthanum and yttrium. These elements, complexed in oxysulfide or oxybromide crystals and embedded in a plastic matrix, have been introduced recently as substitutes for calcium tungstate in intensifying screens. Rare earth screens exhibit not only an increased absorption of diagnostic x rays but also an increased efficiency in the conversion of absorbed x-ray energy to light. Hence, rare earth screens are faster than their calcium tungstate counterparts. This increased speed facilitates one or more of the following changes in radiographic technique:

1. Reduced exposure time and decreased motion unsharpness in the image.
2. Reduced tube current and more frequent use of small focal spots.
3. Reduced tube voltage and improved contrast in the image.
4. Reduced production of heat in the x-ray tube.
5. Reduced patient exposure.

Although some rare earth screens emit blue light and can be used with conventional x-ray film, others emit yellow-green light and must be used with special yellow-green–sensitive film.[8]

The efficiency with which energy in an x-ray beam is converted to light increases with the thickness of the fluorescent layer. Hence, the

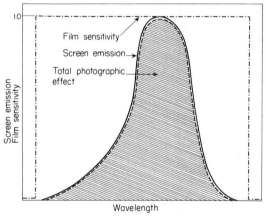

Fig 15-13.—The total photographic effect obtained by combining an intensifying screen and a photographic film with a wavelength sensitivity that extends above and below the emission spectrum for the screen.

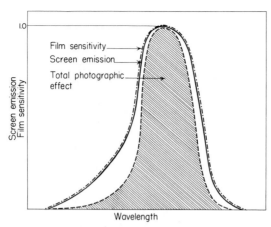

Film sensitivity

Screen emission

Total photographic effect

Wavelength

Fig 15-14. — The total photographic effect is reduced if the spectral sensitivity of the film is matched too closely to the emission spectrum of the intensifying screen.

efficiency of energy conversion is greater for a screen with a thick emulsion (i.e., a fast screen) than for a screen of medium speed (a par-speed screen) or for a slow screen (a detail screen). However, the resolution of the roentgenographic image decreases with increasing speed of the intensifying screen. For example, the maximum resolution is 6–9 lines/mm for a typical fast screen, 8–10 lines/mm for a par-speed screen and 10–15 lines/mm for a detail screen when measured under laboratory conditions. The resolution obtained clinically with these screens usually is considerably less.

The wavelength of light emitted by an intensifying screen should correspond closely with the spectral sensitivity of the film used. Usually, the sensitivity of the film extends to wavelengths both above and below those emitted by the screen (Fig 15-13). The total photographic effect is decreased if the spectral sensitivity of the film is matched too closely to the emission spectrum for the screen (Fig 15-14).

The *intensification factor* of a particular screen-film combination is the ratio of exposures required to produce an optical density of 1.0 without and with the screen in position.

$$\text{Intensification factor} = \frac{\text{Exposure required to produce an } OD \text{ of } 1.0 \text{ without screen}}{\text{Exposure required to produce an } OD \text{ of } 1.0 \text{ with screen}}$$

(15-5)

The intensification factor for a particular screen-film combination varies greatly with the energy of the x rays used for the radiation exposure.

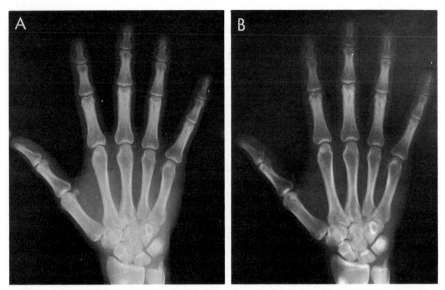

Fig 15-15. — Effect of intensifying screens on exposure time and image detail. **A,** roentgenogram exposed without a screen and requiring 125 mAs. **B,** roentgenogram exposed with a fast calcium tungstate screen and requiring 7 mAs.

Usually, a double-emulsion film is sandwiched in a cassette between two intensifying screens. In some cassettes, the fluorescent layer behind the film is thicker than the layer in front. The resolution of the roentgenographic image is reduced severely if both screens are not in firm contact with the entire surface of the film.

A reduction in exposure time is the major advantage of x-ray intensifying screens. Shorter exposures reduce the loss in resolution caused by voluntary and involuntary motion of the patient. Also, the exposure of the patient to radiation is reduced if a shorter exposure time is used. Shown in Figure 15-15 are roentgenograms obtained with and without a fast calcium tungstate screen. The film exposed without a screen required an exposure of 125 mAs. An exposure of 7 mAs was required for the film exposed with the intensifying screen.

The influence of scattered radiation on the roentgenographic image is reduced somewhat when intensifying screens are used, because scattered x rays with reduced energy are absorbed preferentially in the upper portions of the phosphor layer of the screen. Many of the light photons produced by these scattered x rays are absorbed before they reach the film.

A few precautions are necessary to prevent damage to an intensifying screen. For example, cassettes with intensifying screens should be loaded carefully with film to prevent scratching of the screen surface and accumulation of electric charge, which can produce images of static discharges on the roentgenogram. Moisture on the screen may cause the film to adhere to the screen. When the film and screen are separated, part of the screen may be removed. A screen may be stained permanently by liquids such as developing solution, and care must be taken to insure that liquids are not splashed onto the screen. The surface of the screen must be kept clean and free from lint and other particulate matter. Although screens may be washed with a soap solution or a weak wetting agent, organic solvents should be avoided because the active layer may be softened or otherwise damaged by these materials.

RADIOGRAPHIC GRIDS

Information is transmitted to an x-ray film by unattenuated primary radiation emerging from a patient. Radiation scattered within the patient and impinging on the film tends to conceal this information by producing a general photographic fog on the film. The amount of radiation scattered to a film increases with the volume of tissue exposed to the x-ray beam. Hence, a significant reduction in scattered radiation may be achieved by confining the x-ray beam to just the region of interest within the patient. In fact, proper collimation of an x-ray beam is essential to the production of roentgenograms of highest quality.

Much of the scattered radiation that would reduce the quality of the roentgenographic image may be removed by a radiographic grid between the patient and the x-ray film or screen-film combination. A radio-

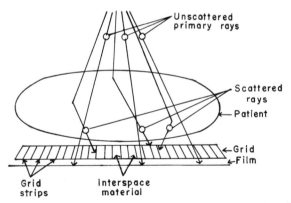

Fig 15-16.—A radiographic grid is used to remove scattered radiation emerging from the patient. Most primary photons are transmitted through the grid without attenuation.

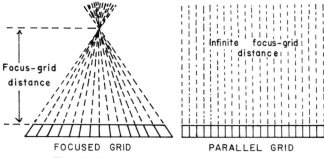

Fig 15-17. — A focused and a parallel grid.

graphic grid is composed of strips of a dense, high-Z material separated by a material that is relatively transparent to x rays. The first radiographic grid was designed by Bucky in 1913. The ability of a grid to remove scattered radiation is depicted in Figure 15-16.

Construction of Grids

Ideally, the thickness of the strips in a radiographic grid should be reduced until images of the strips are not visible in the roentgenographic image. Additionally, the strips should be completely opaque to scattered radiation and should not release characteristic x rays ("grid fluorescence") as scattered x-ray photons are absorbed. These requirements are satisfied rather well by lead foil about 0.05 mm thick, and this material is used for the strips in most radiographic grids. Although grid strips of gold or platinum might have some advantages over lead strips, the high cost of these materials virtually prohibits their use. Grids have been designed with tungsten and uranium strips, but the difficulty of constructing these grids has precluded their use in clinical radiology.[9, 10]

The interspace material between the grid strips may be aluminum, fiber or plastic. Although fiber and plastic transmit primary photons with almost no attenuation, grids with aluminum interspaces are sturdier. Also, grids with aluminum interspaces may furnish slightly greater re-

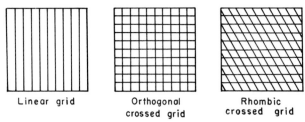

Linear grid   Orthogonal crossed grid   Rhombic crossed grid

Fig 15-18. — Types of focused and parallel grids: linear, orthogonal crossed and rhombic crossed.

duction of the scattered radiation, because scattered x-ray photons that escape the grid strips may be absorbed in the aluminum interspaces.[11]

Types of Grids

Radiographic grids are available commercially with "parallel" or "focused" grid strips in either linear or crossed grid configurations (Figs 15-17 and 15-18). When a focused grid is positioned at the correct distance from the target of an x-ray tube, lines through the grid strips are directed toward a point or "focus" on the target. The focus-grid distance approaches infinity for a grid with parallel strips. With a parallel grid positioned at a finite distance from an x-ray tube, more primary x rays are attenuated along the edge of the roentgenogram than at the center. Consequently, the optical density decreases slightly from the center to the edge of a roentgenogram exposed with a parallel grid. The uniformity of optical density is improved in a roentgenogram exposed with a focused grid, provided the grid is positioned correctly.

A linear grid is constructed with all parallel or focused grid strips in line (Fig 15-18). A crossed grid is made by placing one linear grid on top of another, with the strips in one grid perpendicular to those in the other. In most situations, a crossed grid removes more scattered radiation than a linear grid with the same grid ratio (see below), because a linear grid does not absorb photons scattered parallel to the grid strips. However, a linear grid is easier to use in situations where proper alignment of the x-ray tube, grid and film cassette is difficult.

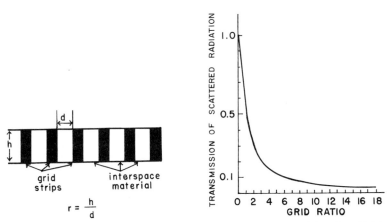

Fig 15-19 (left). — The grid ratio r is the height h of the grid strips divided by the distance between the strips.

Fig 15-20 (right). — The effectiveness of a radiographic grid for removing scattered radiation is pronounced for small grid ratios, but increases only gradually with grid ratios above 8. (Courtesy of S. Ledin and The Elema Shönander Co.)

Describing Radiographic Grids

A grid usually is described in terms of its *grid ratio* (Fig 15-19):

$$\text{Grid ratio} = \frac{\text{Height of grid strips}}{\text{Distance between grid strips}} \qquad (15\text{-}6)$$

$$r = \frac{h}{d}$$

The grid ratio of a crossed grid is $r_1 + r_2$, where r_1 and r_2 are the grid ratios of the linear grids used to form the crossed grid. Radiographic grids are available commercially with grid ratios as high as 16. However, grids with ratios of 8–12 are used most frequently, because the removal of scattered radiation is increased only slightly with grids with a higher ratio. Also, grids with a high grid ratio are difficult to align and require a greater exposure of the patient to radiation. The effectiveness of a radiographic grid for removing scattered radiation is illustrated in Figure 15-20 as a function of grid ratio.

The improvement in radiographic contrast provided by grids with different grid ratios is depicted in Table 15-2. From data in this table, it is apparent that: (1) all grids improve radiographic contrast significantly; (2) the effectiveness of a grid for improving radiographic contrast increases with the grid ratio; (3) the increase in radiographic contrast provided by a grid is less for an x-ray beam generated at a higher voltage; (4) a crossed grid removes scattered radiation more effectively than a linear grid with an equal grid ratio; and (5) the radiation exposure of the patient increases with the grid ratio. The exposure must be increased because the film is exposed to fewer scattered x-ray photons. Also, more primary x-ray photons are absorbed by the grid strips.

TABLE 15-2.—RELATIVE INCREASE IN RADIOGRAPHIC
CONTRAST AND RADIATION EXPOSURE FOR GRIDS WITH
DIFFERENT RATIOS*†

TYPE OF GRID AND GRID RATIO	IMPROVEMENT IN CONTRAST			INCREASE IN EXPOSURE		
	70 kVp	95 kVp	120 kVp	70 kVp	95 kVp	120 kVp
None	1	1	1	1	1	1
5 linear	3.5	2.5	2	3	3	3
8 linear	4.75	3.25	2.5	3.5	3.75	4
12 linear	5.25	3.75	3	4	4.25	5
16 linear	5.75	4	3.25	4.5	5	6
5 cross	5.75	3.5	2.75	4.5	5	5.5
8 cross	6.75	4.25	3.25	5	6	7

*From *Characteristics and Applications of X-Ray Grids*.[12]
†Thickness of the grid strips and interspaces were identical for all grids.

A radiographic grid is not described explicitly by the grid ratio alone, because the grid ratio may be increased by increasing the height of the grid strips or by reducing the width of the interspaces. Consequently, the number of *grid strips per inch* (or per cm) usually is stated with the grid ratio. Grids with many strips ("lines") per inch produce shadows in the roentgenographic image that may be less distracting than those produced by thicker strips in a grid with fewer strips per inch. Grids with as many as 110 strips/in. are available commercially. The *lead content* of the grid in units of grams per square centimeter sometimes is stated with the grid ratio and the number of strips per inch.

The *contrast improvement factor* for a grid is the quotient of the maximum radiographic contrast obtainable with the grid divided by the maximum contrast obtainable with the grid removed. The contrast improvement factor may be used to compare the effectiveness of different grids for removing scattered radiation. The contrast improvement factor for a particular grid varies with the thickness of the patient and with the cross-sectional area and energy of the x-ray beam. Usually, the contrast improvement factor is measured with a water phantom 20 cm thick irradiated by an x-ray beam generated at 100 kVp.[13]

The *selectivity* of a grid is the ratio of primary to scattered radiation transmitted by the grid. The efficiency of a grid for removing scattered radiation is described occasionally as *grid clean-up.* Grids may be described as "heavy" or "light," depending upon their lead content. One popular but rather ambiguous description of grid effectiveness is the *Bucky factor,* defined as the exposure to the film without the grid divided by the exposure to the film with the grid in place and exposed to a wide x-ray field emerging from a thick patient.

Moving Grids

The image of grid strips in a roentgenogram may be distracting to the observer. Also, grid strip shadows sometimes interfere with the identification of small structures such as blood vessels and trabeculae of bone. In 1920, Potter developed the moving grid, referred to as the *Potter-Bucky diaphragm,* which removes the distracting image of grid strips by blurring their image across the film. Early Potter-Bucky diaphragms moved in one direction only. Modern moving grids use a reciprocating motion, with the grid making several transits back and forth during an exposure. The linear distance over which the grid moves is small (1–5 cm) and permits the use of a focused grid. The motion of the grid must not be parallel to the grid strips and must be rapid enough to move the image of a number of strips across each location in the film during exposure. The motion of the grid must be adjusted to prevent synchronization between the position of the grid strips and the rate of pulsation of the x-

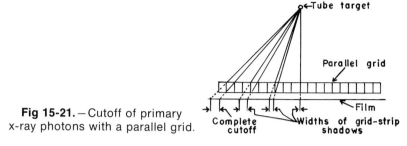

Fig 15-21. — Cutoff of primary x-ray photons with a parallel grid.

ray beam. The direction of motion of the grid changes very rapidly at the limits of grid travel, and the "dwell time" of the grid at these limits is insignificant.

Orthogonal crossed grids are not used often as moving grids. Rhombic crossed grids used in "super-speed recipromatic diaphragms" provide excellent removal of scattered radiation with no image of the grid strips in the roentgenogram. The travel of the grid is very short and does not cause significant off-center cutoff (see below). Most stationary radiographic tables contain a recipromatic Potter-Bucky diaphragm. However, the development of grids with many strips per inch has reduced the need for moving grids. The maintenance cost for reciprocating grids and their poor efficiency for removing the image of grid strips during short exposure times enhance the attractiveness of stationary grids that contain many strips per inch.

The choice of a radiographic grid for a particular examination depends on factors such as the amount of primary and scattered radiation emerging from the patient, the energy of x rays in the x-ray beam and the variety of radiographic techniques provided by the x-ray generator.[12]

Grid Cutoff

The expression "grid cutoff" is used to describe the loss of primary radiation caused by improper alignment of a radiographic grid. With a parallel grid, cutoff occurs near the edges of a large field because grid strips intercept many primary photons along the edges of the x-ray beam. The width of the shadow of grid strips in a parallel grid increases with distance from the center of the grid (Fig 15-21).

The use of a focused grid at an incorrect target-grid distance also causes grid cutoff. This effect is termed *axial decentering* or *off-distance cutoff* and is depicted in Figure 15-22. The optical density of a roentgenogram with off-distance cutoff decreases from the center of the roentgenogram outward. The variation in optical density increases with displacement of the grid from the correct target-grid distance. However, the effect is not objectionable until the displacement exceeds the target-grid distance limits established for the grid. The limits for the target-grid dis-

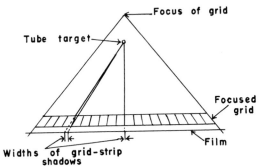

Fig 15-22. — Off-distance cutoff with a focused grid.

tance are narrow for grids with a high grid ratio and wider for grids with a smaller ratio. The effects of off-distance cutoff are more severe when the target-grid distance is shorter than that recommended, and less severe when the target-grid distance is greater.

Lateral decentering or *off-center cutoff* occurs when rays parallel to the strips of a focused grid converge at a location that is displaced laterally from the target of the x-ray tube (Fig 15-23). *Off-level cutoff* results from tilting of the grid (Fig 15-24). Both off-center cutoff and off-level cutoff cause an overall reduction in optical density across the roentgenogram. The importance of correct alignment of the x-ray tube, grid and film increases with the grid ratio.

Air Grids

The amount of scattered radiation reaching an x-ray film or film-screen combination may be reduced somewhat by increasing the distance between the patient and the film. This procedure is referred to as air filtration or using an air grid, and is most effective at low tube voltages, because low-energy x rays are scattered at a wide angle. The use of an air grid is accompanied by magnification of the image and an increase in geometric unsharpness (see chaps. 17 and 18).

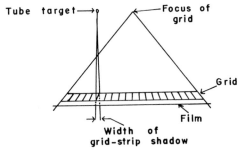

Fig 15-23. — Off-center cutoff with a focused grid.

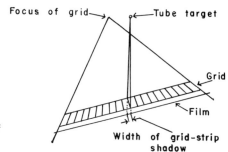

Fig 15-24. — Off-level cutoff with a focused grid.

Moving Slit Radiography

More efficient techniques for removal of scattered radiation have been sought for many years. One technique that has been proposed periodically is moving slit radiography, in which one or more slits in an otherwise x-ray opaque shield move above the patient in synchrony with an equal number of slits in a shield between the patient and the film (Fig 15-25). The long, narrow x-ray beams emerging through the upper slits are scanned across the patient and transmitted to the film through the lower slits below the patient. Radiation scattered by the patient is intercepted by the opaque shield below the patient and does not reach the film. The principal disadvantage of moving slit radiography is the possibility of image distortion due to motion during the time required for the x-ray beam(s) to scan across the patient. This disadvantage is less cumbersome with newer, "fast" x-ray systems using high-mA generators and rare earth intensifying screens.[14]

Fig 15-25. — Moving slit approach to rejection of scattered radiation. (From Hendee, W., Chaney, E., and Rossi, R.: *Radiologic Physics, Equipment and Quality Control* [Chicago: Year Book Medical Publishers, Inc., 1977].)

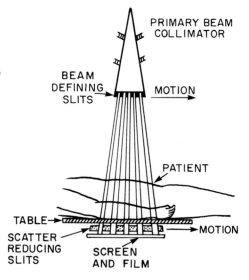

PROBLEMS

°1. Adjacent regions of a roentgenogram have optical densities of 1.0 and 1.5. What is the difference in the transmission of light through the two regions?

°2. Optical densities of 1.0 and 1.5 are measured for adjacent regions of a roentgenogram obtained with x-ray film with a film gamma of 1.0. If the exposure was 40 mR to the region with an optical density of 1.0, what was the exposure to the region with an optical density of 1.5?

3. Explain why poor contact between an intensifying screen and an x-ray film reduces the resolution of the roentgenographic image.

4. The effective atomic number is greater for barium lead sulfate than for calcium sulfate or zinc sulfide. Explain why intensifying screens of barium lead sulfate are particularly useful for roentgenography at higher tube voltages.

5. Explain the meaning of the expressions "grid cutoff," "off-distance cutoff," "off-center cutoff" and "off-level cutoff."

6. Explain why a crossed grid provides a greater contrast improvement factor than a linear grid with the same grid ratio.

7. Discuss the relationships between average gradient, film contrast and latitude.

8. Define film speed and discuss its significance.

9. Describe the principal of moving slit radiography.

10. Describe two reasons why rare earth screens are faster than conventional calcium tungstate screens.

11. Discuss the principal of xeroradiography and ionic radiography.

REFERENCES

1. Ter-Pogossian, M.: *The Physical Aspects of Diagnostic Radiology* (New York: Harper & Row, 1967).

2. Arnold, B., Eisenberg, H., and Bjärngard, B.: Measurements of reciprocity law failure in green-sensitive x-ray films, Radiology 126:493, 1978.

3. Seemann, H.: *Physical and Photographic Principles of Medical Radiography* (New York: John Wiley & Sons, Inc., 1968), p. 69.

4. Jaeger, S., Cacak, R., Barnes, J., and Hendee, W.: Optimization of xeroradiographic exposures, Radiology 128:217, 1978.

5. Coltman, J., Ebbighauser, E., and Altar, W.: Physical properties of calcium tungstate x-ray screens, J. Appl. Phys. 18:530, 1947.

6. Towers, S.: X-ray intensifying screens: Part I, X-Ray Focus 8 (1):2, 1967.

7. Ter-Pogossian, M.: The Efficiency of Radiographic Intensifying Screens, in Moseley, R., and Rust, J. (eds.): *The Reduction of Patient Dose by Diagnostic Radiologic Instrumentation* (Springfield, Ill.: Charles C Thomas, Publisher, 1964), p. 259.

8. Rossi, R., Hendee, W., and Ahrens, C.: An evaluation of rare earth screen/film combinations, Radiology 121:465, 1976.

9. Reiss, K.: Wolfram-viellinienraster, ein neues Hilfsmittel der Röntgendiagnostik, Röntgen-u. Laboratoriumspraxis 14:222, 1961.

10. Ter-Pogossian, M., and Ledin, S.: Uranium x-ray grids, Radiology 75:797, 1960.

11. Hondius-Boldingh, W.: *Grids to Reduce Scattered X-Rays in Medical Ra-*

°For those problems marked with an asterisk, answers are provided on the pages following the appendixes (see pp. 487–488).

diography, Philips Research Reports Supplement 1 (Eindhoven, Netherlands: Philips Research Laboratories, 1964).

12. *Characteristics and Applications of X-Ray Grids* (Cincinnati: Liebel-Flarsheim Co., 1968).

13. International Commission on Radiological Units and Measurements: *Methods of Evaluating Radiological Equipment and Materials.* Recommendations of the ICRU, Report 10f. National Bureau of Standards Handbook 89, 1963.

14. Barnes, G., Cleare, H., and Brezovich, I.: Reduction of scatter in diagnostic radiology by means of a scanning multiple slit assembly, Radiology 120:691, 1976.

16 / Fluoroscopy

INFORMATION ABOUT moving structures within a patient may be obtained with roentgenograms exposed in rapid succession. However, the interval of time between serially exposed films may be too long to provide complete information about dynamic processes within the body. Furthermore, x-ray films must be processed before they can be studied. Consequently, a technique is required to furnish images that reflect instantaneous changes occurring in the patient. This technique is referred to as *fluoroscopy*.

FLUOROSCOPY WITHOUT IMAGE INTENSIFICATION

In early fluoroscopic techniques, x rays emerging from the patient impinged directly on a fluoroscopic screen. Light was emitted from each region of the screen in response to the rate at which energy was deposited by the incident x rays. The light image on the fluoroscopic screen was viewed by the radiologist from a distance of 10 or 15 in. A thin plate of lead glass on the back of the fluoroscopic screen shielded the radiologist from x radiation transmitted by the screen.

Using this fluoroscopic technique, the radiologist perceived a very dim image with poor visibility of detail. In recent years, much effort has been directed toward improvement of the fluoroscopic image. This effort has resulted in development of the image intensifier and the light amplifier, devices that increase the brightness of the fluoroscopic image. Although these components have increased the cost and complexity of fluoroscopic equipment, they also have improved the fluoroscopic image so significantly that fluoroscopy without image intensification is now considered outmoded.

FLUOROSCOPY WITH IMAGE INTENSIFICATION

Radiologists recognized many years ago that the poor visibility of image detail in fluoroscopy was related to the dim image presented by early fluoroscopes.[1, 2] These persons emphasized the need for brighter fluoroscopic images and encouraged the development of the *image intensifier*. Image intensifiers increase the brightness of the fluoroscopic image and permit the observer to use photopic (cone) vision in place of the scotopic (rod) vision required with earlier fluoroscopes. Because of the brighter images, dark adaptation is not required for fluoroscopy with image intensification.

X-Ray Image Intensifier Tubes

An image intensifier tube is diagramed in Figure 16-1. X-ray photons impinge upon a fluorescent screen (input screen) which is 5–12 in. in diameter and slightly convex in shape. The fluorescent emulsion is a thin layer of ZnS:CdS:Ag or, in newer intensifiers, CsI. The principal advantage of CsI over ZnS:CdS:Ag is the increased absorption of x rays because of the presence of higher-Z components in the CsI phosphor, and because of the increased packing density of CsI molecules in the phosphor granules.

For each x-ray photon absorbed, 2,000–3,000 photons of light are emitted by the screen. These light photons are not observed directly. Instead, the light falls on a photocathode composed of Sb-Cs (an S-9 photocathode), Sb-CsO (an S-11 photocathode) or Sb-K-Na-Cs (an S-20 photocathode).[3] Light photons that are released in a direction away from the photocathode are reflected toward the photocathode by an aluminum support on the outside surface of the input screen. If the spectral sensitivity of the photocathode is matched to the wavelength of light emitted by the screen, then 15–20 electrons are ejected from the photocathode for every 100 photons of light received. The number of electrons released from any region of the photocathode depends upon the number of light photons incident upon the region. The electrons are accelerated through a potential difference of 25–35 kV between the photocathode

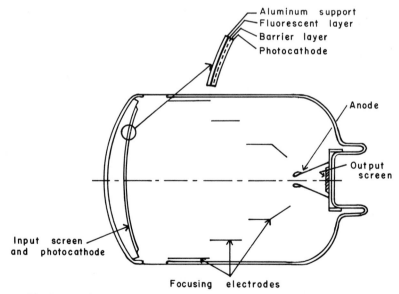

Fig 16-1. — Cross section of a typical x-ray image intensifier tube.

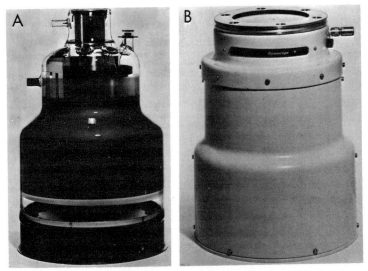

Fig 16-2.—A, image intensifier tube with an input screen 9 in. in diameter. **B,** the tube encased in its housing. (Courtesy of Machlett Laboratories, Inc.)

and the anode of the image intensifier tube. The electrons pass through a large hole in the anode and strike a small fluorescent screen (output screen) mounted on a flat glass support. The emulsion on the output screen resembles that for the input screen, except that the fluorescent granules are much smaller. Diameters of most output screens range from $\frac{1}{2}$ to 1 in. Intensifiers with small output screens are used frequently for television fluoroscopy, because the diameter of the input screen of a television pickup device is small also. A coating of metal, usually aluminum, is deposited on the output screen to prevent the entrance of light from outside the intensifier. The metallic layer also removes electrons accumulated by the output screen.

Electrons from the photocathode are focused on the output screen by cylindrical electrodes positioned between the photocathode and the anode. Usually, three focusing electrodes are used. To protect the input screen from vapors released from the photocathode, a thin (e.g., 0.2 mm) barrier of glass or other transparent material is interposed between the fluorescent screen and the photocathode. The entire assembly is enclosed within an evacuated glass envelope with walls from 2 to 4 mm thick. Residual atoms of gas inside the intensifier are ionized by a sputter ion pump and collected by electrodes before they interfere with the motion of electrons between the photocathode and the anode. The glass envelope is coated to prevent light from entering the tube (Fig 16-2). The glass envelope is contained within a housing of mu metal, an alloy containing iron. The housing attenuates magnetic fields that originate outside the intensifier and prevents these fields from distorting the motion of electrons inside. The motion of electrons and, therefore, the image on the output phosphor still may be distorted by a very strong magnetic field around the intensifier. Also, an intense magnetic field in the vicinity of the image intensifier may magnetize the mu-metal shield and focusing electrodes and cause permanent distortion of the fluoroscopic image. Consequently, image intensifiers should not be located near permanent or transient magnetic fields of high intensity.

With an x-ray image intensifier, four different information carriers transmit information about the patient to the radiologist. The x-ray beam transmits information from the patient to the input screen of the image intensifier. At the input screen, the information carrier is changed from x rays to photons of visible light. As the light photons are absorbed by the photocathode, the information is transferred to an electron beam, which is directed upon the output screen of the intensifier. The information is transmitted as a light image from the output screen to the observer's retina. The information is distorted in each of these stages. Consequently, the resolution of the image is poorer with an image intensifier than with a simple fluoroscopic screen. However, the image intensifier improves the visualization of image detail because the increased brightness of the image permits the radiologist to use photopic vision.

Gain and Conversion Efficiency of Image Intensifiers

The brightness of the image on the output screen of an image intensifier may be compared to the brightness of the image provided by a non-image-intensified fluoroscopic screen (e.g., a Patterson B-2 screen). The image intensifier and the fluoroscopic screen receive identical exposures to radiation and the ratio of the brightness of the two images is termed the *brightness gain* of the image intensifier.[*]

$$\text{Brightness gain} = \frac{\text{Brightness of output screen of image intensifier}}{\text{Brightness of Patterson B-2 screen}} \quad (16\text{-}1)$$

The brightness gain of image intensifiers varies from 1,000 to 6,000, depending on the particular image intensifier used and the fluorescent screen with which it is compared. The gain in brightness results from two independent processes that occur within the intensifier. These processes are *image minification* and *electron acceleration.*

The light image produced as x rays are absorbed in the input screen of an image intensifier is reproduced as a minified image on the output

[*]The luminance or "brightness" of an object is described in units of lamberts. One lambert (L) is the luminance of a perfectly diffusing surface that is emitting or reflecting 1 lumen/sq cm; 1 mL = (1/1,000) L.

screen of the intensifier. Since the output screen is much smaller than the input screen, the amount of light per unit area from the output screen is greater than that from the input screen. The increase in image brightness furnished by minification of the image is referred to as the *minification gain* g_m and is equal to the ratio of the areas of the input and output screens.

$$
\begin{aligned}
g_m &= \frac{\text{Area of input screen}}{\text{Area of output screen}} \\
&= \frac{(\pi/4)(\text{Diameter of input screen})^2}{(\pi/4)(\text{Diameter of output screen})^2} \\
&= \frac{(\text{Diameter of input screen})^2}{(\text{Diameter of output screen})^2}
\end{aligned}
\qquad (16\text{-}2)
$$

For example, the minification gain is 81 for an image intensifier with an input screen 9 in. in diameter and an output screen 1 in. in diameter.

$$
\begin{aligned}
g_m &= \frac{(9 \text{ in.})^2}{(1 \text{ in.})^2} \\
&= 81
\end{aligned}
$$

The brightness of the image on the output screen also is increased because electrons from the photocathode are accelerated as they travel toward the output screen. As these electrons are stopped in the output screen, the number of light photons released varies with the energy of the electrons. The gain in brightness due to electron acceleration is termed the *flux gain* g_f of the image intensifier. A typical image intensifier has a flux gain of about 50.

The *total gain* g in luminance of an image intensifier is the product of the minification gain g_m and the flux gain g_f.

$$
g = (g_m)(g_f) \qquad (16\text{-}3)
$$

For example, the luminance gain g is 4,050 for an image intensifier with a minification gain of 81 and a flux gain of 50.

$$
\begin{aligned}
g &= (81)(50) \\
&= 4,050
\end{aligned}
$$

Two image intensifiers may be compared by describing the conversion factor for each intensifier.[4] The conversion factor G_x is the quotient of the luminance of the output screen of the image intensifier divided by the exposure rate at the input screen. The luminance is expressed in units of candela* per square meter and the exposure rate in milliroentgens per second.

---

*The candela is a unit of luminance and equals $\frac{1}{60}$ of the luminance of a square centimeter of a black body heated to the temperature of solidifying platinum (1,773.5 C). One candela is equivalent to 0.3 millilamberts.

$$G_x = \frac{\text{Luminance of output screen in candela/sq m}}{\text{Exposure rate at input screen in mR/sec}} \qquad (16\text{-}4)$$

The conversion factor for an image intensifier is dependent on the energy of the radiation and should be measured with x radiation from a full-wave rectified or constant potential x-ray generator operated at about 85 kVp. The conversion factor of most image intensifiers ranges from 50 to 100 (candela-sec)/(mR-sq m).

Resolution and Image Distortion with Image Intensifiers

The resolution of an image intensifier is limited by the resolution of the input and output fluorescent screens and by the ability of the focusing electrodes to preserve the image as it is transferred from the input screen to the output screen. The resolution of image intensifiers averages about 2 lines/mm for CdS:ZnS:Ag input screens and up to 4 lines/mm for intensifiers with CsI input screens. Contributions to resolution loss that originate outside the image intensifier include the presence of scattered radiation in the x-ray beam received by the input screen, and unsharpness in the image contributed by patient motion and the finite size of the focal spot. In addition, the quality of the fluoroscopic image is affected by statistical fluctuations in the number of x rays impinging on the input screen. This influence is discussed in Chapter 18.

The resolution, brightness and contrast of an image provided by an image intensifier are greatest in the center of the image and reduced toward the periphery. The decrease in brightness along the periphery usually is less than 25%. The reduction in brightness and image quality along the border of the fluoroscopic image is referred to as *vignetting*. Vignetting is a reflection of the reduced exposure rate along the periphery of the input screen and the reduced precision with which electrons from the periphery of the photocathode strike the output screen. The loss of light from the periphery of the output screen also contributes to vignetting.

Straight lines in an object often appear to curve outward in the fluoroscopic image. This effect is referred to as *pincushion distortion* and is caused by the curvature of the input screen of the image intensifier and by the reduced precision with which electrons from the periphery of the photocathode are focused upon the output screen. Image lag of the input and output screens of an image intensifier may be objectionable during certain procedures such as high-speed cinefluorography.

Size of the Image Intensifier

The diameter of the input screen of an image intensifier ranges from 5 to 12 in. Intensifiers with small input screens are more maneuverable and less expensive. Also, these intensifiers require less exposure of the patient to radiation. A small intensifier furnishes a slight improvement in

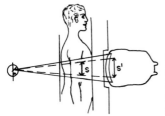

Fig 16-3.—An object of length s has an apparent length s′ on the input screen of an image intensifier. The field of view of an image intensifier is smaller than the size of the input screen.

resolution because electrons from the photocathode strike the output screen with greater precision. However, the region of the patient encompassed by the input screen is restricted with a small intensifier. A larger intensifier is more expensive and less maneuverable but furnishes a larger field of view and greater opportunity for magnification of the image. The high cost and engineering complexity of large image intensifiers have impeded the development of intensifiers larger than about 40 cm in diameter.

The diameter of the input screen of an image intensifier is larger than the diameter of the region studied within the patient. In Figure 16-3, for example, an object of length s has a length s′ in the image on the input screen. If d is the distance from the target of the x-ray tube to the object and d' is the distance from the target to the input screen, then the apparent length s′ of an object of actual length s is

$$s' = s\left(\frac{d'}{d}\right) \tag{16-5}$$

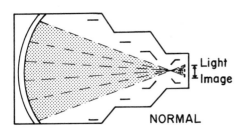

Fig 16-4.—A dual-field image intensifier. By changing the voltage on the focusing electrodes, two different electron crossover points are produced, corresponding to normal and magnified modes of viewing.

Light
Image

NORMAL

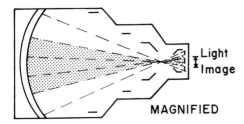

Light
Image

MAGNIFIED

The magnification M of the image is

$$M = \frac{s'}{s} \tag{16-6}$$

Example 16-1

An x-ray tube is positioned 45 cm below a fluoroscopic table. The input screen of an image intensifier is 15 cm in diameter and 30 cm above the table. What is the maximum length s of an object that is included completely on the screen? What is the magnification of the image? The object is 10 cm above the table.

$$s' = s\left(\frac{d'}{d}\right) \tag{16-5}$$

$$s = s'\left(\frac{d}{d'}\right)$$

$$= (15 \text{ cm})\left(\frac{10 \text{ cm } + 45 \text{ cm}}{30 \text{ cm } + 45 \text{ cm}}\right)$$

$$= 11 \text{ cm}$$

$$M = \frac{s'}{s} \tag{16-6}$$

$$= \frac{15 \text{ cm}}{11 \text{ cm}}$$

$$= 1.36$$

Dual- and Triple-Field Intensifiers

Many image intensifiers permit magnified viewing of the central region of the input screen. These intensifiers are termed *dual-field* intensifiers if one mode of magnified viewing is provided, and *triple-field* intensifiers if two magnified viewing modes are offered. The operation of a dual-field intensifier is diagramed in Figure 16-4. In the normal mode of viewing, electrons from the photocathode converge upon the electron crossover point at the location nearest the output screen and strike only the region of the output screen visible to the observer. Hence, the observer views the entire input screen of the intensifier. When the intensifier is operated in magnified mode, the voltage on the focusing electrodes is changed and electrons converge upon a crossover point farther from the output screen. Under this condition, electrons originating from the periphery of the input screen strike the output screen outside the region viewed by the observer. Only the central region of the input screen is viewed, and this region is seen as a magnified image. In a 22.5-cm (9-in.) dual-field image intensifier, only the central 15 cm (6 in.) of the input screen are seen in the magnified viewing mode.

If the voltage on the focusing electrodes is changed again, electrons from the photocathode can be forced to converge upon a crossover point even farther from the output screen. In this manner, a second mode of magnified viewing is presented to the observer. An intensifier with two magnified viewing modes is termed a *triple-field image intensifier*. Many 22.5-cm triple-field image intensifiers provide an image of the entire input screen in the normal viewing mode, and an image of the central 15 cm (6 in.) and 11 cm (4.5 in.) of the input screen during magnified viewing.

In the magnified viewing mode, the image on the output screen is produced by electrons from only the central portion of the input screen. Since fewer electrons are used to produce the image, the brightness of the image would be reduced unless the exposure rate to the input screen is increased. This increase in exposure rate is accomplished automatically as the viewing mode is switched from normal to magnified.

Solid-State Image Intensifiers

Considerable effort has been directed toward the replacement of image intensifier tubes with solid-state image intensifiers, referred to as *image intensifier panels*. One type is diagramed in Figure 16-5. An alternating voltage is applied across the photoconducting surface (CdS or CdSe) and the electroluminescent layer (ZnS or ZnSSe). These components are separated by an insulator opaque to light. The thickness of the photoconducting surface is about $\frac{1}{2}$ mm, and the thickness of the electroluminescent layer is about 50 μ. In regions where the intensity of incident x rays is high, the electric resistance of the photoconductor is reduced, and more of the alternating voltage is applied across the corresponding region of the electroluminescent layer. In regions of the photoconductor where the x-ray intensity is lower, less voltage is applied

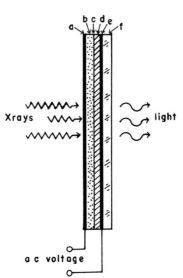

Fig 16-5. — Cross section of a solid-state image intensifier: *a* and *e*, conducting electrodes; *b*, photoconducting layer; *c*, insulator opaque to light; *d*, electroluminescent layer; *f*, glass plate.

across the electroluminescent layer. Hence, the variation in voltage across the electroluminescent layer reflects the variation in intensity across the x-ray beam. Each region of the electroluminescent layer emits yellow-green light in response to the potential difference across (i.e., the electric current through) the particular region. Consequently, the intensifier panel furnishes a light image that corresponds to variations in intensity across the x-ray beam.

Until recently, solid-state intensifying panels had not been developed that solved problems such as undesirable image persistence and less-than-expected brightness gain. Recent advances in the design of these panels and the use of microchannel plate electron multipliers and proximity-type intensifier tubes suggest that these problems may be nearing solution.[5, 6]

Light Amplifiers

A light amplifier differs from an image intensifier only in the placement of the fluorescent screen. The screen of an image intensifier is placed inside the vacuum envelope. With a light amplifier, the screen is positioned between the vacuum envelope of the image intensifier and the patient. The screen is coupled optically by concentric mirrors to the photocathode inside the envelope (Fig 16-6). Flat fluorescent screens used with light amplifiers resemble those used for conventional fluoroscopy. The "Cinelix image intensification system" uses a light amplifier to enhance the brightness of the image. With this approach, a large light amplifier is not required for a large field of view, because the image may be reduced optically before it is admitted into the light amplifier. However, the set of mirrors between the fluorescent screen and the light

Fig 16-6.—A light amplifier is used with a flat fluorescent screen and an optical system.

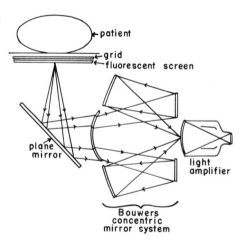

amplifier makes the resulting system large and bulky. Light amplifiers are relatively inexpensive to replace, and the fluorescent screen may be changed rapidly if a screen with coarser or finer granularity is desired.

Advantages of Image Intensification

Advantages of image intensification fluoroscopy over conventional fluoroscopy include:

1. Increased visibility of detail because photopic vision is used.
2. Elimination of the need for dark adaptation.
3. A slight reduction (usually) of exposure of the patient to radiation. This reduction would be much greater if the observer were willing to accept an image comparable to that provided by non-image-intensified fluoroscopy. In practice, the radiation exposure of the patient during fluoroscopy with image intensification is not much less than the exposure during earlier modes of fluoroscopy. However, the image is much brighter.
4. The availability of cinefluorography and television viewing.

Disadvantages of fluoroscopy with image intensification include:

1. Slight increase in expense and maintenance.
2. Limited access to the patient because of the space occupied by the image intensifier.
3. Restriction of the observer's movement when using the mirror or optical viewer.
4. Reduction of the field of view.

OPTICS FOR IMAGE INTENSIFICATION

The small image on the output screen of an image intensifier must be enlarged with mirrors and lenses to a size convenient for viewing. The image may be reflected into the observer's eyes by a plane mirror after the image has been enlarged to a size sufficient to encompass both eyes of the observer. With a few image intensifiers, a smaller image is observed through an ocular viewer.

Exit Pupil

The exit pupil is the cone of light that emerges from an optical system in the direction of the observer (Fig 16-7). To see the image on the output screen of an image intensifier, at least one eye of the observer must be enclosed within the exit pupil for the optical system coupled to the output screen. If binocular vision is desired, then both eyes must be enclosed within the cone of light. To encompass both eyes, the exit pupil must have a diameter of at least 10 cm at a viewing distance of 25–40 cm. An image is blurred if viewed at a distance less than about 25 cm, because the eye is unable to accommodate sufficiently to provide a focused

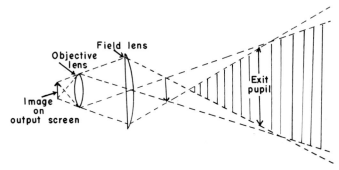

Fig 16-7.—Optical system and exit pupil for viewing the image on the output screen of an image intensifier.

image on the retina. If the exit pupil has a diameter greater than the distance of separation of the observer's eyes, then the observer can shift position slightly without "losing" the image.

Lenses

The image on the output screen of an image intensifier is magnified by the optical system that follows the intensifier. The image seldom is magnified to life size, because the size of the exit pupil decreases as the magnification of the image increases. Instead, the magnified image usually is 10–30% smaller than the corresponding region within the patient, and represents a compromise between magnification and the size of the exit pupil required for convenient viewing.

The objective lens (Fig 16-7) directs light from the output screen into the optical system. The greater the speed of the objective lens, the more light is gathered from the output screen. The speed of a lens is denoted by its *f-number*, where

$$\text{f-number} = \frac{\text{Focal length of lens}^*}{\text{Effective diameter of lens}^*} \tag{16-7}$$

As the f-number of a lens is increased, the speed of the lens is reduced. A fast or high-speed objective lens accompanies most image intensifiers because it provides the greatest magnification for an exit pupil of given size.

The field lens (Fig 16-7) forms an exit pupil of the desired size. This lens also may be used to increase the image magnification. The image

---

*The *focal length of a lens* is the distance from the center of the lens to the focal point, which is the location where parallel rays of light converge to a point after passing through the lens. The *effective diameter of a lens* is the diameter of the part of the lens that receives light. The effective diameter usually is limited by an aperture of fixed or variable diameter positioned immediately in front of the lens.

may be projected by the field lens onto a plane mirror, which is directed toward the observer. Full magnification of the image is possible if the field lens projects the image instead into a third lens, which is part of an ocular viewer. With an ocular viewer, the eye of the observer is confined to the viewer. A third lens may be inserted between the objective lens and the field lens. This permits magnification of the image to almost life size without restriction of the exit pupil to an unacceptably small size.

To deflect part of the light toward a cinefluorographic camera, a partially silvered (semireflective) mirror may be positioned between the objective lens and the field lens. This mirror is moved into position when the cinefluorographic camera is used and is removed when the image is viewed directly or by a television camera. A very small, fully reflective mirror may be used in place of the partially silvered mirror to deflect a small amount of light to the pickup device or cinefluorographic camera.

Room light incident upon the viewing mirror may pass through the optical system and fall on the output screen of the image intensifier. This light reduces the contrast and visibility of detail in the image. Also, room light may produce a glare in the viewing mirror which distracts the observer. For these reasons, room light that is directed onto the viewing mirror should be minimized during fluoroscopy.

TELEVISION DISPLAY OF THE FLUOROSCOPIC IMAGE

The image furnished by an image intensifier may be televised by viewing the intensifier output screen with a television camera. The signal from the camera is transmitted by cable to a television monitor. This method for transmission and display of an image is referred to as *closed-circuit television*, because the signal is transmitted from the television camera to the monitor by a coaxial cable rather than by air (Fig 16-8).

Television Cameras

Television cameras, sometimes referred to as television pickup tubes, average about 15 cm in length and 3 cm in diameter (Fig 16-9). A thin layer of photoconducting material [usually antimony trisulfide (SbS_3) in the vidicon camera and lead monoxide (PbO) in the plumbicon camera] is plated on the inner surface of the face of a glass envelope and is sepa-

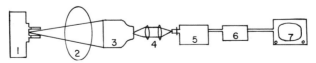

Fig 16-8.—Typical system for television fluoroscopy: *1,* x-ray tube; *2,* patient; *3,* image intensifier; *4,* optical system; *5,* television camera; *6,* camera control unit; *7,* television monitor.

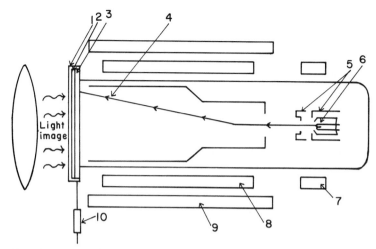

Fig 16-9. — A vidicon television pickup tube. *1,* glass envelope; *2,* transparent conducting layer; *3,* photoconducting layer; *4,* scanning electron beam; *5,* grids; *6,* electron gun; *7,* alignment coil for scanning beam; *8,* horizontal and vertical deflection coils; *9,* focusing coils; *10,* load resistor.

rated from the glass by a thin, transparent conducting layer. The side of the photoconducting layer nearest to the face of the glass envelope is 20–60 V positive with respect to the cathode of the electron gun. The photoconducting layer is an electric insulator when not exposed to light. When light from the output screen of the image intensifier falls upon the photoconducting layer, the resistance across the layer decreases; that is, the resistance across any region of an illuminated photoconducting layer depends on the amount of light incident on the region.

The scanning electron beam from the electron gun deposits electrons on the photoconducting layer. Some of the electrons migrate toward the positive side of the layer and are collected by the conducting layer. In any region, the number of electrons that migrate to the positive side depends on the resistance and, consequently, the illumination of the region. Electrons collected by the conducting layer furnish an electric signal that fluctuates in response to variations in the illumination of the photoconducting layer. This signal is amplified and used to control the intensity of the electron beam that is scanned across the fluorescent screen of the television monitor in synchrony with the scanning electron beam in the camera. Hence, the image on the television monitor corresponds closely to the image on the output screen of the image intensifier.

Advantages of vidicon and plumbicon television cameras include:[7]

1. Low cost and simplicity.
2. Ruggedness.
3. Satisfactory performance over a wide range of temperatures.

4. Only minor distortion of the image from statistical fluctuations in the x-ray beam or from other carriers of information. The distortion is low because the vidicon and plumbicon exhibit some image persistence and average the response over a finite interval of time.

Disadvantages of the vidicon and plumbicon television cameras include:
1. Relatively low sensitivity, so that a fairly bright image is required on the output screen of the image intensifier.
2. Persistence of the image. With early cameras, image persistence or lag was a major disadvantage; the persistence has been reduced considerably with newer vidicons and plumbicons.
3. Reduced contrast in the image with vidicons, because the modulation of the electric signal is not exactly proportional to the illumination of the photoconducting layer. The reduction in image contrast is less noticeable with plumbicons.

Television Scanning of Fluoroscopic Image

As the scanning electron beam moves horizontally across the photoconducting layer of the television camera, the signal from the conducting layer is modulated in response to the illumination of each photoconducting element in the path of the scanning electron beam. This motion of the scanning electron beam is termed an *active sweep*. As the electron beam is scanned horizontally in the opposite direction *(retrace sweep)*, no information is transmitted to the television monitor. The retrace sweep is about five times faster than the active sweep. As the next active sweep is initiated, it is displaced slightly below the preceding sweep. The number of active sweeps of the scanning electron beam across the image may be 525, 625, 837, 875, 945 or 1,024. Hence, the image is divided into 525, 625, 837, 875, 945 or 1,024 horizontal lines on the screen of the television monitor. (This number of lines must be reduced slightly because of the vertical retrace; see below.) Images with a large number of horizontal scan lines provide better vertical resolution than those formed with a smaller number of lines.[8]

To prevent brightness flicker in the image, the electron beam of the television camera first scans the photoconducting layer along even-numbered sweeps (2, 4, 6, 8, . . .). The resulting set of horizontal scan lines or *field* then is interlaced with sweeps of the electron beam along odd-numbered lines (1, 3, 5, 7, . . .). The final image produced by two interlaced sets of scan lines is referred to as a *frame*. A frame is completed in $1/30$ second with voltage alternating at 60 cps, and in $1/25$ second with voltage alternating at 50 cps. The rather uncommon 1,024-line image is produced by scanning the image three times and interlacing all three sets of scan lines.

After the entire photoconducting layer has been scanned once to compose a television field, the electron beam is returned to the top of the image to begin the next set of interlaced scan lines. The return of the scanning beam requires about 10^{-4} seconds and is referred to as the *vertical retrace*. Because of the time required for the vertical retrace, not all of the scan lines theoretically available are realized in practice. In a television system with 525 possible lines, for example, the image is actually formed with about 490 horizontal lines.[9] The remaining 35 lines are lost during the time required for the vertical retrace.

The vertical resolution of a television image is determined primarily by the number of active sweeps of the electron beam across the anode or photoconducting layer and by the *Kell factor*. The Kell factor is the fraction of the active sweeps that actually are effective in preserving detail in the image. The Kell factor is about 0.7 for most television systems.[10]

Vertical resolution = (Number of active sweeps/frame)(Kell factor) (16-8)

If the number of active sweeps is increased, then the visibility of detail may be improved in the vertical direction across the television image. Of course, a camera with more active sweeps will not improve the vertical resolution if the detail is not available initially in the image on the output screen of the image intensifier.

The horizontal resolution of a television image is determined primarily by the number of resolution elements available across a single horizontal scan line. The number of resolution elements available depends primarily upon the number of scan lines per frame and upon the range of frequencies transmitted by the electronic circuitry between the television camera and monitor. The highest frequency of signal modulation that is transmitted undistorted from the television camera to the television monitor is referred to as the *frequency bandpass* or *bandwidth* of the television system. Bandwidths for closed-circuit television circuits used in radiology range from 3.5 MHz (3.5 megacycles/sec) to 12 MHz. Although television systems with bandwidths up to 20 MHz and higher are available, they are expensive and are not used routinely. A bandwidth of 3.5 MHz is used in broadcast television. The influence of bandwidth in the resolution of the television image is illustrated in the simplified problem in Example 16-2.

Example 16-2

A 525-line television system provides about 490 active sweeps per frame and a vertical resolution of

Vertical resolution = (Number of active sweeps/frame)(Kell factor)

(16-8)

= (490 active sweeps/frame)(0.7)

= 343 lines

What minimum bandwidth is required to provide equal horizontal (343 resolution elements per line) and vertical (343 lines per frame) resolution in the image?

Number of resolution
elements transmitted = (343 resolution elements/Line)(343 lines/Frame)
per second   (30 frames/sec)
      = 3.53 × 10⁶ resolution elements/sec

To transmit this number of resolution elements per second, a television system is required with a bandwidth of at least 3.53 × 10⁶ Hz. That is, a system bandwidth of 3.5 MHz is barely adequate for this application and may sacrifice some image detail for very closely spaced structures in the object.

An exact expression for the horizontal resolution in resolution elements per line is[9]

$$\text{Horizontal resolution} = \frac{2(\text{Bandwidth})(\text{Horizontal fraction})(\text{Aspect ratio})}{(\text{Frames/second})(\text{Lines/frame})}$$

(16-9)

In equation (16-9), (1) the bandwidth is expressed in hertz; (2) the horizontal fraction is the quotient of the time required to complete one active sweep of the scanning electron beam divided by the time required for both the active and the retrace sweeps; (3) the number of frames per second usually is 30; (4) the lines per frame is the number of horizontal scanning lines per frame; (5) the aspect ratio is the ratio of the width of a television frame to its height and (6) the expression is multiplied by 2 because resolution is described in terms of the total number of resolution elements, both light and dark, that are visible in the television image. If the number of horizontal scanning lines per frame is increased, as in a high-resolution television system, then the visibility of detail in the image may be increased in the vertical direction. However, an increase in bandwidth is required if the image detail is to be maintained or improved in the horizontal direction. Most television systems provide an image with about equal horizontal and vertical resolution.

Example 16-3

An image of light and dark vertical and horizontal lines is presented on the output screen of an image intensifier. This image is transmitted to a television monitor by a 525-line television camera. The bandwidth is 3.5 MHz for the television chain. The framing time of the camera is 1/30 second. What is the maximum number of light and dark lines on the output screen that are duplicated without distortion on the television monitor?

With an aspect ratio of 1 and a horizontal fraction of 0.83 (since the retrace sweep is five times as rapid as the active sweep), the horizontal resolution may be computed with equation (16-9)

$$\text{Horizontal resolution} = \frac{2(\text{Bandwidth})(\text{Horizontal fraction})(\text{Aspect ratio})}{(\text{Frames/second})(\text{Lines/frame})}$$

$$= \frac{2(3.5 \times 10^6 \text{ Hz})(0.83)(1.0)}{(30 \text{ frames/second})(525 \text{ lines/frame})}$$
$$= 370 \text{ lines}$$

The image will be transmitted undistorted if it is composed of no more than 185 dark lines separated by 185 light lines. As described in Example 16-2, the vertical resolution for a 525-line camera is 343 lines. Hence, the vertical and horizontal resolutions are about equal.

Data in Table 16-1 show the bandwidths required for different television systems to furnish equal resolution in the vertical and horizontal directions. These data were computed for an aspect ratio of 1.0 and a horizontal fraction of 0.83.

TABLE 16-1.—BANDWIDTH REQUIRED FOR VARIOUS
TELEVISION SYSTEMS TO PROVIDE EQUAL
RESOLUTION IN HORIZONTAL AND VERTICAL
DIRECTION ACROSS THE IMAGE

NO. OF SCAN LINES/FRAME	FRAMES/SEC	VERTICAL AND HORIZONTAL RESOLUTION (LINES)	BANDWIDTH (MEGAHERTZ)
525	30	343	3.3
625	25	408	3.8
837	30	547	8.3
875	30	571	9.1
945	30	617	10.5
1,024	16.7	670	6.9

Attempts to construct a television pickup device that is sensitive directly to x rays have not been very successful.[11] With one method (the x-ray–sensitive vidicon), x rays impinge directly upon a PbO photoconducting plate that is 8–12 in. in diameter. Changes in resistance across the PbO plate reflect variations in photon flux density across the x-ray beam. The photoconducting plate is scanned by an electron beam to furnish a modulated electric signal. To furnish an image of acceptable quality, the photoconducting plate of PbO must be very thin. Consequently, only a few of the incident x rays are absorbed, and the x-ray–sensitive vidicon is relatively insensitive. Also, the sensitivity appears to decrease with use.[12] Exposure rates that provide an acceptable image on the television monitor are too high for clinical radiology. Also, persistence of the image is severe with x-ray–sensitive vidicons developed so far.

ADVANTAGES OF TELEVISION FLUOROSCOPY

The advantages of television fluoroscopy over fluoroscopy with an image intensifier equipped with a mirror or ocular viewer include:

1. The convenience of observing the image on a television monitor.
2. Observation of the image by a large number of persons simultaneously.
3. Alteration of image brightness and contrast electronically. In general, the contrast control on the television monitor should be adjusted until noise becomes apparent in the image. The contrast then should be reduced slightly and the brightness decreased until the darkest areas in the image are black.
4. The possibility of recording the image on videotape or video disk. With the original information recorded on tape or disk, the image may be altered for viewing without distortion or destruction of the original information.
5. Reversal of blacks and whites in the image, and inversion of the image.
6. Transmission of the image to remote television monitors.

Disadvantages of television fluoroscopy include:
1. Increased cost, complexity and maintenance.
2. Some degradation in image quality.

PROBLEMS

°1. An image intensifier has an input screen 9 in. in diameter and an output screen 1 in. in diameter. The flux gain of the intensifier is 40. What is the total gain in luminance?
2. In an image intensification system with a mirror viewer, trace the information and its carrier from the x-ray beam emerging from the patient to the visual image on the observer's retina. Describe the factors that contribute to resolution loss at each stage of this transformation.
°3. A patient 12 in. thick is positioned on a table 15 in. from the target of an x-ray tube. The region of interest in the patient is 6 in. in diameter and 3 in. above the table. Can the entire region be displayed at once with an image intensifier with an input screen 9 in. in diameter?
°4. A television system with 875 scan lines per frame provides 815 active sweeps per frame. If the Kell factor is 0.7, the horizontal fraction is 0.83, the aspect ratio is 1.0 and the frame rate is 30 fps, what bandwidth is required to provide equal resolution horizontally and vertically?
5. What is meant by vignetting in an image furnished by image intensification fluoroscopy? What is meant by "pincushion distortion"?

REFERENCES

1. Chamberlain, W.: Fluoroscopes and fluoroscopy, Radiology 38:383, 1942.
2. Sturm, R., and Morgan, R.: Screen intensification systems and their limitations, Am. J. Roentgenol. 62:617, 1959.
3. Niklas, W.: Conversion Efficiencies of Conventional Image Amplifiers, in Janower, M. (ed.): *Technological Needs for Reduction of Patient Dosage*

°For those problems marked with an asterisk, answers are provided on the pages following the appendixes (see pp. 487–488).

from Diagnostic Radiology (Springfield, Ill.: Charles C Thomas, Publisher, 1963), p. 271.

4. International Commission on Radiological Units and Measurements: *Methods of Evaluating Radiological Equipment and Materials.* Recommendations of the ICRU, Report 10f. National Bureau of Standards Handbook 89, 1963, p. 3.

5. Balter, S., et al.: A microchannel plate x-ray converter and intensifier tube, Radiology 110:673, 1974.

6. Wang, S., Robbins, C., and Bates, C.: A Novel Proximity X-Ray Image Intensifier Tube, in Hendee, W., and Gray, J. (eds.): *Proceedings SPIE Applications of Optical Instrumentation in Medicine V* (Bellingham, Wash.: Soc. Photo-Optical Instrumentation Engr, Publisher, 1977), p. 188.

7. Gebauer, A., Lissner, J., and Schott, O.: *Roentgen Television* (New York: Grune & Stratton, Inc., 1967).

8. Moseley, R., and Rust, J.: *Television in Diagnostic Radiology* (Birmingham, Ala.: Aesculapius Publishing Co., 1969).

9. Templeton, A., et al.: Standard and high-scan line television systems, Radiology 91:725, 1968.

10. Kell, R., Bedford, A., and Fredendall, G.: A determination of optimum number of lines in a television system, RCA Rev. 5:8, 1940.

11. Jacobs, J., and Beyer, H.: Large-area photoconductive x-ray pick-up tube performance, Elect. Engineering 75:158, 1956.

12. Bigdow, J., and Haq, K.: Significance of fatigue in lead oxide vidicon target, J. Appl. Phys. 33:2980, 1962.

17 / Special Imaging Techniques

CINERADIOGRAPHY

THE ACQUISITION of roentgenographic images separated only slightly in time is termed *cineradiography* or *serial radiography.* In cineradiography, an automatic film or cassette changer is used to position cut or roll film automatically in the x-ray beam between exposures.

Automatic Cassette Changers

An automatic cassette changer transfers a cassette loaded with cut film from a shielded storage bin to a position for exposure to the x-ray beam (Fig 17-1). Cassettes with exposed film are stored under the cassette with unexposed film and are shielded by a lead sheet on the back of each overlying cassette. Cassette changers may contain up to 20 cassettes for 14 by 14 in. film and may expose as many as 12 films each second.[1]

Roll-Film Changers

Film cassettes are bulky and difficult to move. Hence, serial roentgenograms often are obtained with a changer that transports cut or roll film from a shielded container into a position for exposure between intensify-

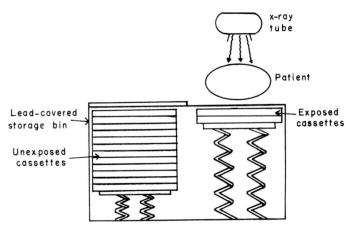

Fig 17-1.—An automatic cassette changer. Between exposures, a cassette is moved from the shielded storage bin to a position for exposure during the next x-ray pulse. Exposed cassettes are stored below the cassette positioned for exposure and are protected from radiation by a sheet of lead on the back of each overlying cassette.

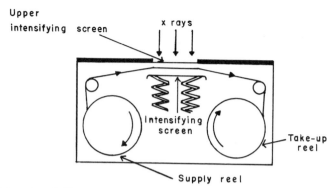

Fig 17-2.—A roll-film changer, illustrating the supply reel, the intensifying screens and the take-up reel.

ing screens. In the roll-film changer (Fig 17-2), the bottom intensifying screen is lowered between exposures to permit the film to move easily. After an unexposed segment of film has been placed into position for exposure, the motion of the film is stopped and the bottom intensifying screen is raised into firm contact with the film. Each frame of film is 12 by 12 in. or 12 by 14 in. Roll-film changers may be loaded with up to 80 ft of film to furnish 65–75 frames. Most roll-film changers have a film-advance mechanism with which the operator may select the number of frames exposed each second. With some changers, as many as 12 frames of film may be exposed each second.[2] With a programmable changer, the operator may vary the time between successive exposures in a series. For example, many frames may be exposed during the first few seconds of an examination. As the examination continues, the exposures may be

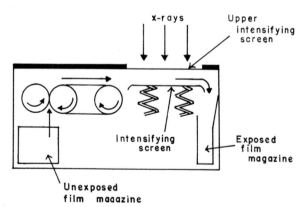

Fig 17-3.—A cut-film changer, illustrating the storage magazine for unexposed film, the intensifying screens and the storage magazine for exposed film.

separated by longer intervals. Roll film requires special equipment for development and processing. Although cut film may be processed more conveniently, fewer frames of cut film can be exposed each second.

Cut-Film Changers

In the cut-film changer (Fig 17-3), rubber-covered wheels move unexposed film into position for exposure. When the film is positioned for exposure, the bottom intensifying screen is raised into firm contact with the film and the film is exposed. In some changers, film as large as 14 by 17 in. may be transported and exposed at rates up to 6 films/second.[2] Cutfilm changers hold up to 30 films, and some changers permit the operator to program the interval of time between successive exposures. Cut films may be exposed, removed from the changer and processed individually.

CINEFLUOROGRAPHY

The image on the output screen of an image intensifier may be photographed with a 16-mm or 35-mm movie camera or with a camera containing 70-, 90- or 105-mm film. In Figure 17-4, a partially silvered mirror

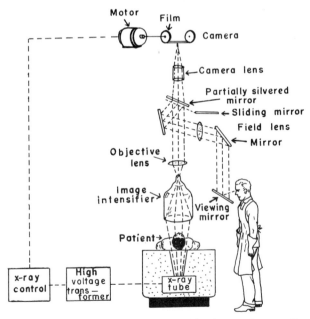

Fig 17-4.—Optical system for simultaneous viewing and recording of the fluoroscopic image. Most (85–95%) of the light from the output screen of the image intensifier is transmitted by the partially silvered mirror and is directed upon film in the cinefluorographic camera. The remaining 5–15% is reflected to the mirror viewer. A small, fully silvered mirror that intercepts part of the transmitted light may be substituted for the partially silvered mirror.

transmits part of the light from the output screen into the cinefluorographic camera. The remainder of the light is reflected into a mirror that is viewed directly by the observer. Alternately, a small, fully silvered mirror may be used to reflect part of the light to the viewing mirror. Light that is not reflected by the fully silvered mirror is collected and transmitted to the camera. The partially or fully silvered mirror is removed from the light beam when a cinefluorographic recording is not desired.

Cinefluorography became practical in clinical radiology only with the advent of image intensification. Images on a conventional fluoroscopic screen were too dim to furnish photographs of acceptable quality. Increasing the brightness of these images improved the quality of the photograph, but raised the radiation exposure of the patient to an unacceptable level. Although the exposure to the patient also increases significantly during cinefluorography with image intensification, the exposure increase is much less than that which would be required for cinefluorography without image intensification.

SYNCHRONIZATION OF FILM MOVEMENT AND X-RAY EXPOSURE

During cinefluorography, the film must be shielded from light after exposure of each frame of film to permit the next unexposed frame to be moved into position for exposure. In early cinefluorographic units, light shielding was furnished by a shutter on the cinefluorographic camera. The circular shutter, with approximately equal open and closed portions, rotated at constant speed in front of the cinefluorographic camera. Hence, the film was shielded from light about as often as it was exposed, and a frame of unexposed film was moved into position for exposure each time the shutter was closed. By energizing the x-ray tube only when the shutter was open, the exposure of the patient to radiation could be reduced to about half that received if x rays were generated continuously. Also, higher tube currents could be used during exposure without overloading the x-ray tube. In such a synchronized cinefluorographic system, the camera shutter actually is unnecessary since the x-ray beam is on only when the film is in proper position for exposure. Consequently, newer synchronized cinefluorographic systems do not use a camera shutter.

In a cinefluorographic system supplied with single-phase power, uniform exposure of successive frames of film can be achieved only if the frame rate is a submultiple of the frequency of the alternating voltage applied to the x-ray tube. For this reason, typical cinefluorographic cameras designed for use with single-phase power in the United States furnish frame rates of 7.5, 15, 30 and 60 frames per second. With three-phase power, cinefluorographic frame rates are not confined to submultiples of the frequency of the applied voltage.

Three methods have been used to synchronize the x-ray exposure with the position of the film in the cinefluorographic camera. The *Dynapulse circuit* uses a grid-controlled switching tube in the high-voltage circuit of the x-ray generator. The voltage across the secondary winding of the high-voltage transformer is applied across capacitors in parallel with the x-ray tube. The bias voltage on the grid of the switching tube is controlled by a pulse-shaping and timing circuit that is linked to the drive mechanism for film in the cinefluorographic camera. Current is conducted through the switching tube when the bias voltage is removed from the grid, and energy stored in the capacitors is delivered to the x-ray tube. The Dynapulse circuit has been used for cinefluorography and for examinations such as serial angiography that require very short exposure times (e.g., 1 msec).

The technique of *primary pulsing* also has been used to apply voltage across the x-ray tube in synchrony with the film position in the cinefluorographic camera. In this method, two switching tubes in the primary circuit of the x-ray generator apply voltage to the primary winding of the high-voltage transformer when the cinefluorographic film is ready for exposure.

Grid-controlled x-ray tubes have essentially replaced the preceding methods for synchronization of the x-ray exposure with the cinefluorographic film. With these x-ray tubes, the bias voltage on the focusing cup surrounding the filament is regulated by a timing circuit that is synchronized with the film-supply mechanism of the cinefluorographic camera. Electrons flow across the x-ray tube only when the cinefluorographic film is in position for exposure.

"Flickering" of the image in the viewing mirror is noticeable during cinefluorography with a synchronized cinefluorographic unit operated at frame rates slower than about 30 frames per second. The rate at which the image flickers depends on the number of frames of film exposed per second.

Cinefluorographic Film

The photographic film used for cinefluorography must be sensitive to the wavelength of light from the output screen of the image intensifier. Orthochromatic emulsions (sensitive to all visible light except red light) and panchromatic emulsions (sensitive to all wavelengths of visible light) are used for cinefluorography. A relatively high-speed film with high inherent contrast should be used for cinefluorography. The film should be able to record fine detail. No single film satisfies all these re-

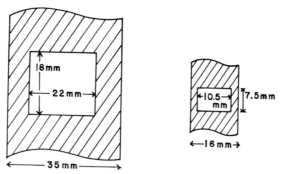

Fig 17-5.—Dimensions of single frames of 16-mm and 35-mm cinefluorographic film.

quirements, and a compromise must be reached when a particular film is chosen for a cinefluorographic examination.

Both 16-mm and 35-mm film are used for cinefluorography. Each frame of 16-mm film is 10.5 mm wide and 7.5 mm long (Fig 17-5), with 40 frames available per linear foot of film. Each frame of 35-mm film is 22 mm wide and 18 mm long and furnishes 16 frames per linear foot. Although 16-mm film is less expensive and easier to project, 35-mm film usually provides higher-quality images because the area of a frame of 35-mm film is four times that for a 16-mm frame. If all the detail present in the image on the output screen can be captured on 16-mm film, then the quality of the image is not improved with 35-mm film.

Each frame of 16-mm and 35-mm film is rectangular rather than square. If the size of the recorded image is restricted to the smaller dimension of a frame, then the frame is not exposed at the borders along the larger dimension. Expanding the image to fill the larger dimension of the film is referred to as *overframing*. Overframing causes the loss of part of the image at the borders along the shorter dimension of the frame. If the lost portion of the image is not important clinically, then overframing is useful because it expands the image over a larger area of film and may increase the image detail that is recorded.

Example 17-1

An image intensifier provides a resolution of 2 lines/mm on an input screen 6 in. in diameter. The smaller dimension of a 16-mm frame is 0.75 cm. Without overframing, the minification of the image on a frame of 16-mm cinefluorographic film is

$$\frac{(6 \text{ in.})(2.54 \text{ cm/in.})}{0.75 \text{ cm}} = 20$$

Therefore, the film should provide a resolution of

$$(2 \text{ lines/mm})(20) = 40 \text{ lines/mm}$$

Commercial 16-mm film provides this resolution, and 35-mm film furnishes no improvement in image detail.

Example 17-2
An image intensifier provides a resolution of 3 lines/mm on an input screen 9 in. in diameter. Without overframing, the minification of the image on 16 mm cinefluorographic film is

$$\frac{(9 \text{ in.})(2.54 \text{ cm/in.})}{0.75 \text{ cm}} = 30$$

Therefore, the film should provide a resolution of

$$(3 \text{ lines/mm})(30) = 90 \text{ lines/mm}$$

Cinefluorographic film will not provide this level of resolution.

Example 17-3
If the image on the image intensifier in Example 17-2 is overframed, then the dimension of the image on the cinefluorographic film is 1.05 cm. The minification of the image is

$$\frac{(9 \text{ in.})(2.54 \text{ cm/in.})}{1.05 \text{ cm}} = 21.7$$

Therefore, the film should provide a resolution of

$$(3 \text{ lines/mm})(21.7) = 65 \text{ lines/mm}$$

Some types of cinefluorographic film provide this level of resolution.

Example 17-4
If 35-mm film is substituted for 16-mm film in Example 17-2, then the smaller dimension of a single frame is 1.8 cm and the minification is

$$\frac{(9 \text{ in.})(2.54 \text{ cm/in.})}{1.8 \text{ cm}} = 12.5$$

The film should provide a resolution of

$$(3 \text{ lines/mm})(12.5) = 40 \text{ lines/mm}$$

This resolution is provided by cinefluorographic film, and 35-mm film furnishes an image with resolution greater than that provided by 16-mm film.

Cinefluorographic Cameras

Motion-picture cameras used in cinefluorography are similar to those used for professional and amateur cinematography. The mechanism for film transport is shown in Figure 17-6. Some cameras, particularly those that hold large amounts (e.g., 400 linear ft) of film, possess a double sprocket that moves the film continuously by engaging perforations on each side of the film. Film is moved into position for exposure by a "pulldown mechanism," which is operated only when the shutter is closed. Loops of film above and below the pulldown mechanism collect film that is unrolled continuously by the supply reel and store exposed film that is supplied by the pulldown mechanism. A "pressure plate" positions each frame and holds it firmly in position during exposure.

Cinefluorographic Projectors

Projectors for cinefluorographic film (1) should run in either direction; (2) should provide projection rates up to at least 16 frames per second; (3) should change instantaneously between forward and reverse travel of the film; (4) should project stationary single frames; (5) should furnish flicker-free viewing at low frame rates; and (6) should possess a "fire gate" which drops into position automatically during single-frame projection or during projection at low rates of film travel to protect the film from heat generated by the high-intensity projection bulb.[3]

Image detail is sacrificed if cinefluorographic images are projected onto a conventional beaded screen. In place of a conventional beaded screen, a radiographic intensifying screen or a screen with very fine beads should be used.

Radiation Dose in Cinefluorography

During cinefluorography, the current through the x-ray tube is increased many times more than that required for routine fluoroscopy with

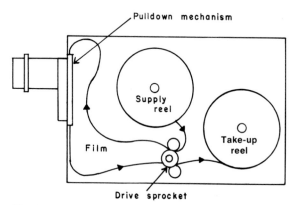

Fig 17-6. — The film-transport mechanism in a cinefluorographic camera.

an image intensifier. The increased current is necessary to provide an image on the output screen that is bright enough to expose each frame of cinefluorographic film. This exposure requires an exposure rate of 10–40 μ R/frame at the input screen of the image intensifier,[4] and an exposure rate 100–1,000 times this value at the entrance surface of the patient. Since the exposure rate increases linearly with current through the x-ray tube, the exposure of the patient to radiation also is increased many times during a cinefluorographic examination.[5-7]

Photospot Images

Spot photographs of the image on the output screen of an image intensifier may be substituted for spot roentgenograms (spot films) obtained by interposing full-size x-ray film between the patient and the input screen of the image intensifier. Compared to full-size roentgenograms, the smaller photospot images obtained with 70-, 90- or 105-mm film are less expensive and easier to store. Also, photospot images require less exposure of the patient to radiation.[8] Although the image quality of a 105-mm photospot image may be slightly less than that furnished by a conventional spot film, the image should be satisfactory for most examinations.[9]

AUTOMATIC BRIGHTNESS CONTROL

In x-ray image intensification fluoroscopy, an automatic brightness control (ABC) unit is used to maintain an image of constant brightness on the output screen of the intensifier, irrespective of changes in the attenuation of the x-ray beam in the patient. An image of constant brightness is achieved by automatic adjustment of exposure technique variables (e.g., peak kilovoltage, milliamperes and x-ray pulse width) in response to fluctuations in brightness of the output screen. For purposes of discussion, an ABC unit may be separated into two components: (1) the brightness-sensing element, with an output used to control (2) the machine's technique variables, which are adjusted automatically to maintain constant image brightness.[10, 11]

Brightness-Sensing Elements

The earliest technique to monitor image brightness was continuous measurement of the image intensifier photocathode-anode current. With this approach there is no simple way to compensate for bright edge effects at the periphery of the image that are caused by x rays unattenuated by the patient. Compensation for variable collimation usually is provided by a shutter compensation control, which reduces the ABC's response as the field size is decreased.

In systems that offer television viewing of the fluoroscopic image, a second approach is available to monitor the brightness of the entire image on the output screen. This approach uses the intensity of the television signal as an indication of output screen brightness. In some recent installations the portion of the image actually monitored can be selected electronically. If the center of the image is monitored, bright edge and collimation effects are eliminated.

The most common method of brightness sensing uses a photomultiplier tube to monitor the brightness of the output screen of the intensifier. The area monitored can be defined optically with lenses and diaphragms, thereby eliminating edge and collimation effects. This approach has the advantage of less sensitivity to noise and image intensifier aging effects and, along with the television method, is not influenced greatly by x-ray energy.

Technique Variables Controlled by the ABC

Three variables that can be controlled by an ABC unit are the peak kilovoltage, the tube current and the width of the x-ray pulses in x-ray units with variable pulse width.

KVP VARIABILITY.—With systems of this type, the mA is selected by a continuous or fixed-step mA control and the kVp is selected automatically to provide an image of desired brightness. In the automatic mode, the selected mA exerts some influence on the kVp required to furnish a satisfactory image; that is, high mA lowers kVp, and low mA raises kVp. On some machines, the kVp control establishes the maximum kVp that the ABC can select. On units with an Automatic/Manual control, the manual setting disables the ABC unit and permits the operator to select both the mA and the kVp. X-ray systems with kVp-variable ABC units usually have a faster response time than mA-variable machines, because the ABC unit functions by mechanical rather than thermal means. Also, kVp-variable units provide a wider dynamic range of brightness control.

MA VARIABILITY.—An mA-variable ABC control offers the advantage of operator control of kVp during ABC operation. At the kVp selected, however, the tube current must be sufficiently variable to furnish an image of adequate brightness over a wide range of x-ray beam attenuation. Usually, the dynamic range of an mA-variable unit is less than that of a kVp-variable unit. Units with variable mA have a relatively long response time because they depend on the thermal characteristics of the x-ray tube filament.

KVP-MA VARIABILITY.—Some ABC units vary both the kVp and the mA, with both technique variables changed in the same direction (i.e., either increased or decreased). This approach offers a wide dynamic range but provides little control over the kVp selected for the examination. For this reason, some kVp-mA–variable systems offer the option of manual selection of either kVp or mA. With these options, operation is identical to that described above for mA- or kVp-variable units.

PULSE WIDTH VARIABILITY. — Machines equipped with cine cameras sometimes use grid-controlled x-ray tubes to vary the width (time) of the voltage pulse across the x-ray tube. In this manner, the brightness of the image can be kept constant during fluoroscopy. In most units of this type, the mA is set at a fixed value, and the pulse width of the x-ray beam is varied up to some maximum limit. Many of the units furnish some indication of pulse width in milliseconds. In earlier versions of this approach to ABC operation, pulse widths were limited from about 0.2 to 8 msec. At least one recent unit provides a range from 20 μsec to 4 msec in the fluoroscopic mode, and a kVp override circuit which increases the kVp above that selected if an image of adequate brightness is not achieved at maximum pulse width. The pulse width variable type of control has the distinct advantages of instantaneous response and, with the latter circuit described, a very wide dynamic range.

COMBINATION CIRCUITS. — Any combination of the above approaches to ABC operation is possible, but the one most commonly used, other than kVp-mA variability, is the kVp override capability. This method may be applied to either mA- or pulse-width-variable machines. The kVp override approach provides automatic compensation if the selected kVp is not adequate to furnish an image of desired brightness.

VIDEO RECORDING

Videotape is a plastic tape 1 or 2 in. wide. An emulsion about 1 mm thick on one side of the tape contains magnetizable particles, usually

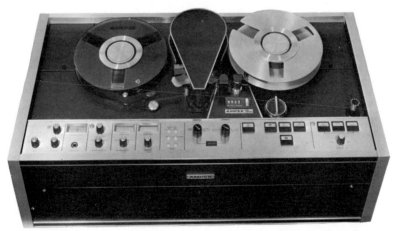

Fig 17-7. — A videotape recorder. (Courtesy of Ampex Corp.)

iron oxide. In the videotape recorder, the particles are magnetized by a varying magnetic field produced by the modulated electric signal from the television camera. The electric signal from the camera is recorded in a zigzag pattern from side to side and along the length of a "track" in the videotape. When the videotape is played back in the videotape recorder, the magnetization along the tape induces a varying current within a small coil. This current is transmitted to the television monitor and is used to regulate the intensity of the electron beam that is scanned across the fluorescent screen of the monitor. The resulting image resembles the image on the output screen of the image intensifier.

A photograph of a videotape recorder is furnished in Figure 17-7. The read-write head moves rapidly (e.g., 30 m/sec) with respect to the tape, which moves from 10 to 300 cm/sec. To record all the information carried by the video signal, the frequency response of the videotape recorder must be at least equal to the frequency bandwidth of the television system. In addition to the recording track for the signal from the television camera, videotape furnishes two channels for audio signals.

Advantages of recording images on videotape include: (1) immediate playback of the image; (2) superimposition of sound (e.g., radiologists' comments or patient's heartbeat) on the video signal; (3) playback at slower speeds; (4) capability for single framing; (5) recording of images at no increase in patient dose; (6) repeated playback of the recorded image; and (7) the capability of videotape to withstand up to 400 recordings and erasures. Disadvantages include: (1) slight degradation of image quality and (2) increased (although moderate) cost.

The video disk recorder resembles the videotape recorder except that the television signal is recorded on both sides of a rigid disk rather than on one side of a flexible tape. The advantages of video disk over videotape recorders include improved resolution and their usefulness in pulsed fluoroscopic techniques that provide intermittent fluoroscopic images with significant reductions in patient dose.[12, 13]

STEREOSCOPIC RADIOGRAPHY

Two roentgenograms exposed with the x-ray tube in slightly different positions and viewed with a stereoscopic viewer provide an image with an illusion of depth. The procedure outlined below may be followed to obtain a pair of stereoscopic roentgenograms:

1. The patient, cassette and x-ray film are positioned as if a single film were to be exposed.

2. The x-ray tube is shifted parallel to the film by one-half the distance indicated in Table 17-1. If a grid is used, then the tube is shifted parallel to the grid strips.

3. The x-ray film is exposed.

TABLE 17-1.—TUBE SHIFTS IN INCHES FOR
VARIOUS EXPOSURE AND VIEWING DISTANCES
FOR STEREOSCOPIC RADIOGRAPHY°†

TARGET-FILM DISTANCE (IN.)	EYE-FILM DISTANCE		
	25 IN.	28 IN.	30 IN.
25	2⁹/₁₆	2¹/₄	2¹/₁₆
30	3³/₁₆	2³/₄	2⁹/₁₆
36	3⁷/₈	3⁷/₁₆	3¹/₈
42	4⁵/₈	4¹/₁₆	3³/₄
48	5³/₈	4¹¹/₁₆	4⁵/₁₆
60	6¹³/₁₆	6	5¹/₂
72	8⁵/₁₆	7¹/₄	6¹¹/₁₆

°From Seemann.[14]
†If the target-film distance equals the eye-film distance, then the
tube-shift distance equals the interpupillary distance of 2⁹/₁₆ in.

4. Steps 1–3 are repeated with a tube shift in the opposite direction.
The patient must remain stationary between exposures.

5. The x-ray films are subjected to identical processing conditions.

6. The roentgenograms are viewed in a stereoscopic viewer.

The direction of tube shift should be perpendicular to prominent features in the patient. For stereoscopic roentgenograms of the chest, for example, the tube shift is parallel to the vertebral column because the borders of the ribs furnish the dominant lines. For anatomical parts containing long bones, the tube shift is perpendicular to the long axes of the bones. The direction of tube shift is not important for stereoscopic roentgenograms of the skull.

One type of stereoscopic viewer is described in Figure 17-8. The left roentgenogram is viewed by the left eye and the right roentgenogram is viewed by the right eye. The radiologist coalesces the images mentally to obtain an image with an illusion of depth. Stereoscopic roentgeno-

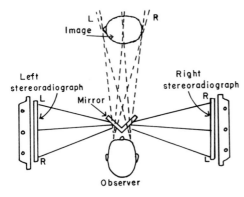

Fig 17-8.—One type of viewer for stereoscopic radiography. The images viewed by the radiologist are integrated mentally to provide an illusion of depth.

grams obtained with a horizontal tube shift are viewed as though the patient were standing; those obtained with a vertical tube shift are viewed as though the patient were lying down.

Many radiologists are able to perceive depth in superimposed stereoscopic roentgenograms without the use of a stereoscopic viewer. The techniques they use include those referred to as "cross-eyed stereoscopy" and "objective stereoscopy."[15]

SUBTRACTION RADIOGRAPHY AND FLUOROSCOPY

In roentgenographic studies using a contrast medium, information that is not required for diagnosis may be subtracted from an image by the

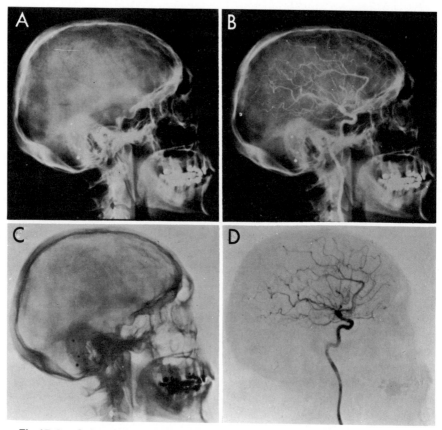

Fig 17-9. — Subtraction radiography. **A,** roentgenogram obtained before introduction of contrast medium; **B,** roentgenogram obtained after introduction of contrast medium; **C,** subtraction mask of first roentgenogram; **D,** subtraction image obtained by combining the second roentgenogram with the subtraction mask. (From Ziedses des Plantes, B.: The electronic subtraction method, Electromedica 1:23, 1968.)

technique of *radiographic subtraction* developed originally by Ziedses des Plantes.[16, 17] If the subtraction method is used properly, only structures containing contrast medium are outlined in the final image. To obtain a subtraction roentgenogram, x-ray films are exposed before and after the contrast medium is administered to the patient. The patient must not move between exposures. A positive print (the *subtraction mask*) of the first roentgenogram is superimposed on the second roentgenogram and a photograph is made of the combination. Except for structures containing contrast medium, dark areas on the second roentgenogram are matched with light areas on the subtraction mask, and vice versa. This matching of light and dark areas produces a final photograph that is relatively uniform over all regions except those that display the image of structures containing contrast medium. The subtraction image of the skull in Figure 17-9 exhibits structures that are less noticeable in the original roentgenogram.

Requirements for subtraction roentgenography include:[18]

1. The film used as a subtraction mask should have an average gradient close to 1.

2. All parts of the image to be subtracted should have an optical density of at least 0.25 and should fall within the straight-line portion of the film's characteristic curve.

3. The subtraction image must be a positive image with a high contrast and should provide a homogeneous background with an optical density of about 1.

MAGNIFICATION ROENTGENOGRAPHY

If x rays are assumed to originate from a single point on the target of the x-ray tube, then the magnification of a roentgenographic image is:

$$\text{Magnification} = \frac{\text{Image size}}{\text{Object size}} = \frac{\text{Target-film distance}}{\text{Target-object distance}}$$

If the distance between the target of the x-ray tube and the x-ray film is constant, then the ratio of image to object size may be increased by moving the object toward the x-ray tube. This method of image enlargement is referred to as *object-shift enlargement* (Fig 17-10). If the distance between target and object is constant, then the ratio of image size to object size may be increased by moving the film farther from the object. This technique of image enlargement is referred to as *image-shift enlargement*.

The amount of enlargement possible without significant loss of image detail should be determined when radiologic images are magnified. With the image receptor close to the patient, the visibility of image detail usually is determined primarily by the unsharpness of the intensifying

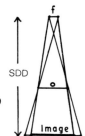

Fig 17-10. — Principle of enlargement radiography; *f* is the apparent focal spot of the x-ray tube, *o* is the object size and *SDD* represents the distance between the image receptor and the target of the x-ray tube.

screen. As the distance between the screen and the patient is increased by object-shift or image-shift enlargement, no change occurs in the contribution of screen unsharpness to the visibility of image detail. However, the contribution of geometric unsharpness increases steadily with increasing distance between patient and image receptor. At some patient-receptor distance, geometric unsharpness equals screen unsharpness. Beyond this distance, the visibility of image detail deteriorates steadily as geometric unsharpness increasingly dominates image unsharpness. As a general rule, the image should not be magnified beyond the point at which geometric and screen unsharpness are about equal.

An image also may be magnified by optical enlargement of a processed roentgenogram. This technique may enhance contrast but offers no improvement in resolution. For most procedures, magnification roentgenograms obtained directly by geometric enlargement of the image are preferred over those obtained by optical enlargement.[19, 20]

MICRORADIOGRAPHY

For small, thin sections of an object, magnification much greater than that furnished by enlargement radiography may be obtained by either contact microradiography or projection microradiography.

Contact Microradiography

Contact microradiographs are obtained by placing a thin (i.e., $100-1,000\ \mu$) section of the object in close contact with the emulsion of a film with very fine grain. This composite is exposed to an x-ray beam generated at $1-20$ kVp in an x-ray tube with a thin beryllium window. The focal spot of the target of the x-ray tube is very small, and the region between the target and the object is evacuated. A vacuum cassette with a thin window opaque to light is used to provide intimate contact between sample and film. The image recorded on the fine-grained film may be enlarged up to 500 times without significant loss of image detail.

Projection Microradiography

In projection microradiography, a magnified image is obtained directly rather than by optical enlargement. A thin specimen is mounted on or placed close to a metal foil used as the target for an electron beam accelerated through 1–20 kV. The film is positioned some distance away and is exposed to x rays generated in the metal foil and transmitted by the specimen. A very small focal spot (e.g., 0.001 mm) should be used for projection microradiography.[14]

TOMOGRAPHY

In a conventional roentgenogram, all structures within the region of the patient exposed to x rays are recorded "in focus" on the film. Often, the image of a particular structure within a patient is obscured by objects above or below. To improve the visualization of this structure, the image of overlying and underlying objects may be blurred by moving the x-ray tube and film during exposure about an axis through the structure of interest. The extent to which images of overlying and underlying structures are blurred depends largely on the angle subtended by the motion of the x-ray tube and film. The blurring of undesired images by movement of the x-ray tube and film is referred to as *tomography*. Tomography sometimes is referred to as *body-section radiography, planigraphy, stratigraphy, laminography* and *zonography*. Although these terms may be used to distinguish among minor variations in technique, the principles of tomography are applicable to all procedures.

The principle of *linear tomography* is diagramed in Figure 17-11. The axis L_2 for the motion of the x-ray tube and film is positioned in a plane that contains the region of interest in the patient. With the x-ray tube and film at the beginning of the path of motion (i.e., at the origin of the "track"), images of structures L_1, L_2 and L_3 are projected to points L_1', L_2' and L_3' at the left, center and right of the film, respectively. Rays through L_1, L_2 and L_3 continue to strike the film at the locations L_1', L_2' and L_3' as the x-ray tube and film move toward the end of the track. Consequently, images are in focus on the film for structures such as L_1, L_2 and L_3 in a

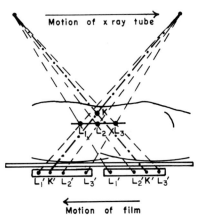

Motion of x ray tube

L_1' K' L_2' L_3' L_1' $L_2'K'$ L_3'

Motion of film

Fig 17-11.—The principle of a linear tomographic unit. The motion of the x-ray tube and film about the axis L_2 in the patient produces blurred images of structures above and below the plane of section through L_2.

plane that contains the axis and is parallel to the motion of the x-ray tube and film. With the tube and film at the origin of the track, a ray through structure K above the axis projects to the location K' on the right side of the film. Toward the end of the track, the ray through K strikes the left side of the film. Hence, images of structure K (and of all other structures above the axis) are projected to different parts of the film, and these images are blurred. Similarly, the images of structures below the axis are not apparent on the film. Images of structures are displayed clearly in the tomographic image only if the structures are positioned within a *plane of section* containing the axis of motion for the x-ray tube and film. The depth of the plane of section within the patient is varied by raising or lowering the patient with respect to the axis of motion.

Tomographic images for planes of section at different depths within the patient may be obtained with a series of exposures. The patient is raised or lowered slightly between each exposure. To reduce the exposure of the patient to radiation, a cassette may be designed to hold several films. The x-ray films are sandwiched between intensifying screens and are separated by spacers. The distance from the patient to the film is different for each film in the cassette, and images that are in focus on one film are not in focus on the other films. Consequently, structures in different planes of section through the patient are portrayed in focus on different films in the multifilm cassette. The sensitivity of the screen-film combinations in the cassette must increase from top to bottom, because the exposure rate decreases as the radiation traverses overlying screens and films. The rate of decrease in exposure rate through the cassette varies with the energy of the radiation. Consequently, a particular multifilm cassette should be used with x rays generated over a limited range of tube voltage.

A linear tomographic unit blurs the image of structures that are located above or below the plane of section and are oriented in any manner other than parallel to the motion of the x-ray tube and film. The images of structures outside the plane of section and oriented parallel to the motion of the x-ray tube and film are elongated and distorted but are not blurred enough to be indiscernible in the resulting tomographic image (tomogram). These distorted images (shadows) interfere with the visibility of image detail. To reduce or eliminate the influence of these shadows, motions such as curvilinear, circular, elliptical, spiral and hypocycloidal have been devised for tomography. The ideal motion for a tomographic unit is one that causes the x-ray beam to originate from an infinite number of locations during an exposure. In this situation, the motion of the x-ray tube is perpendicular to all structures in the patient during at least part of the exposure. Undesired images are eliminated more successfully with the hypocycloidal path of motion than with most of the other motions for which mechanical linkage has been developed.

TABLE 17-2.—TYPES OF MOTION, ANGLE OF TUBE
MOTION, LENGTH OF TRAJECTORY AND
THICKNESS OF CUT (PLANE OF SECTION) FOR
THE MASSIOT-PHILIPS POLYTOME*

TYPE OF MOTION	ANGLE OF TUBE MOTION (DEGREES)	LENGTH OF TRAJECTORY (CM)	THICKNESS OF CUT (MM)
Linear	29	56	2.3
	36	69	1.8
	40	77	1.6
	48	92	1.3
	60	115	1.0
Circular	29	176	2.3
	36	217	1.8
Elliptical	40	186	1.6
Hypocycloidal	48	451	1.3

*Used with permission of Medical Systems Division, North American Philips Corp.

The plane of section is the *slice* or *cut* within the patient that contains structures in focus in the tomographic image. The width of the plane of section is reduced as the angle subtended by the x-ray tube and film is increased.[21-23] If a thick plane of section is desired, then angles of motion smaller than 5 degrees should be used. Tomographic procedures that use small angles of motion are termed *small-angle zonography*. The relationship between the thickness of the plane of section and the angle of tube motion is described in Table 17-2 for the Massiot-Philips "Polytome."

NEUTRON RADIOGRAPHY

Radiographs obtained by exposing objects to slow neutrons (kinetic energy $\simeq 0.025$ eV) are remarkably dissimilar from those obtained by exposing the same objects to x rays. Slow neutrons are attenuated primarily during interactions with low-Z nuclei. In tissue, neutrons are attenuated more rapidly in muscle and fat than in bone, because the concentration of low-Z nuclei (primarily hydrogen) is greater in muscle and fat. Neutron radiographs display excellent contrast between air and soft tissue and between soft tissue and structures that contain a contrast agent (e.g., Gd_2O_3) for slow neutrons. The contrast is poor between fat and muscle but may be improved by exposing the specimen to heavy water (water with an increased concentration of deuterium).[24] Bone transmits slow neutrons readily, and neutron radiographs of regions containing bone furnish excellent detail of soft tissue without the distracting image of surrounding bone. A slow neutron radiograph of a rat leg, paw and tail is compared in Figure 17-12 with a conventional roentgenogram

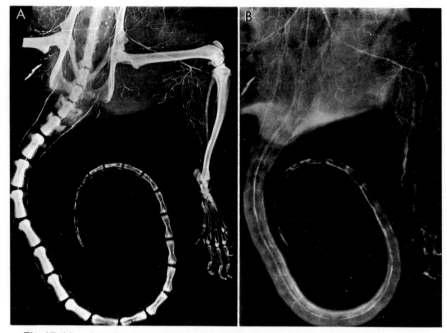

Fig 17-12. — Arteriograms of a rat leg, paw and tail, utilizing Gd_2O_3 as the contrast medium: **A,** radiograph obtained with 20-kVp x rays; **B,** slow neutron radiograph exposed with an antiscatter grid. (From Brown, M., Allen, J., and Parks, P.: Slow neutron imaging of fatty tissues through deuteration with heavy water, Biomed. Sci. Instrum. 6, 1969.)

obtained with 20-kVp x rays. A number of technical problems associated with neutron radiography have delayed the application of this technique to clinical radiology.[25]

PROBLEMS

1. Explain why the exposure rate required for cinefluorography is much greater than the exposure rate required for image intensification fluoroscopy.
2. Explain the influence of the following variables on patient dose during cinefluorography: (a) frame rate; (b) film speed; (c) lens aperture opening (f stop); (d) speed of objective lens and (e) patient thickness.
3. Discuss the advantages and disadvantages of spot photographs with 70-mm or 105-mm film compared with spot radiographs with conventional x-ray film.
4. Explain the various modes of operation of an automatic brightness control unit. Why is such a system necessary for cinefluorography and photospot recording of images?
5. Why is the maximum magnification without significant loss of image detail

greater for fluoroscopy with image intensification than for radiography with intensifying screens?
6. Discuss the production of "shadows" in tomographic images. How can they be reduced or eliminated?

REFERENCES

1. Ridgway, A., and Thumm, W.: *The Physics of Medical Radiography* (Reading, Mass.: Addison-Wesley Publishing Co., Inc., 1968).
2. England, I.: Angiography: Choice of equipment, X-Ray Focus 6:4, 1965.
3. Dreisinger, F.: Analytical Projectors for Cinefluorography, in Cornwell, W., et al. (eds.): *Cinefluorography* (Springfield, Ill.: Charles C Thomas, Publisher, 1960), p. 151.
4. International Commission on Radiation Units and Measurements: *Cameras for Image Intensifier Fluorography*, ICRU Report 15, Washington, D.C., 1969.
5. Addison, S., Hendee, W., Whitaker, F., and Rossi, R.: Diagnostic x-ray survey procedures for fluoroscopic installations — Part III: Cinefluorographic units, Health Phys. 35:845, 1978.
6. Hale, J., et al.: Physical Factors in Cinefluorography, in Moseley, R., and Rust, J. (eds.): *The Reduction of Patient Dose by Diagnostic Radiologic Instrumentation* (Springfield, Ill.: Charles C Thomas, Publisher, 1964), p. 78.
7. Henny, G.: Dose Aspects of Cinefluorography, in Janower, M. (ed.): *Technical Needs for Reduction of Patient Dosage from Diagnostic Radiology* (Springfield, Ill.: Charles C Thomas, Publisher, 1963), p. 319.
8. Carlson, C., and Kaude, J.: Integral dose in 70-mm fluorography of the gastroduodenal tract, Acta Radiol. (Diagnosis) 7:84, 1968.
9. Olsson, O.: Comparison of Image Quality: 35 mm, 70 mm and Full Size Films, in Moseley, R., and Rust, J. (eds.): *Diagnostic Radiologic Instrumentation* (Springfield, Ill.: Charles C Thomas, Publisher, 1965), p. 370.
10. Hendee, W., and Chaney, E.: Diagnostic x-ray survey procedures for fluoroscopic installations — Part I: Undertable units, Health Phys. 29:331, 1975.
11. Whitaker, F., Addison, S., and Hendee, W.: Diagnostic x-ray survey procedures for fluoroscopic installations — Part II: Automatic brightness controlled units, Health Phys. 32:61, 1977.
12. Hendee, W., Chaney, E., and Rossi, R.: *Radiologic Physics, Equipment and Quality Control* (Chicago: Year Book Medical Publishers, Inc., 1977), p. 141.
13. Sashin, D., Porti, A., Heinz, E., and Sternglass, E.: Video techniques in diagnostic radiology, Proc. SPIE 35:147, 1972.
14. Seemann, H.: *Physical and Photographic Principles of Medical Radiography* (New York: John Wiley & Sons, Inc., 1968).
15. Daves, M., and Dalrymple, G.: Objective stereoscopy, Radiology 78:802, 1962.
16. Ziedses des Plantes, B.: Subtraktion: Eine röntgenographische Methode zur separaten Abbildung bestimmter Teile des Objekts, Fortschr. Geb. Röntgenstrahlen 52:69, 1935.
17. Ziedses des Plantes, B.: The electronic subtraction method, Electromedica 1:23, 1968.
18. Hardstedt, C., and Welander, U.: Photographic subtraction, Acta Radiol. [Diagn.] 16:559, 1975.
19. Enlargement radiography, a review of 0.3 mm techniques with bibliography, Cathode Press 24:32, 1967.

20. Isard, H., et al.: *An Atlas of Serial Magnification Roentgenography*, Cathode Press Supplement (Stamford, Conn.: Machlett Laboratories, Inc.).
21. Littleton, J.: Some blurring characteristics of small angle tomography, Medicamundi 10:10, 1964.
22. Hodes, P., DeMoor, J., and Ernst, R.: Body-section radiography: Fundamentals, Radiol. Clin. North Am. 1:229, 1963.
23. International Commission on Radiological Units and Measurements: *Methods of Evaluating Radiological Equipment and Materials*. Recommendations of the ICRU, Report 10f. National Bureau of Standards Handbook 89, 1963.
24. Brown, M., Allen, J., and Parks, P.: Slow Neutron Imaging of Fatty Tissues through Deuteration with Heavy Water, in *Biomedical Sciences Instrumentation*, Vol. 6, Proc. 7th National ISA/UM Biological Sciences Instrumentation Symposium on Imagery in Medicine, Ann Arbor, Mich., May 19–22, 1969.
25. Brown, M., and Parks, P.: Neutron radiography in biological media: Techniques, observations and implications, Am. J. Roentgenol. 106:254, 1969.

18 / Quality of the Radiologic Image

THE IMAGE furnished by a radiographic, fluoroscopic, nuclear medicine or ultrasound imaging system is useful only if it furnishes sufficient information with adequate clarity. In other words, the image is satisfactory only if the *visibility of anatomical detail* is satisfactory. The visibility of anatomical detail depends on properties of the image such as the degree of image unsharpness, the level of image noise and the contrast of the image. Image contrast refers to the difference in optical density or brightness between adjacent regions in the image and is influenced by *subject contrast* and *detector contrast*. Subject contrast describes differences in the number of x or γ rays emerging from adjacent regions of a

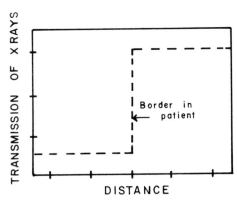

Fig 18-1. — *Subject contrast* describes the variation in exposure across a beam of x- or γ-ray photons emerging from a patient. This variation in exposure is converted by the detector into an image with image contrast. *Image contrast* is defined for film as the difference in optical density between adjacent regions of the image. *Image unsharpness* describes the distance in an image that corresponds to a sharp border in the object. Image detail is improved as this distance is reduced.

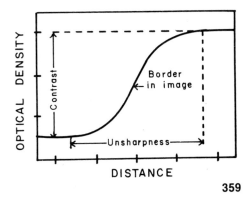

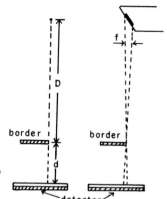

Fig 18-2. — Geometric unsharpness caused by the finite size of the focal spot of an x-ray tube.

patient and reflects differences in effective atomic number, density and thickness of the adjacent regions. Detector contrast describes the ability of a detector to convert differences in the number of x or γ rays across an x-ray beam into differences in optical density or brightness in the image. A detector may enhance or suppress subject contrast. If film is used as the radiation detector, then detector contrast is called *film contrast* and is described by the average gradient of the film.

Image *detail* (also termed *definition, resolution* and *sharpness*) describes the exactness with which differences in the attenuation of x or γ rays in adjacent regions of the patient are displayed in the image. Detail is the opposite of image *unsharpness*, which refers to blurred images of sharp borders in the object. Radiologic contrast and unsharpness are depicted in Figure 18-1.

PHYSICAL FACTORS AFFECTING IMAGE QUALITY

Geometric Unsharpness

Geometric unsharpness in a roentgenogram refers to the loss of image detail caused by the finite size of the focal spot of the x-ray tube. In Figure 18-2, a sharp border in the patient is projected undistorted onto the detector by x rays from a "point" focal spot. When the focal spot is increased to finite size, however, the image of the sharp border is expanded over a finite distance on the detector. This distance is a measure of geometric unsharpness in the image. As the focal spot is increased in size, the unsharpness is increased and the detail present in the image is decreased. As shown in equation (18-1), the geometric unsharpness increases with focal spot size and object-detector distance and decreases with target-object distance. The increase in geometric unsharpness with object-film distance is the principal factor limiting the amount of useful magnification in magnification roentgenography.

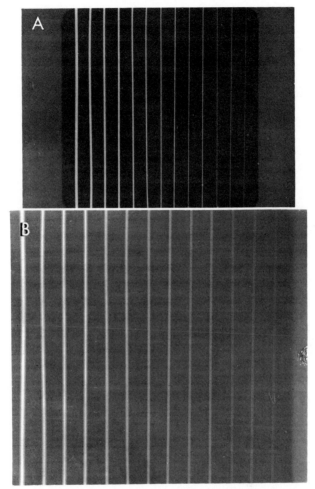

Fig 18-3.—A, contact roentgenogram of a series of parallel wires spaced 1/8 in. apart. The diameters of the wires decrease from left to right. **B,** roentgenogram of phantom with magnification factor of 3.15. (Figures 18-3 and 18-4 from Friedman, P., and Greenspan, R.: Observations on magnification radiography, Radiology 92:549, 1969.)

$$\text{Geometric unsharpness} = f\left(\frac{d}{D}\right) \qquad (18\text{-}1)$$

where

f = Size of apparent focal spot.
d = Object-detector distance.
D = Target-object distance.

Shown in Figure 18-3 are roentgenograms of a phantom containing

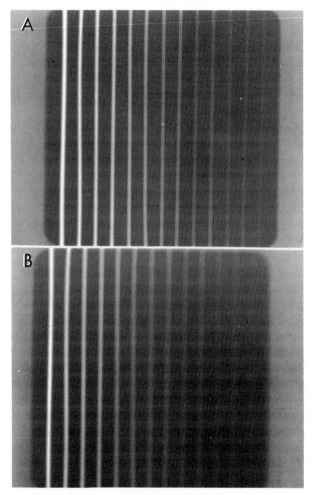

Fig 18-4.—Roentgenograms of the wire phantom of Figure 18-3, obtained with a Machlett Dynamax 40 x-ray tube with an apparent focal spot of 1.0 × 1.7 mm. **A,** wires positioned parallel to the cathode-anode axis; **B,** wires positioned perpendicular to the cathode-anode axis.

steel wires of various diameters spaced ⅛ in. apart.[1] The roentgenogram in Figure 18-3, *A*, was exposed with the x-ray film in contact with the phantom. The roentgenogram in Figure 18-3, *B*, was exposed with the x-ray film displaced below the phantom to provide a magnification factor of 3.15. In *B*, geometric unsharpness blurs the edges of the images of the wires. The images of the smaller wires exhibit higher contrast along the edges than at the center. The enhanced contrast along the image borders

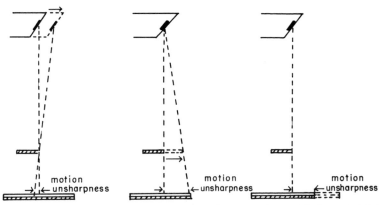

Fig 18-5. — Motion unsharpness resulting from motion of *(left to right)* the x-ray tube, the patient and the film cassette.

results primarily from the nonuniformity of radiation from the focal spot of the x-ray tube and is more apparent when the wires are parallel rather than perpendicular to the cathode-anode axis of the x-ray tube (Fig 18-4).

Motion Unsharpness

Motion of the x-ray tube, patient or detector contributes to unsharpness in the roentgenographic or fluoroscopic image (Fig 18-5). Usually, voluntary or involuntary movement by the patient is the major cause of motion unsharpness. Image unsharpness is affected more by small movements of the patient or detector than by similar movements of the x-ray tube. Motion unsharpness may be reduced by supporting the x-ray tube and the film cassette or fluoroscopic system firmly and by instructing the patient to remain still during the examination. Image unsharpness caused by involuntary motion may be reduced by using very rapid exposures (e.g., < $\frac{1}{30}$ second).

Screen Unsharpness

Unsharpness of the roentgenographic image also is caused by lateral diffusion of light between its origin in the intensifying screen and its

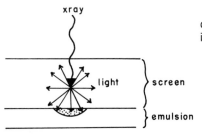

Fig 18-6. — Loss of image detail caused by lateral diffusion of light in an intensifying screen.

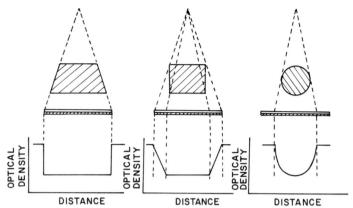

Fig 18-7.—Effect of the shape of a structure on the sharpness of the image of its borders.

absorption in the x-ray film (Fig 18-6). The amount of diffusion and therefore the screen unsharpness increase with the thickness of the fluorescent layer of the screen and, to a lesser extent, with the average size of fluorescent granules in the screen. The active layer of detail screens often is tinted to reduce the lateral diffusion of light. The resolution varies from 6–9 lines/mm for images made with fast screens to as many as 10–15 lines/mm for images obtained with detail screens under laboratory conditions. Resolutions this high are seldom realized clinically. The resolution is much poorer (2–4 lines/mm) for fluoroscopic images obtained with an image intensifier. Screen unsharpness increases greatly if the intensifying screen and film are not in intimate contact.

Film Unsharpness

The contribution of film to the unsharpness of a roentgenographic image almost always is negligible in comparison with geometric, motion and screen unsharpness. Film unsharpness is important only when x-ray film is exposed directly to x rays and when motion and geometric unsharpness are exceptionally small. The primary contribution of film to image clarity is its effect on quantum mottle, with images recorded with high-speed film displaying more quantum mottle because of the reduced number of x rays used in forming the image. Film unsharpness is greater for double-emulsion films than for films with a single emulsion.

Effects of Object Shape on Radiographic Detail

Illustrated in Figure 18-7 is the effect of the shape of a structure on the visibility of its borders in the image. Images of borders are sharper for the truncated pyramid on the left than for the sphere on the right, because the attenuation of the x-ray beam increases gradually from the edge toward the center of the spherical object.

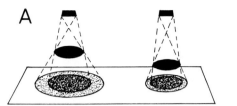
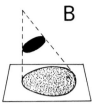
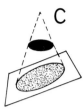

Fig 18-8. — Some causes of distortion in the radiographic image: **A,** distortion between images of structures at different depths within the patient; **B,** distortion of the image of a structure tilted with respect to a plane perpendicular to the central axis of the x-ray beam; **C,** distortion caused by improper alignment of source and detector.

Radiologic Distortion

Some structures within a patient are near the x-ray film or fluoroscopic screen, and other structures are farther away. Hence, the magnification of the image varies for different structures in the patient. These differences in magnification are described as radiographic distortion. The image is distorted also if a structure is tilted with respect to a plane perpendicular to the x-ray beam central axis, or if the detector is tilted with respect to a particular structure within the patient (Fig 18-8).

STATISTICAL FACTORS AFFECTING IMAGE QUALITY

At every location in an x-ray beam, the photon flux density varies with time according to a Poisson probability law (Chapter 12); that is, the number of x rays per unit area of the x-ray beam fluctuates continually at every location in the beam. As the sensitivity of a detector (e.g., x-ray film or a fluoroscopic screen) is increased, a response is elicited by fewer x rays per unit area. Consequently, the relative differences increase among the photon fluences that impinge upon different regions of the more sensitive detector. The variation in x-ray fluence across an intensifying screen, x-ray film or fluoroscopic screen contributes to *radiologic mottle* or *image noise*, expressions that describe the mottled "salt and pepper" appearance of roentgenograms and fluoroscopic images.

Suppose one region of a patient transmits 10% less radiation than an adjacent region. If the photon fluence is 100 photons/sq. mm through the first region, then the expected photon fluence through the adjacent region is 110 photons/sq mm. However, the photon fluence is subject to statistical fluctuations. The estimated standard deviations of the fluences are $\sqrt{100}$ photons/sq mm = 10 photons/sq mm and $\sqrt{110}$ photons/sq mm = 10.5 photons/sq mm. The probability density curve for the number of photons transmitted by each region is shown in Figure 18-9. The upper curves overlap greatly, suggesting that the probablity is only 40–50% that the image will depict the adjacent regions clearly. That is, fluctuations in photon fluence across the x-ray beam tend to obscure differences

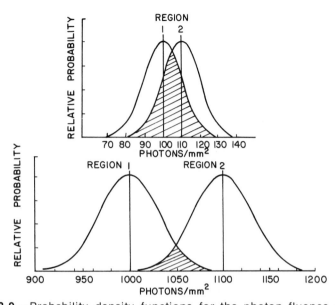

Fig 18-9.—Probability density functions for the photon fluence emerging from adjacent regions of a patient with a 10% difference in transmission. The lower curves reflect a tenfold increase in the photon fluence over that depicted in the upper curves. Fluctuations in photon fluence across the x-ray beam are more significant when fewer photons are required for a radiographic image.

in the transmission of x-ray photons through adjacent regions of the patient, especially if these differences are not very great (i.e., low subject contrast). If the photon fluence transmitted by the adjacent regions is increased tenfold (1,000 photons/sq mm and 1,100 photons/sq mm, respectively), then the probability is increased greatly that the regions are distinguishable in the image (Fig 18-9, *bottom*). However, a tenfold increase in the photon fluence requires a tenfold decrease in the sensitivity of the detector.

Fluctuation in the photon fluence across a beam of x-ray photons limits the sensitivity of a detector used to obtain a roentgenographic or fluoroscopic image. Most x-ray film exposed with conventional intensifying screens requires a photon fluence of at least 10^5 rays/sq mm to produce an acceptable image, and image noise does not contribute significantly to the loss of image quality in roentgenography with these screens. With more sensitive rare earth screens, images may be noticeably affected by image noise.

During fluoroscopy with an image intensifier, as few as 40 photons/sq mm may be received by the input screen during the integrating time of the eye (approximately 0.2 second). In this case, fluctuations in photon

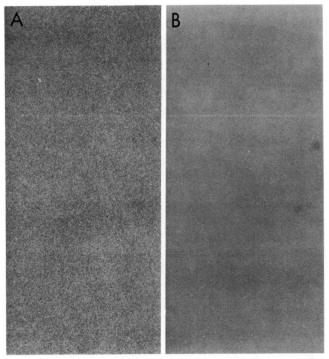

Fig 18-10.—Radiologic mottle in roentgenograms exposed with intensifying screens. **A,** roentgenogram exposed with firm contact between screens and film, **B,** roentgenogram exposed with a separation of 1/16 in. between film and screens. (From Cleare, H., Splettstosser, H., and Seemann, H.: An experimental study of the mottle produced by x-ray intensifying screens, Am. J. Roentgenol. 88:168, 1962.)

fluence across the x-ray beam are one of the major contributors to loss of image quality.

In nuclear medicine and computed tomographic imaging, *image noise* also is a significant factor in the overall quality of the image. Image noise is illustrated in Figure 18-10, *A,* in which a roentgenogram exposed with

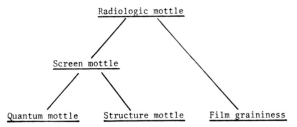

Fig 18-11.—Constituents of radiologic mottle (image noise).

Fig 18-12. — Image noise in Eastman Kodak Royal Blue film for "flash" exposures at 70 kVp with calcium tungstate screens: **A,** roentgenogram obtained with medium-speed screens; **B,** roentgenogram obtained with fast screens. (Figures 18-12 to 18-16 from Rossmann, K.: Some physical factors affecting image quality in medical radiography, J. Photo. Sci. 12:279, 1964.)

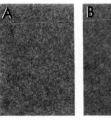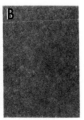

intensifying screens is reproduced. The roentgenogram in Figure 18-10, *B,* was exposed after the intensifying screens were displaced ¹⁄₁₆ in. above and below the film. This displacement increases the diffusion of light from the screens and decreases the capability of the film to record the unevenness in light flashes across the screens.[2] The mottled appearance of the roentgenogram in *B* is attributable primarily to the size of granules in the film emulsion, and is described as *film graininess.* The increased mottle of the roentgenogram in *A* is described as *screen mottle* and is caused primarily by fluctuation of the flashes of light in the active layer of the screen. The fluctuation of the light flashes reflects the irregular structure of the screen emulsion *(structure mottle)* and the randomness with which x-ray photons are absorbed in the intensifying screens *(quantum mottle).* Radiologic mottle is a reflection of both screen mottle and film graininess (Fig 18-11). Usually, screen mottle is the more important constituent, primarily because of the presence of quantum mottle.

The lateral diffusion of light from the active layer increases with the thickness of an intensifying screen. Hence, screens with thick active layers (fast screens) reduce the effect of quantum mottle.[3] That is, the optical density is more uniform across a roentgenogram exposed with a thick, fast screen than across a roentgenogram exposed with a slower screen. Fast screens do not improve the quality of the roentgenographic image, however, because structures are defined less sharply. The influence of screen speed upon radiologic mottle is illustrated in Figure 18-12.

DESCRIBING THE QUALITY OF A RADIOLOGIC IMAGE

A number of phantoms have been developed to test the resolution of radiologic imaging devices. For radiographic units, phantoms often contain opaque wires or strips with separations that diminish gradually from one side of the phantom to the other. The resolution of a roentgenographic or fluoroscopic unit is described as the maximum number of lines per millimeter visible in the image.

The resolution furnished by a radiographic system may be evaluated

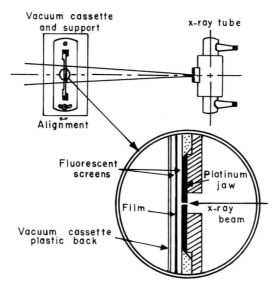

Fig 18-13. — Test object for evaluating the resolution of a radiographic system.

with a test object developed originally by VanAllen and Morgan.[4] In this test object, two metal jaws opaque to x rays are separated by a slit of adjustable width (Fig 18-13). A screen-film combination or a fluoroscopic screen is exposed with the test object positioned between the film cassette or fluoroscopic screen and the x-ray tube. Results are shown in Figure 18-14 for different combinations of intensifying screens and film exposed to radiation transmitted by the test object.

The sharpness of the image of the slit between the metal jaws of the test object may be described by the *line spread function*. The line spread function is determined from measurements of the transmission of light at increments across the image of the slit. Line spread functions, normalized to a transmission of 1.0 at the center of the slit, are plotted in Figure 18-15 for roentgenograms exposed with medium and fast calcium tungstate screens. The image of the slit is less sharp in the roentgenogram ob-

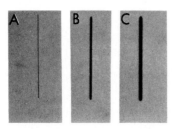

Fig 18-14. — Roentgenograms of a 10-μ slit on Kodak Royal Blue medical x-ray film exposed: **A,** without intensifying screens; **B,** with medium-speed calcium tungstate screens; **C,** with fast calcium tungstate screens.

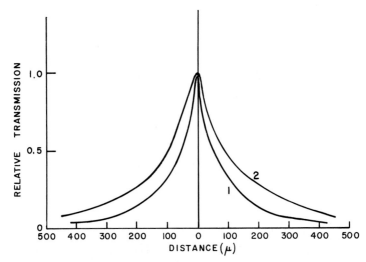

Fig 18-15.—Normalized line spread functions for slit images obtained with calcium tungstate screens. Curve *1*, two medium-speed screens; curve *2*, two fast screens.

tained with fast screens. Consequently, structures in a patient also are recorded less sharply if fast screens are used.

Modulation transfer functions (MTF) may be computed from normalized line spread functions.[5-7] The modulation transfer function for a radiographic system describes the capability of the system to furnish an im-

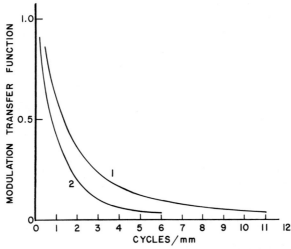

Fig 18-16.—Modulation transfer functions computed from the line spread functions in Figure 18-15. Curve *1*, slit images obtained with medium-speed screens; curve *2*, slit images obtained with fast screens.

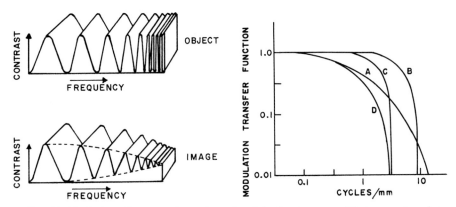

Fig 18-17 *(left).* —Suppression of contrast in the image with increasing frequency of variation in transmission of x rays through an object.

   Fig 18-18 *(right).* —Modulation transfer functions for components of a roentgenographic system and the composite modulation transfer function for the entire system. Curve *A, MTF* for screen-film combination; Curve *B, MTF* for a 1-mm focal spot with 90 cm between the focal spot and the object and 10 cm between the object and the film; Curve *C, MTF* for 0.3-mm motion of the object during exposure; Curve *D,* composite *MTF* for the entire system. (From Morgan, R.: The frequency response function, Am. J. Roentgenol. 88:175, 1962.)

age that varies in optical density or brightness in exactly the same way that a test object or patient varies in the transmission of x radiation. The modulation transfer function sometimes is termed the *sine-wave response, contrast transmission function* or *frequency response function;* however, the expression "modulation transfer function" has been recommended by the International Committee for Optics.[8]

   Modulation transfer functions for the line spread functions depicted in Figure 18-15 are plotted in Figure 18-16. The modulation transfer functions in Figure 18-16 describe the capability of two different screen-film combinations to provide discrete images of the thin slit in a test object as the number of slits per millimeter (lines or cycles per millimeter) increases.

   For an object with a sinusoidal variation in transmission of x radiation, the radiographic image may be distorted in several ways. *Amplitude distortion* refers to the suppression of contrast in the image with increasing frequency (lines/mm) of variation in the transmission of radiation through the object (Fig 18-17). Usually, amplitude distortion is the major contributor to reduction in the modulation transfer function. *Harmonic distortion* refers to the introduction into the image of variations in contrast which do not reflect differences in transmission through the object. Harmonic distortion in roentgenography is caused primarily by the nonlinear response of x-ray film to light from an intensifying screen. *Phase*

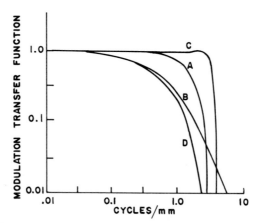

Fig 18-19.—Modulation transfer functions for components of a fluoroscopic system and the composite *MTF* for the entire system. Curve *A*, *MTF* for a 1-mm apparent focal spot with a ratio of 3 between target-object distance and object-screen distance; Curve *B*, *MTF* for the image intensifier; Curve *C*, *MTF* for a 525-line television system; Curve *D*, composite *MTF* for the entire system. (From Morgan, R.: Physics of Diagnostic Radiology, in Glasser, O., et al. (eds.): *Physical Foundations of Radiology* [3d ed.; New York: Harper & Row, 1961].)

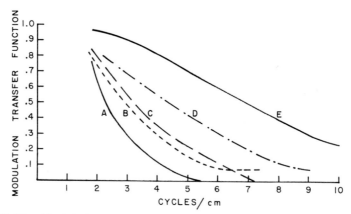

Fig 18-20.—Modulation transfer functions for various isotope-imaging devices. Curve *A*, *MTF* for Picker Magnascanner with a 3 in. crystal and a #2102A 31-hole intermediate focus collimator; Curve *B*, *MTF* for Nuclear Chicago Pho/Gamma II single-crystal scintillation camera equipped with a multihole collimator; Curve *C*, *MTF* for Picker Magnascanner with a 3-in. crystal and a #2107 19-hole collimator; Curve *D*, *MTF* for Argonne Cancer Research Hospital brain scanner with an isoresponse collimator designed for ^{203}Hg; Curve *E*, *MTF* for Picker Magnascanner with a 3-in. crystal and a #2102 31-hole fine focus collimator.

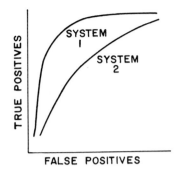

Fig 18-21.—Relative operating characteristics (ROC) curves for two imaging systems, with System 1 yielding superior results.

distortion refers to the blurring of boundaries in the image caused by the inability of the screen-film combination to reproduce sinusoidal variations in transmission of radiation through the object. Phase distortion usually is not important in roentgenography but may cause severe distortion of fluoroscopic and nuclear medicine images.

For a complete radiologic imaging system, the modulation transfer function is the product of the modulation transfer function for each component of the system. In Figure 18-18, the *MTF* for a complete roentgenographic system (curve *D*) is the product of the *MTF* for the screen-film combination (curve *A*), the *MTF* for the focal spot of the x-ray tube (curve *B*) and the *MTF* for the motion of the object (curve *C*).[9] The modulation transfer function for a fluoroscopic system with an image intensifier and a television monitor is shown in Figure 18-19.[10] Modulation transfer functions for selected nuclear medicine imaging devices are shown in Figure 18-20.[11]

Although the modulation transfer function is an elegant description of the resolution of an imaging system, it is not a complete assessment of the ability of an imaging system to furnish high-quality images. One obvious omission from the modulation transfer function is the effect of image noise. Another omission is the transfer of information from the image to the radiologist, a very important step in successful utilization of the information. To encompass these factors as well as image resolution, an approach known as *relative operating characteristics* (ROC) analysis has been used. In the application of this approach to the assessment of radiologic imaging systems, a series of images obtained with each of the systems is shown to a group of viewers. Each of the images may or may not contain an abnormality. If a viewer detects the abnormality in an image, the result is scored as a "true positive." If a viewer detects the abnormality when it is not present in an image, the result is scored as a "false positive." A plot of true positives versus false positives (Fig 18-21) reveals the relative performance of the imaging systems in terms of their ability to yield accurate diagnoses, with the superior system occupying the more elevated position in the upper left quadrant of the plot.

QUANTUM LEVELS AND CONVERSION EFFICIENCIES

The number of x-ray photons or light photons per unit area may be described at each stage of transformation of information in an x-ray beam into a visual image. These numbers are termed *quantum levels*. For example, a typical roentgenogram may require an exposure of 3×10^7 x-ray photons per sq cm to the intensifying screen (Fig 18-22). About 30% of the x-ray photons may be absorbed in the screen. For each x-ray photon absorbed, 1,000 photons of light may be liberated. About 50% of these light photons escape from the screen and interact in the emulsion of the x-ray film. In a typical photographic emulsion, 200 photons of light are absorbed for each photographic granule affected. In curve A of Figure 18-22, the number of photons per unit area is lowest at the stage of absorption of x-ray photons in the intensifying screen. This stage is termed the *quantum sink*. The quantum sink determines the major influence of quantum mottle upon the resolution of the roentgenographic image.

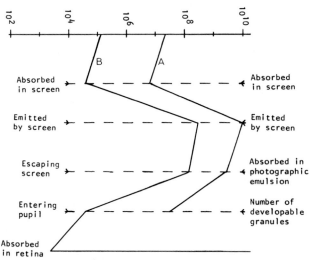

Fig 18-22.—Quantum levels for stages of information conversion in roentgenography and fluoroscopy. Curve *A*, roentgenogram with intensifying screens; Curve *B*, conventional fluoroscopy. (Figures 18-22 and 18-23 from Ter-Pogossian, M.: *The Physical Aspects of Diagnostic Radiology* [New York: Harper & Row, 1967].)

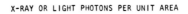

X-RAY OR LIGHT PHOTONS PER UNIT AREA

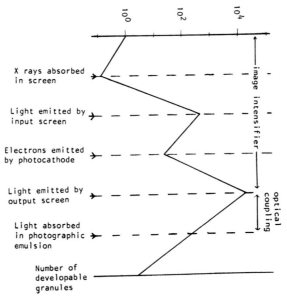

Fig 18-23. — Quantum levels for stages of information conversion in a typical cinefluorographic system.

Quantum levels for stages in fluoroscopy without an image intensifier are depicted also in Figure 18-22. The x-ray photon fluence is 2×10^5 photons/sq. cm on the fluoroscopic screen during the integrating time (0.2 second) of the eye. In this mode of fluoroscopy (and in fluoroscopy with image intensification), the quantum sink is the stage of absorption of light photons in the observer's retina. In Figure 18-22, only 4×10^3 light photons are absorbed in each square centimeter of the retina during the integrating time. Consequently, the effect of quantum mottle upon image resolution is more pronounced in fluoroscopy than in roentgenography.

Quantum levels for stages of a cinefluorographic system are depicted in Figure 18-23. The quantum sink is the stage of absorption of x-ray photons by the input screen of the image intensifier.

PROBLEMS
1. Illustrate by diagrams the change in geometric unsharpness with:
    a. Size of the apparent focal spot of the x-ray tube.
    b. Distance between the object and the detector.
    c. Distance between the x-ray tube and object.
2. Define the expressions "subject contrast," "detector contrast" and "image

contrast." Discuss the influence of subject contrast and detector contrast upon image contrast.

3. Discuss the concept of quantum mottle and how quantum mottle limits the useful brightness gain of an image intensifier used for fluoroscopy.
4. Describe the influence of each contribution to radiologic mottle in (a) image intensification fluoroscopy and in (b) roentgenography with intensifying screens.
5. Discuss the meaning of the expression "image detail" or "image resolution," and one method for measuring the resolution of a roentgenographic or fluoroscopic system.

REFERENCES

1. Friedman, P., and Greenspan, R.: Observations on magnification radiography, Radiology 92:549, 1969.
2. Cleare, H., Splettstosser, H., and Seemann, H.: An experimental study of the mottle produced by x-ray intensifying screens, Am. J. Roentgenol. 88:168, 1962.
3. Rossmann, K.: Some physical factors affecting image quality in medical radiography, J. Photo. Sci. 12:279, 1964.
4. VanAllen, W., and Morgan, R.: Measurement of resolving powers of intensifying screens, Radiology 47:166, 1946.
5. Rossmann, K.: Measurement of the modulation transfer function of radiography systems containing fluorescent screens, Phys. Med. Biol. 9:551, 1964.
6. Gregg, E.: Assessment of radiologic imaging, Radiology 97:776, 1966.
7. Lubberts, G.: The line spread-function and the modulation transfer function of x-ray fluorescent screen-film systems: Problems with double-coated films, Am. J. Roentgenol. 105:909, 1969.
8. Rossmann, K.: Modulation transfer function of radiographic systems using fluorescent screens, J. Opt. Soc. Am. 52:774, 1962.
9. Morgan, R.: The frequency response function, Am. J. Roentgenol. 88:175, 1962.
10. Morgan, R.: Physics of Diagnostic Radiology, in Glasser, O., et al.: (eds.): *Physical Foundations of Radiology* (3d ed.; New York: Harper & Row, 1961), p. 117.
11. Gottschalk, A.: Modulation Transfer Function Studies with the Gamma Scintillation Camera, in Gottschalk, A., and Beck, R. (eds.): *Fundamental Problems in Scanning* (Springfield, Ill.: Charles C Thomas, Publisher, 1968), p. 314.

19 / Computed Tomography

IN CONVENTIONAL ROENTGENOGRAPHY, subtle differences of a few percent in subject contrast (i.e., x-ray attenuation in the body) are not visible in the image for the following reasons:

1. The projection of three-dimensional anatomical information onto a two-dimensional image receptor obscures subtle differences in x-ray transmission through structures aligned parallel to the x-ray beam. Although conventional tomography resolves this problem to some degree, structures above and below the tomographic section may remain visible in the image if they differ significantly in their x-ray attenuating properties from structures in the section.

2. Conventional image receptors (i.e., film, intensifying and fluoroscopic screens) are not able to resolve small differences (1–2%) in the intensity of incident radiation.

3. Large-area x-ray beams used in conventional roentgenography produce considerable scattered radiation that interferes with the display of subtle differences in subject contrast.

To a significant degree, each of these difficulties is eliminated in computed tomography (CT), and differences in subject contrast of a few tenths of a percent are revealed in the image. Although the spatial resolution of 1–2 mm provided by computed tomography is notably poorer than that obtained by conventional roentgenography, the superior visualization of subject contrast, together with the display of anatomy across planes (e.g., cross sectional) that is not accessible by conventional imaging techniques, makes computed tomography exceptionally useful for visualizing the anatomy in the head and promising for visualizing anatomy in many other regions of the body.

HISTORY

The image reconstruction techniques used in computed tomography were developed for use in radio astronomy,[1] electron microscopy[2,3] and optics.[4,5] In 1961, Oldendorf explored the principle of computed tomography with an apparatus using an ^{131}I source.[6] Shortly thereafter, Kuhl and colleagues developed emission and [241]Am transmission CT imaging systems and described the application of these systems to brain imaging.[7,8] In spite of these early efforts, computed tomography remained unexploited for clinical imaging until the announcement by EMI Ltd. in

1972 of the first commercially available x-ray transmission CT unit designed exclusively for studies of the head.[9] The prototype for this unit had been studied since 1970 at Atkinson-Morley Hospital in England, and the first commercial unit was installed in the United States in 1973. The same year, Ledley and colleagues announced the development of a whole body CT scanner.[10] In 1974, Ohio Nuclear Inc. also developed a whole body CT scanner, and clinical models of both units were installed in 1975. By 1977, 16 or so commercial companies were marketing more than 30 models of transmission CT scanners, and two companies had developed emission scanners for use in nuclear medicine, principally for positron imaging. This commitment by commercial organizations reflects the proven value of computed tomography in neuroradiologic diagnosis and the potential of this technique for radiologic diagnosis in many other anatomical regions. The commitment reflects also the large investment of the medical community in computed tomography, as each transmission CT unit costs $100,000 to $1 million. In all likelihood, the advent of computed tomography represents the beginning of a transition in diagnostic radiologic imaging from direct film recording methods to quantitative imaging processes using electronic radiation detectors and computer data processing.[11, 12]

PRINCIPLE OF COMPUTED TOMOGRAPHIC IMAGING

In earlier CT imaging devices ("scanners") a narrow beam of x rays is scanned across a patient in synchrony with a radiation detector on the opposite side of the patient (Fig 19-1). If the beam is monoenergetic or nearly so, the transmission of x rays through the patient is given by the equation (see Chap. 6)

$$I = I_0 e^{-\mu x}$$

where the patient is assumed to be a homogeneous medium. If the x-ray

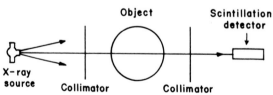

Fig 19-1. — Principle of operation of a first-generation computed tomographic scanner in which x-ray transmission measurements are accumulated while an x-ray source and detector are translated and rotated in synchrony on opposite sides of the patient. (From Brooks, R. A., and DiChiro, G.: Principles of computer assisted tomography [CAT] in radiographic and radioisotopic imaging, Phys. Med. Biol. 21:723, 1976. Copyright 1976 by The Institute of Physics. Reprinted with permission.)

beam is intercepted by two regions with attenuation coefficients μ_1 and μ_2 and thickness x_1 and x_2, the x-ray transmission is

$$I = I_0 e^{-(\mu_1 x_1 + \mu_2 x_2)}$$

If many (n) regions with different linear attenuation coefficients occur along the path of x rays, the transmission is

$$I = I_0 e^{-\Sigma_{i=1}^n \mu_i x_i}$$

where $-\Sigma_{i=1}^n \mu_i x_i = -(\mu_1 x_1 + \mu_2 x_2 + \ldots + \mu_n x_n)x$, and the fractional transmission I/I_0 is

$$e^{-\Sigma_{i=1}^n \mu_i x_i}$$

With a single transmission measurement, the separate attenuation coefficients cannot be determined because there are too many unknown values of μ_i in the equation. However, with multiple transmission measurements at different orientations of the x-ray source and detector, the separate coefficients can be distinguished so that a cross-sectional display of coefficients is obtained across the plane of transmission measurements. By assigning gray levels to different ranges of attenuation coefficients, a gray scale image can be obtained that represents various structures in the patient with different x-ray attenuation characteristics. This gray scale display of attenuation coefficients constitutes a CT image.

In earlier (first-generation) CT scanners, multiple x-ray transmission measurements are obtained by scanning a pencil-like beam of x rays and a NaI detector in a straight line on opposite sides of the patient (Fig 19-2, A). During this translational scan of perhaps 40 cm in length, multiple (e.g., 160) measurements of x-ray transmission are obtained. Next, the angular orientation of the scanning device is incremented 1 degree and a second translational scan of 160 transmission measurements is performed. This process of translational scanning separated by 1 degree increments is repeated through an arc of 180 degrees, so that $160 \times 180 = 28,800$ x-ray transmission measurements are accumulated. These measurements are transmitted to a computer equipped with a mathematical package for reconstructing an image of attenuation coefficients across the anatomical plane defined by the scanning x-ray beam.

RECONSTRUCTION ALGORITHMS

The foundation of the mathematical package for image reconstruction is the reconstruction algorithm, which may be one of four types.[13]

1. *Simple back projection.* — In this method, each x-ray transmission path through the body is divided into equally spaced elements, and each element is assumed to contribute equally to the total attenuation along the x-ray path. By summing the attenuation for each element over all x-

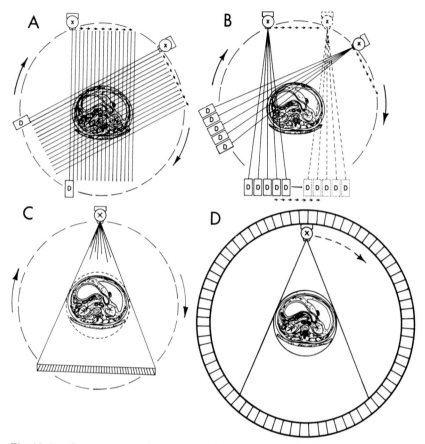

Fig 19-2.—Scan motions in computed tomography: **A,** first-generation scanner using a pencil x-ray beam and a combination of translational and rotational motion; **B,** second-generation scanner with a fan x-ray beam, multiple detectors and a combination of translational and rotational motion; **C,** third-generation scanner using a fan x-ray beam and smooth rotational motion of x-ray tube and detector array; and **D,** third-generation scanner with rotational motion of the x-ray tube within a stationary circular array of 600 or more detectors. (**A, B** and **C** from Brownell, G.: *New Instrumentation for Computerized Tomography,* in Proc. Conference on Computerized Tomography in Radiology, St. Louis, Missouri, April 25–28, 1976 [Chicago: American College of Radiology, 1976], p. 15. Reprinted with permission.)

ray paths that intersect the element at different angular orientations, a final summed attenuation coefficient is determined for each element. When this coefficient is combined with the summed coefficients for all other elements in the anatomical section scanned by the x-ray beam, a composite image of attenuation coefficients is obtained. Although the simple back projection approach to reconstruction algorithms is straight-forward, it produces blurred images of sharp features in the object.

2. *Integral equations.*—This reconstruction algorithm was pioneered by Radon[14] and uses a one-dimensional integral equation for the reconstruction of a two-dimensional image. In the convolution method of using an integral equation, a deblurring function is combined (convolved) with the x-ray transmission data to remove most of the blurring before the data are back-projected. The most common deblurring function is a frequency filter that removes the high-frequency components of the x-ray transmission data. These components are responsible for most of the blurring in the composite image. One of the advantages of the convolution method of image reconstruction is that the image can be reconstructed while x-ray transmission data are being collected. The convolution method is the most popular reconstruction algorithm used today in computed tomography.

3. *Fourier transform.*—In this approach, the x-ray attenuation pattern at each angular orientation is separated into frequency components of various amplitudes, similar to the way a musical note can be divided into relative contributions of different frequencies. From these frequency components, the entire image is assembled in "frequency space" and then reconstructed by an inverse Fourier transform process into a spatially correct image. For high-resolution images, the Fourier transform reconstruction process requires a computer of considerable size.

4. *Series expansion.*—In this technique, variations of which are known as ART (algebraic reconstruction technique) and SIRT (simultaneous iterative reconstruction technique), x-ray attenuation data at one angular orientation are divided into equally spaced elements along each of several rays. These data are compared to similar data at a different angular orientation, and differences in x-ray attenuation at the two orientations are added equally to the appropriate elements. This process is repeated for all angular orientations, with a decreasing fraction of the attenuation differences added each time to insure convergence of the reconstruction data. In this method, all x-ray attenuation data must be available before the reconstruction process can begin.

SCAN MOTIONS

Early (first-generation) CT scanners used a pencil beam of x rays and a combination of translational and rotational motion to accumulate the many transmission measurements required for image reconstruction (see Fig 19-2, *A*). Although this approach yields satisfactory images of stationary objects, considerable time (4–5 minutes) is required for data accumulation, and the images are subject to motion blurring. Soon after the introduction of pencil beam scanners, fan-shaped x-ray beams were introduced so that multiple measurements of x-ray transmission could be made simultaneously (see Fig 19-2, *B*). Fan beam geometries with increments of a few degrees for the different angular orientations (e.g., a 30-degree fan beam and 10-degree angular increments) reduced the scan time to 20–60 seconds and improved the image quality by reducing the effects of motion. Computed tomographic scanners with x-ray fan beam geometries and multiple radiation detectors constitute the second generation of CT scanners.

In late 1975, the third generation of CT scanners was introduced. These scanners eliminate the translational motion of previous scanners and rely exclusively upon rotational motion of the x-ray tube and detector array (see Fig 19-2, *C*) or upon rotational motion of the x-ray tube within a stationary circular array of 600 or more detectors (see Fig 19-2, *D*). With these scanners, data accumulation times as fast as 2 seconds are achievable.

The three generations of CT scanners that have evolved over the six years since CT scanning was introduced reflect improvements in scanner design (e.g., elimination of translational motion) and in the x-ray source used for data accumulation (e.g., substitution of rotating-anode for stationary-anode x-ray tubes). Further major reductions in scan time are not foreseeable in the immediate future because the present scanners are constrained by fundamental limitations such as x-ray fluence and detector response time rather than by the time required for motion of the x-ray source and detector. It is conceivable that CT scanners with multiple x-ray sources and detectors might be used to reduce the CT data accumulation time into the millisecond range, and research currently is under way to investigate this possibility.[15]

X-RAY SOURCES

Both stationary- and rotating-anode x-ray tubes are used in CT scanners. Many of the translate-rotate CT scanners have an oil-cooled, stationary-anode x-ray tube with a focal spot on the order of 2×16 mm. The limited output of these x-ray tubes necessitates a sampling time of about 5 msec for each measurement of x-ray transmission. This sampling time, together with the time required to move and rotate the source and detector, limit the speed with which data can be accumulated with CT units using translational and rotational motion.

To reduce the sampling time to 2–3 msec, most fast-scan CT units use rotating-anode x-ray tubes, often with a pulsed x-ray beam, to achieve higher x-ray outputs. Even with rotating-anode tubes, the heat-storage capacity of the anode may be exceeded if cooling periods are not observed between sets of successive images.

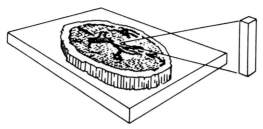

Fig 19-3. — Display of a three-dimensional volume of tissue (voxel) as a two-dimensional element in the CT image (pixel). (From McCullough, E.: Factors affecting the use of quantitative information from a CT scanner, Radiology 124: 99, 1977. Reprinted with permission.)

COLLIMATION

After transmission through the patient, the x-ray beam is collimated to confine the transmission measurement to a slice with a thickness of a few millimeters and to reduce scattered radiation to less than 1% of the primary beam intensity. The height of the collimator defines the thickness of the CT slice. This height, when combined with the area of a single picture element (pixel) in the display, defines the three-dimensional volume element (voxel) in the patient corresponding to the two-dimensional pixel of the display (Fig 19-3). A voxel encompassing a boundary between two tissue structures (e.g., muscle and bone) yields an attenuation coefficient for the pixel that is intermediate between the values for the two structures. This "partial volume artifact" may be reduced by narrowing the collimator to yield thinner slices. However, this approach reduces the number of x rays incident upon the detector, and the resulting detector signals are subject to greater statistical fluctuations, yielding a noisier image in the final display.

X-RAY DETECTORS

To reduce the detector response time, all detectors used in CT scanning are operated in current rather than pulse mode. Also, rejection of scattered radiation is assigned to the detector collimators rather than to pulse height analyzers. Detectors for CT scanning are chosen on the basis of detection efficiency (greater than 50%), short response time and stability of operation, and are either gas-filled ionization chambers or solid scintillation detectors. Scintillation detectors include NaI (Tl) and CsI crystals and newer bismuth germanate (BiGeO) detectors chosen for their high detection efficiency and low fluorescence decay time. Ionization chambers used so far contain xenon pressurized up to 25 atm to improve the x-ray detection efficiency. With any detector, the stability of response from one transmission measurement to the next is essential for the production of artifact-free reconstruction images. With a pure rotational source and detector geometry, for example, detector instability gives rise to ring-shaped artifacts in the image. Minimum energy dependence of the detectors over the energy range for the CT x-ray beam also is important if corrections for beam hardening are to be applicable to all patient sizes and configurations.

VIEWING SYSTEMS

The numbers computed by the reconstruction algorithm are not exact values of attenuation coefficients. Instead, they are integers termed *CT numbers*, which are related to attenuation coefficients. On most newer CT units, the CT numbers range from $-1,000$ for air to $+1,000$ for bone, with the CT number for water set at 0. CT numbers normalized in this manner are termed *Hounsfield units* and provide a range of several CT numbers for a 1% change in attenuation coefficient.

To portray the CT numbers as a gray scale visual display, a storage oscilloscope or television monitor may be used. This viewing device contains a contrast enhancement feature that superimposes the shades of gray available in the display device (i.e., the dynamic range of the display) over the range of CT numbers of diagnostic interest. Control of image contrast with the contrast enhancement feature is essential in x-ray computed tomography, because the electron density and therefore

TABLE 19-1.—ELECTRON DENSITIES OF
VARIOUS BODY TISSUES*

TISSUE	ELECTRON DENSITY (ELECTRONS/CC)	PHYSICAL DENSITY (gm/cc)
Water	3.35×10^{23}	1.00
Bone	3.72–5.59	1.2–1.8
Spleen	3.52	1.06
Liver	3.51	1.05
Heart	3.46	1.04
Muscle	3.44	1.06
Brain		
White matter	3.42	1.03
Gray matter	3.43	1.04
Kidney	3.42	1.05
Pancreas	3.40	1.02
Fat	3.07	0.92
Lung	0.83	0.25

*Data were calculated from the atomic composition and physical density. (From Geise, R., and McCullough, E.: The use of CT scanners in megavoltage photon-beam therapy planning, Radiology 124:133, 1977. Reprinted with permission.)

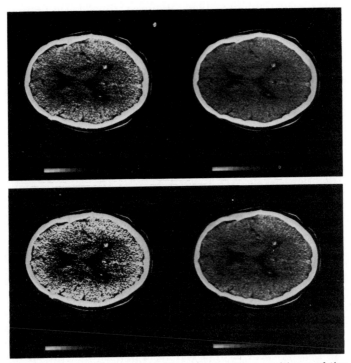

Fig 19-4.—Display of x-ray attenuation data at four positions of the window level of the contrast enhancement control.

the x-ray attenuation are remarkably similar for most tissues of diagnostic interest. This similarity is apparent from the data in Table 19-1. The same cross-sectional CT data displayed at different settings of the "window" of the contrast enhancement control are illustrated in Figure 19-4. In addition, the viewing console of the CT scanner may contain auxiliary features such as image magnification, quantitative and statistical data display, and patient identification data. Also, many scanners permit the display of coronal and sagittal images by combining reconstruction data for successive slices through the body.

PATIENT DOSE

The radiation dose delivered during a CT scan is somewhat greater than that administered for an equivalent roentgenographic image. A CT image of the head requires a dose of about 1–2 rad, for example, whereas an abdominal image usually requires a dose of 3–5 rad. These doses would have to be increased significantly to improve the contrast and spatial resolution of CT images. The relationship between resolution and dose is expressed as

$$D = \alpha\left(\frac{s^2}{e^3 h}\right) \qquad (19\text{-}1)$$

where D = patient dose, s = signal/noise ratio, e = spatial resolution, h = slice thickness and α = constant. From equation (19-1), it is apparent that:

1. A twofold improvement in the signal/noise ratio (contrast resolution) requires a fourfold increase in patient dose.

2. A twofold improvement in spatial resolution requires an eightfold increase in patient dose.

3. A twofold reduction in slice thickness requires a twofold increase in patient dose.

EMISSION-COMPUTED TOMOGRAPHY

The principles of computed tomography may also be applied to imaging the distribution of radioactive nuclides in the body. A number of investigators have explored this application,[16-18] and at least two emission-computed tomographic units are available commercially.

Perhaps the most promising application of emission tomography is for imaging the distribution of positron-emitting radionuclides in the body. In this application, each detector is operated along with a number of detectors on the opposite side of the body. This arrangement facilitates the precise localization of the origin of 511-keV annihilation radiation released in the body as positrons emitted by the nuclide are annihilated. Among the more promising nuclides for positron imaging are cyclotron-produced ^{11}C, ^{13}N and ^{15}O, which can be labeled isotopically into compounds of biologic interest, and generator-produced ^{68}Ga, which is formed by decay of its longer-lived parent ^{68}Ge.

ULTRASOUND-COMPUTED TOMOGRAPHY

Another application of computed tomography is in ultrasound imaging of certain anatomical structures, including the breast.[19, 20] To obtain an ultrasound-computed tomographic image, a transmitting transducer on one side of the patient is moved in synchrony with a receiving transducer on the opposite side of the patient in a manner identical with the motion of the x-ray tube and detector in an x-ray CT scanner. By measuring the intensity of the transmitted ultrasound at multiple positions of the transducers, an attenuation image is obtained that is similar to that for x-ray transmission tomography. An ultrasound CT image of a young female breast with some development of fibrocystic disease is shown in Figure

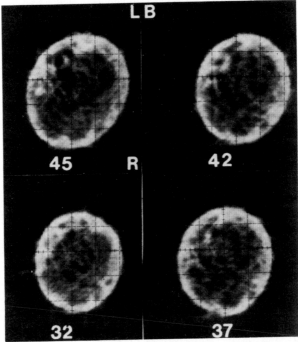

Fig 19-5. — Transmission ultrasound-computed tomographic image of successive planes through the breast of a young woman with some indications of fibrocystic development.

19-5. Alternately, the transducers can be used to measure the time of flight of ultrasound beams through the body. These data can be used to reconstruct a speed-of-sound image. In this type of image, the speed of sound through different structures in a cross section of the patient's anatomy may be portrayed as shades of gray.

PROBLEMS

1. Compare the spatial and contrast resolution of conventional roentgenographic and CT images.
2. List three reasons why contrast resolution is improved in CT imaging compared with conventional roentgenographic imaging.
3. Describe the mechanical features of the three generations of CT scanners.
4. Briefly describe the simple back-projection approach to image reconstruction, and explain how the convolution method improves these images.
5. What are the two major constraints on further reductions in CT scan time?
6. Explain the relationship between a voxel and a pixel.
7. What types of detectors are used in CT scanners?

8. Define a Hounsfield unit and explain the purpose of contrast enhancement in a CT viewing device.
9. Explain how image noise and patient dose in CT scanning are influenced by the signal/noise ratio, the size of each resolution element and the slice thickness.

REFERENCES

1. Bracewell, R.: Strip integration in radio astronomy, Aust. J. Phys. 9(2):198, 1956.
2. DeRosier, D., and Klug, A.: Reconstruction of three dimensional structures from electron micrographs, Nature 217:130, 1968.
3. Gordon, R., Bender, R., and Herman, T.: Algebraic reconstruction techniques (ART) for three-dimensional electron microscopy and x-ray photography, J. Theor. Biol. 29:471, 1970.
4. Rowley, P.: Quantitative interpretation of three-dimensional weakly refractive phase objects using holographic interferometry, J. Opt. Soc. Am. 59:1496, 1969.
5. Berry, M., and Gibbs, D.: The interpretation of optical projections, Proc. R. Soc. A 314:143, 1970.
6. Oldendorf, W.: Isolated flying spot detection of radiodensity discontinuities—displaying the internal structural pattern of a complex object, IRE Trans. Biomed. Elec., BME-8:68, 1961.
7. Kuhl, D., and Edwards, R.: Image separation radioisotope scanning, Radiology 80(4):653, 1963.
8. Kuhl, D., Hale, J., and Eaton, W.: Transmission scanning: A useful adjunct to conventional emission scanning for accurately keying isotope deposition to radiographic anatomy, Radiology 87:278, 1966.
9. Hounsfield, G.: Computerized transverse axial scanning (tomography): Part I. Description of system, Br. J. Radiol. 46:1016, 1973.
10. Ledley, R., DiChiro, G., Lussenhop, A., and Twigg, H.: Computerized transaxial x-ray tomography of the human body, Science 186:207, 1974.
11. Swindel, W., and Barrett, H.: Computerized tomography: taking sectional x rays, Phys. Today 32:32, 1977.
12. McCullough, E., and Payne, J.: X-ray transmission computed tomography, Med. Phys. 4:85, 1977.
13. Brooks, R., and DiChiro, G.: Principles of computer assisted tomography (CAT) in radiographic and radioisotopic imaging, Phys. Med. Biol. 21:689, 1976.
14. Radon, J.: Ueber die Bestimmung von Funktionen durch ihre integralwerte laengs gewisser Mannigfaltigkeiten (on the determination of functions from their integrals along certain manifolds). Berichte Saechsische Akademie der Wissenschaften (Leipzig) Mathematische-Physische Klasse 69:1917, 262.
15. Robb, R., Harris, L., and Ritman, E.: Computerized x-ray reconstruction tomography in stereometric analysis of cardiovascular dynamics, Proc. Soc. Photoopt. Instrum. Engineering 89:69, 1976.
16. Ter-Pogossian, M., Phelps, M., Brownell, G., Cox, J., Davis, D., and Evens, R. (eds.): *Reconstruction Tomography in Diagnostic Radiology and Nuclear Medicine* (Baltimore: University Park Press, 1977).
17. Hoffman, E., Phelps, M., Mullani, N., Higgins, C., and Ter-Pogossian, M.: Design and performance characteristics of a whole-body positron transaxial tomography, J. Nucl. Med. 17:493, 1976.

18. Correia, J., Chesler, D., Hoop, B., Ahluwaliz, B., Walters, T., and Brownell, G.: Transverse section reconstruction with positron emitters and the MGH positron camera, J. Nucl. Med. 17:551, 1976.
19. Carson, P., Oughton, T., Hendee, W., and Ahuja, A.: Imaging soft tissue through bone with ultrasound transmission tomography by reconstruction, Med. Phys. 4:302, 1977.
20. Greenleaf, J., Johnson, S., Sarnayoa, W., and Duck, F.: Reconstruction of Material Characteristics from Highly Refraction Distorted Projections by Ray Tracing, in *Image Processing for 2-D and 3-D Reconstruction from Projections* (Stanford, Calif.: Stanford University Press, 1975), p. MA2.

20 / Ultrasound Waves

ULTRASOUND is a mechanical disturbance that is propagated as a wave through a medium. When the medium is a patient, the propagation of the wavelike disturbance is the basis for use of ultrasound as a diagnostic tool. Hence, an appreciation of the characteristics of ultrasound waves and their behavior in various media is essential to understanding the use of diagnostic ultrasound in clinical medicine.[1-6]

WAVE MOTION

A fluid medium is a collection of particles such as atoms or molecules that are in continuous random motion. The particles are represented as filled circles in Figure 20-1. When no external force is applied to the medium, the particles are distributed more or less uniformly throughout the medium. When the medium is acted upon by a force (represented by movement of the piston from left to right in Figure 20-1, B), the particles are concentrated in the region in front of the piston. The region of increased particle density is termed a *zone of compression*. Because of the forward motion imparted to the particles by the piston, the region of increased particle density begins to migrate away from the piston and through the medium. That is, a mechanical disturbance introduced into the medium travels through the medium in a direction away from the source of the disturbance. In clinical applications of ultrasound, the piston is replaced by an ultrasound transducer.

As the zone of compression begins its migration through the medium, the piston might be withdrawn from right to left, creating a region of reduced particle density immediately behind the compression zone. Particles from the surrounding medium move into this region to restore it to normal particle density, and a second region, termed a *zone of rarefaction*, begins to migrate away from the face of the piston (Fig 20-1, C). That is, the compression zone is followed by a zone of rarefaction also moving through the medium.

If the piston is displaced again to the right, a second compression zone is established and follows the zone of rarefaction through the medium. If the piston oscillates continuously, alternate zones of compression and rarefaction are propagated through the medium, as illustrated in Figure 20-1, D. The propagation of these zones establishes a wave disturbance in the medium, which is termed a *longitudinal wave* because the motion

390

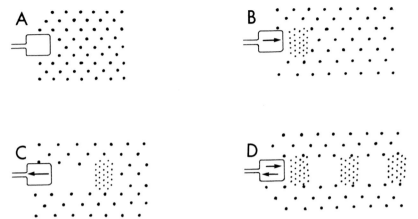

Fig 20-1. — Production of an ultrasound wave: **A,** uniform distribution of particles in a medium. **B,** movement of the piston to the right produces a zone of compression. **C,** withdrawal of the piston to the left produces a zone of rarefaction. **D,** alternate movements of the piston to the right and left establish a longitudinal wave in the medium.

of the particles in the medium is parallel to the direction of wave propagation. One compression zone followed by a zone of rarefaction is referred to as a *wave cycle*, and the number of these cycles established in the medium each second is termed the *frequency* of the wave. A wave with a frequency between about 20 and 20,000 cycles per second or hertz (Hz) is a sound wave that is audible to the human ear. An infrasonic wave is a sound wave below 20 Hz that is not audible to the human ear. An ultrasound (or ultrasonic) wave has a frequency greater than 20,000 Hz and also is inaudible. In clinical diagnosis, ultrasound waves of frequencies between 1 and 20 million cycles per second [1–20 megahertz (MHz)] are used.

As a longitudinal wave moves through a medium, particles at the edge of the wave slide past one another. Resistance to this shearing effect causes these particles to move somewhat in a direction away from the moving longitudinal wave. This transverse motion of particles along the edge of the longitudinal wave establishes shear waves that radiate transversely from the longitudinal wave. In general, shear waves are significant only in a rigid medium such as a solid. In biologic tissues, bone is the only medium in which shear waves are significant.

WAVE CHARACTERISTICS

A zone of compression and an adjacent zone of rarefaction are termed one *cycle* of an ultrasound wave. A cycle may be represented diagrammatically in a graph of particle density versus distance in the direction of

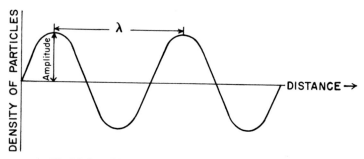

Fig 20-2. – Characteristics of an ultrasound wave.

the ultrasound wave (Fig 20-2). The distance covered by one cycle is termed the *wavelength* λ of the ultrasound wave. The number of cycles introduced into the medium each second is referred to as the *frequency ν* of the wave, expressed in units of hertz (Hz), kilohertz (kHz) or mega-hertz (MHz). The maximum height of the cycle in Figure 20-2 is the amplitude of the ultrasound wave. The product of the frequency and the wavelength is the velocity *c* of the wave; that is,

$$c = \nu\lambda$$

In most soft tissues, the velocity of ultrasound is roughly 1,540 m/sec, and frequencies of 1 MHz and greater are required to furnish ultrasound wavelengths suitable for diagnostic imaging (i.e., wavelengths on the order of 1 mm or less).

ULTRASOUND WAVEFRONTS

Often the centers of compression zones of an ultrasound wave are rep-resented by lines perpendicular to the motion of the the particles and the ultrasound wave in the medium. These lines are referred to as *wave-fronts*. For an ultrasound source of large dimensions (i.e., a large-diame-ter transducer), ultrasound wavefronts are represented as equally spaced straight lines such as those in Figure 20-3, A. Wavefronts of this type are termed *planar* wavefronts, and the ultrasound wave they represent is termed a *planar* or *plane* wave. At the other extreme, an ultrasound wave originating from a source of very small dimensions (i.e., a point source) is represented by wavefronts that describe spheres of increasing diameter at increasing distance from the source. Spherical wavefronts for a point source are diagramed in Figure 20-3, B.

For the practical case of ultrasound production for diagnostic use, sources of exceptionally small or large dimensions are not used routine-ly. Instead, sources with finite dimensions are used. These sources can be considered as a collection of point sources, each radiating spherical

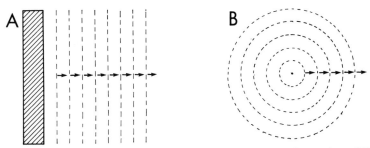

Fig 20-3. — Ultrasound wavefronts from a source of large dimensions **(A)** and a source of small dimensions **(B)**.

wavefronts (termed *wavelets*) into the medium, as shown in Figure 20-4, A. In regions where compression zones for one wavelet intersect compression zones for another, a condition of constructive interference is established. With constructive interference, the wavelets reinforce each other and the total pressure in the region is the sum of the pressures contributed by each wavelet. In regions where compression zones for one wavelet intersect zones of rarefaction for another wavelet, a condition of destructive interference is established. In these regions, the particle density is reduced.

With many spherical wavelets radiating from a transducer of reasonable size (i.e., the diameter of the transducer is considerably larger than the ultrasound wavelength), many regions of constructive and destructive interference are established in the medium. In Figure 20-4, B, these regions are represented as intersections of lines depicting compression zones of individual wavelets. From this figure it is apparent that the reinforcement and cancellation of individual wavelets are most noticeable in the region near the source of ultrasound, and are progressively less dra-

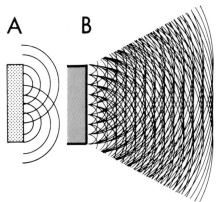

Fig 20-4. — **A,** ultrasound sources may be considered as a collection of point sources, each radiating spherical wavelets into the medium. **B,** interference of the spherical wavelets establishes a characteristic pattern for the resulting net wavefronts.

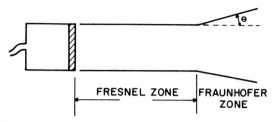

Fig 20-5. — Divergence of the ultrasound beam in the Fraunhofer region. The angle θ is the Fraunhofer divergence angle.

matic with increasing distance from the ultrasound source. The region near the source where the interference of wavelets is most apparent is termed the *Fresnel* (or *near*) *zone*. For a disk-shaped transducer of radius r, the length D of the Fresnel zone is

$$D_{Fresnel} = \frac{r^2}{\lambda}$$

where λ is the ultrasound wavelength. Within the Fresnel zone, most of the ultrasound energy is confined to a beam width no greater than the transducer diameter. Beyond the Fresnel zone, some of the energy es-

TABLE 20-1. — TRANSDUCER RADIUS AND ULTRA-
SOUND FREQUENCY AND THEIR RELATIONSHIP
TO FRESNEL ZONE DEPTH AND
BEAM DIVERGENCE

FREQUENCY (MHz)	WAVELENGTH (cm)	FRESNEL ZONE DEPTH (cm)	FRAUNHOFER DIVERGENCE ANGLE (DEGREES)
Transducer radius constant at 0.5 cm			
0.5	0.30	0.83	21.5
1.0	0.15	1.67	10.5
2.0	0.075	3.33	5.2
4.0	0.0325	7.80	2.3
8.0	0.0163	15.33	1.1

RADIUS (cm)	FRESNEL ZONE DEPTH (cm)	FRAUNHOFER DIVERGENCE ANGLE IN WATER (DEGREES)
Frequency constant at 2 MHz		
0.25	0.83	10.6
0.5	3.33	5.3
1.0	13.33	2.6
2.0	53.33	1.3

capes along the periphery of the beam, producing a gradual divergence of the ultrasound beam described by

$$\sin \theta = 0.612 \left(\frac{\lambda}{r} \right)$$

where θ is the Fraunhofer divergence angle in degrees (Fig 20-5). The region beyond the Fresnel zone is termed the *Fraunhofer* (or *far*) *zone*.

For medical applications of ultrasound, beams with little lateral dispersion of energy (i.e., a long Fresnel zone) are preferred. Hence, a reasonably high ratio of transducer radius to wavelength (r/λ) is required. This requirement can be satisfied by using ultrasound of short wavelengths (i.e., high frequencies). Unfortunately, the absorption of ultrasound energy increases at higher frequencies, and ultrasound frequencies for clinical imaging are limited to 2–20 MHz. At these frequencies, a transducer radius of 10λ or more usually furnishes an ultrasound beam with adequate directionality for medical use. The relationship of transducer radius and ultrasound frequency to the depth of the Fresnel zone and the amount of beam divergence is illustrated in Table 20-1.

VELOCITY OF ULTRASOUND

The velocity of an ultrasound wave varies with the physical properties of the medium transmitting the wave. In low-density media, such as air and other gases, particles may move a considerable distance before they influence neighboring particles. In these media, the velocity of an ultrasound wave will be relatively low. In solids, particles of the medium are constrained in their motion, and the velocity of ultrasound waves is rela-

TABLE 20-2.—APPROXIMATE VELOCITIES OF ULTRA-
SOUND IN SELECTED MATERIALS

NONBIOLOGIC MATERIAL	VELOCITY (m/sec)	BIOLOGIC MATERIAL	VELOCITY (m/sec)
Acetone	1,174	Fat	1,475
Air	331	Brain	1,560
Aluminum (rolled)	6,420	Liver	1,570
Brass	4,700	Kidney	1,560
Ethanol	1,207	Spleen	1,570
Glass (Pyrex)	5,640	Blood	1,570
Acrylic plastic	2,680	Muscle	1,580
Mercury	1,450	Lens of eye	1,620
Nylon (6-6)	2,620	Skull bone	3,360
Polyethylene	1,950	Soft tissue (mean value)	1,540
Water (distilled), 25 C	1,498		
Water (distilled), 50 C	1,540		

tively high. Velocities intermediate between those in gases and those in solids are attained by ultrasound waves moving through liquids. With the notable exceptions of lung and bone, the velocity of ultrasound in biologic tissues is roughly similar to the velocity of ultrasound in liquids. In different media, changes in velocity are reflected in changes in wavelength of the ultrasound waves, with the frequency remaining relatively constant. In ultrasound imaging, variations in the velocity of ultrasound in different media introduce artifacts into the image, with the major artifacts attributable to bone, fat and, in ophthalmologic applications, the lens of the eye. The velocities of ultrasound in various media are listed in Table 20-2.

It is important to distinguish the velocity of an ultrasound wave from the velocity of particles in the medium whose displacement into zones of compression and rarefaction constitutes the wave. The particle velocity describes the velocity of the individual particles of the medium, whereas the wave velocity describes the velocity of the ultrasound wave through the medium. Properties of ultrasound such as reflection, transmission and refraction are characteristic of the wave velocity of the ultrasound, rather than the particle velocity.

ULTRASOUND INTENSITY

The intensity I of an ultrasound wave is the rate at which energy is transmitted by the wave, described usually in units of watts per square centimeter. The intensity usually is described relative to some reference intensity I_0 and expressed in units of decibels (dB). The ratio of intensities of two ultrasound waves is described as

$$\text{Intensity ratio (dB)} = 10 \log \left(\frac{I}{I_0}\right)$$

where I and I_0 are the intensities of the two waves. If two ultrasound waves differ in intensity by a factor of 10, then the intensity ratio is 10 dB, since

$$\text{Intensity ratio (dB)} = 10 \log \left(\frac{1}{10}\right) = 10 \log (10^{-1}) = -10$$

where the negative sign indicates that the intensity I is less than the intensity I_0. Similarly, two waves differing in intensity by a factor of 100 have an intensity ratio of 20 dB:

$$\text{Intensity ratio (dB)} = 10 \log \left(\frac{1}{100}\right) = 10 \log (10^{-2}) = -20$$

The rate of energy transmission (i.e., the intensity) of an ultrasound wave is related to the maximum particle velocity V_m and the maximum wave pressure P_m by the expressions

$$I = \frac{\rho c V_m^2}{2} = \frac{P_m^2}{2\rho c}$$

where ρ is the density of the undisturbed medium and c is the wave velocity of ultrasound in the medium. Substitution of these expressions for intensity in the expression for the intensity ratio yields

$$\text{Intensity ratio (dB)} = 20 \log \left[\frac{V_m}{(V_m)_0} \right] = 20 \log \left[\frac{P_m}{(P_m)_0} \right]$$

where $(V_m)_0$ and $(P_m)_0$ are the maximum particle velocity and wave pressure of the reference ultrasound wave.

The decibel notation of intensity difference is particularly useful in describing the attenuation of an ultrasound wave as it moves through a medium. For example, suppose that the intensity of an ultrasound wave is reduced by a factor of 10 in moving through a particular medium. The attenuation of the wave is 10 dB. An intensity ratio of 0 dB implies no attenuation of ultrasound. Occasionally, the attenuating characteristics of a medium are described in terms of the half-power thickness, defined as the thickness of attenuating medium required to reduce the intensity of the wave to half. A half-power thickness corresponds to a reduction in intensity of 3 dB.

Attenuation of an ultrasound wave also may be described in units of nepers per centimeter:

$$\text{Attenuation (nepers/cm)} = \ln \left(\frac{I}{I_0} \right)$$

ACOUSTIC IMPEDANCE

In most diagnostic applications of ultrasound, use is made of ultrasound waves reflected from interfaces between different tissues in the patient. The fraction of the impinging energy reflected from an interface depends on the difference in acoustic impedance of the media on opposite sides of the interface. The acoustic impedance Z of a medium is the product of the density ρ of the medium and the velocity of ultrasound in the medium:

$$Z = \rho c$$

The acoustic impedances of several materials are listed in Table 20-3.

The larger the difference in acoustic impedance between two media (i.e., the larger the impedance mismatch), the greater is the fraction of

TABLE 20-3.—APPROXIMATE ACOUSTIC IMPEDANCES OF
SELECTED MATERIALS

NONBIOLOGIC MATERIAL	ACOUSTIC IMPEDANCE $(\text{kg-m}^{-2} - \sec^{-1}) \times 10^{-4}$	BIOLOGIC MATERIAL	ACOUSTIC IMPEDANCE $(\text{kg-m}^{-2} - \sec^{-1}) \times 10^{-4}$
Air at standard		Fat	1.38
temperature and		Aqueous and	
pressure	0.0004	vitreous	
Water	1.50	humor of eye	1.50
Polyethylene	1.85	Brain	1.55
Plexiglas	3.20	Blood	1.61
Aluminum	18.0	Kidney	1.62
Mercury	19.5	Human soft	
Brass	38.0	tissue,	
		mean value	1.63
		Spleen	1.64
		Liver	1.65
		Muscle	1.70
		Lens of eye	1.85
		Skull bone	6.10

impinging ultrasound energy that is reflected at the interface. For an ultrasound wave incident perpendicularly upon an interface, the fraction α_R of the incident energy that is reflected is

$$\alpha_R = \left[\frac{Z_2 - Z_1}{Z_2 + Z_1}\right]^2$$

where Z_1 and Z_2 are the acoustic impedances of the two media, and the fraction reflected is known as the *reflection coefficient* α_R. The fraction of the incident energy that is transmitted across an interface is described by the *transmission coefficient* α_T:

$$\alpha_T = \frac{4Z_1 Z_2}{(Z_1 + Z_2)^2}$$

Obviously, $\alpha_T + \alpha_R = 1$.

With a large impedance mismatch at an interface, much of the energy of an ultrasound wave is reflected, and only a small amount is transmitted across the interface. For example, ultrasound beams are reflected strongly at air-tissue and air-water interfaces because the impedance of air is much less than that of tissue or water. At a muscle-air interface, $Z_1 = 1.65$ and $Z_2 = 0.0004$ (both multiplied by 10^{-4} with units of kg-m^{-2} – sec^{-1}).

$$\alpha_R = \left[\frac{1.65 - 0.0004}{1.65 + 0.0004}\right]^2 \qquad \alpha_T = \frac{4(1.65)(0.0004)}{(1.65 + 0.0004)^2}$$
$$= 0.9995 \qquad\qquad\qquad = 0.0005$$

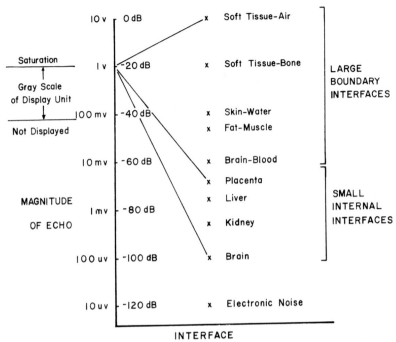

Fig 20-6.—Range of magnitudes of echoes from biologic interfaces and selection of internal echoes to be displayed over the major portion of the gray scale of an ultrasound display unit. (Reprinted with permission from Kossoff, G., Garrett, W., Carpenter, D., Jellins, J., and Dadd, M.: Principles and classification of soft tissues by grey scale echography, Ultrasound Med. Biol. 2:90, 1976.)

So 99.95% of the ultrasound energy is reflected at the air-muscle interface and only 0.05% of the energy is transmitted. At a muscle-liver interface where values of Z_1 and Z_2 are typically 1.70 and 1.65,

$$\alpha_R = \left[\frac{1.70 - 1.65}{1.70 + 1.65}\right]^2 \qquad \alpha_T = \frac{4(1.70)(1.65)}{(1.70 + 1.65)^2}$$
$$= 0.015 \qquad\qquad = 0.985$$

At a muscle-liver interface, slightly more than 1% of the incident energy is reflected, and about 99% of the energy is transmitted across the interface. Even though the reflected energy is small, it often is sufficient for visualization of the liver border. The magnitudes of echoes from various interfaces in the body are described in Figure 20-6.

Because of the high value of the coefficient of ultrasound reflection at an air-tissue interface, water paths and various creams and gels are used during ultrasound examinations to remove air pockets (i.e., to obtain good acoustic coupling) between the ultrasound transducer and the pa-

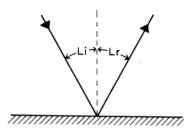

Fig 20-7. — Reflection of ultrasound at an interface, where the angle of incidence L_i equals the angle of reflection L_r.

tient's skin. With adequate acoustic coupling, the ultrasound waves will enter the patient with little reflection at the skin surface. Similarly, strong reflections of ultrasound occur at the boundary between the chest wall and the lungs and at the millions of air-tissue interfaces within the lungs. Because of the large impedance mismatch at these interfaces, efforts to use ultrasound as a diagnostic tool for the lungs have been unrewarding. The impedance mismatch also is high between soft tissues and bone, and the use of ultrasound to identify tissue characteristics in regions behind bone has had limited success.

The discussion of ultrasound reflection above assumes that the ultrasound beam strikes the reflecting interface at a right angle. In the body, ultrasound impinges upon interfaces at all angles. For any angle of incidence, the angle at which the reflected ultrasound energy leaves the interface equals the angle of incidence of the ultrasound beam; that is

Angle of incidence = Angle of reflection

This relationship is depicted in Figure 20-7.

In a typical medical examination that uses reflected ultrasound and a transducer that both transmits and detects ultrasound, very little reflected energy will be detected if the ultrasound strikes the interface at an angle more than about 3 degrees from perpendicular. A smooth reflecting interface must be essentially perpendicular to the ultrasound beam to permit visualization of the interface.

REFRACTION

As an ultrasound beam crosses an interface obliquely between two media, its direction is changed (i.e., the beam is bent). If the velocity of ultrasound is higher in the second medium, then the beam enters this medium at a more oblique angle. This behavior of ultrasound transmitted obliquely across an interface is termed *refraction* and is illustrated in Figure 20-8. The relationship between incident and refraction angles is described by Snell's Law:

$$\frac{\text{Sine of incidence angle}}{\text{Sine of refraction angle}} = \frac{\text{Velocity in incidence medium}}{\text{Velocity in refractive medium}}$$

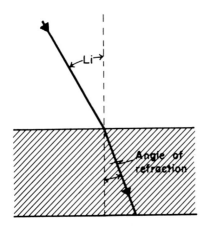

Fig 20-8. — Refraction of ultrasound at an interface, where the ratio of the velocities of ultrasound in the two media is related to the sine of the angles of incidence and refraction.

For example, an ultrasound beam incident obliquely upon an interface between muscle (velocity = 1,580 m/sec) and fat (velocity = 1,475 m/sec) will enter the fat at a steeper angle.

If an ultrasound beam impinges very obliquely upon a medium in which the ultrasound velocity is increased, the beam may be refracted so that no ultrasound energy enters the medium. The incidence angle at which refraction causes no ultrasound to enter a medium is termed the *critical angle.* For any particular interface, the critical angle depends on the velocity of ultrasound in the two media separated by the interface.

Refraction is a principal cause of artifacts in clinical ultrasound images. For example, the ultrasound beam in Figure 20-9 is refracted at a steeper angle as it crosses the interface between medium 1 and 2 ($c_1 > c_2$). As the beam emerges from medium 2 and reenters medium 1, it resumes its original direction of motion. The presence of medium 2 simply

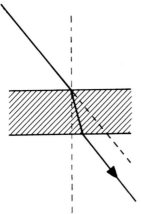

Fig 20-9. — Lateral displacement of an ultrasound beam as it traverses a slab interposed in an otherwise homogeneous medium.

displaces the ultrasound beam laterally for a distance that depends upon the difference in ultrasound velocity in the two media and upon the thickness of medium 2. Suppose a small structure below medium 2 is visualized by reflected ultrasound. The position of the structure would appear to the viewer as an extension of the original direction of the ultrasound through medium 1. In this manner, refraction adds spatial distortion and resolution loss to ultrasound images.

ATTENUATION OF ULTRASOUND

As an ultrasound beam penetrates a medium, energy is removed from the beam by processes such as absorption, scattering and reflection. As illustrated in Figure 20-10, the energy remaining in the beam decreases approximately exponentially with the depth of penetration of the beam into the medium. The reduction in energy (i.e., the decrease in ultrasound intensity) may be described in decibels, as noted earlier. For example, an energy attenuation of 1 dB/cm indicates a 90% reduction in the intensity of an ultrasound beam traversing 10 cm of medium. The attenuation of ultrasound in a material is described by the attenuation coefficient α in units of decibels per centimeter. Values of α for common biologic materials are listed in Table 20-4. Many of the values in Table 20-4 are known only approximately and vary significantly with both the particular sample chosen for measurement and the conditions of the sample at the time of measurement.[7] From Table 20-4, it is apparent that the attenuation of ultrasound is very high in bone. This property, together with the large reflection coefficient of a tissue-bone interface, make it difficult to visualize structures lying behind bone. Little attenuation occurs in water, and this medium is a very good transmitter of ultrasound energy. To a first approximation, the attenuation coefficient of

Fig 20-10. – Energy remaining in an ultrasound beam as a function of the depth of penetration of the beam into a medium.

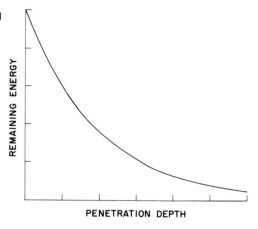

TABLE 20-4.—ATTENUATION COEFFICIENTS
α FOR 1-MHz ULTRASOUND

MATERIAL	α (dB/cm)	MATERIAL	α (dB/cm)
Blood	0.18	Lung	40
Fat	0.6	Liver	0.9
Muscle		Brain	0.85
(across fibers)	3.3	Kidney	1.0
Muscle		Spinal cord	1.0
(along fibers)	1.2	Water	0.0022
Aqueous and vitreous		Castor oil	0.95
humor of eye	0.1	Lucite	2.0
Lens of eye	2.0		
Skull bone	20		

most soft tissues can be approximated as 0.9ν, where ν is the frequency of the ultrasound in units of megahertz. This expression implies that the attenuation of ultrasound energy increases with frequency in biologic tissues. That is, higher-frequency ultrasound is attenuated more readily and is less penetrating than ultrasound of lower frequency.

The energy loss in a medium composed of layers of different materials is the sum of the energy loss in each layer. For example, suppose that a block of tissue consists of 2 cm of fat, 3 cm of muscle (ultrasound propagated parallel to the fibers) and 4 cm of liver. The total energy loss is

$$
\begin{aligned}
\text{Total energy loss} &= (\text{Energy loss in fat}) + (\text{Energy loss} \\
&\quad \text{in muscle}) + (\text{Energy loss in liver}) \\
&= (0.6\text{ dB/cm})(2\text{ cm}) + (1.2\text{ dB/cm})(3\text{ cm}) \\
&\quad + (0.9\text{ dB/cm})(4\text{ cm}) \\
&= 1.2\text{ dB} + 3.6\text{ dB} + 3.6\text{ dB} \\
&= 8.4\text{ dB}
\end{aligned}
$$

For an ultrasound beam that traverses the block of tissue and, after reflection, returns through the tissue block, the total attenuation is twice 8.4 dB or 16.8 dB.

ATTENUATION PROCESSES

Relaxation processes are the primary mechanism of energy dissipation for an ultrasound beam traversing tissue. These processes involve removal of energy from the ultrasound beam and eventual dissipation of this energy primarily as heat. As discussed earlier, ultrasound is propagated by displacement of particles of a medium into regions of compression and rarefaction. The displacement of a particle into a compression zone requires energy, which is provided to the medium by the source of ultrasound. As the particle attains maximum displacement from an equilibri-

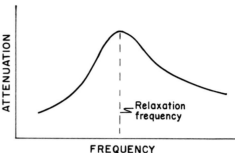

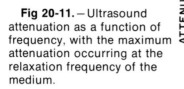

Fig 20-11. – Ultrasound attenuation as a function of frequency, with the maximum attenuation occurring at the relaxation frequency of the medium.

um position, its motion stops and the energy of the particle is translated from kinetic energy associated with the particle's motion to potential energy associated with the particle's position in the compression zone. From this position, the particle begins to move in the opposite direction, and potential energy is transformed gradually into kinetic energy. The maximum kinetic energy (i.e., the highest particle velocity) is achieved when the particle passes through its original equilibrium position, where the displacement and potential energy are zero. If the kinetic energy of the particle at this position equals the energy absorbed originally from the ultrasound beam, then no dissipation of the particle's energy has occurred and the medium is an ideal transmitter of ultrasound energy. Actually, the conversion of kinetic to potential energy (and vice versa) always is accompanied by some dissipation of the energy. Therefore, the energy of the ultrasound beam is gradually reduced as it passes through the medium. The rate at which the beam energy decreases is a reflection of the energy attenuation properties of the medium.

An analogy to the propagation of ultrasound in a medium is the oscillation that occurs when a stretched spring is released (i.e., relaxed). A spring that oscillates for a long time with little reduction in amplitude experiences only a gradual dissipation of energy from the energy conversion process. A spring that exhibits a rapid dampening of the oscillation indicates a more rapid loss of energy. This energy loss, termed *relaxation energy loss*, occurs as the spring is stretched and relaxed. The same term is used to describe similar energy loss mechanisms that occur as an ultrasound beam traverses a medium.

In any medium, the rate of energy loss varies with the frequency of an ultrasound beam. This dependence of energy loss on frequency is illustrated in Figure 20-11. Frequencies at which maximum attenuation occurs are termed the *relaxation frequencies* of the medium. At frequencies ν well below a relaxation frequency, the dissipation varies with ν^2; at frequencies near the relaxation frequency, the dissipation varies more nearly with ν. Hence, ultrasound may be attenuated more strongly in one

TABLE 20-5.—VARIATION OF ULTRASOUND
ATTENUATION COEFFICIENT α WITH
FREQUENCY ν IN MHz, WHERE α_1 IS THE
ATTENUATION COEFFICIENT AT 1 MHz

TISSUE	FREQUENCY VARIATION	TISSUE	FREQUENCY VARIATION
Blood	$\alpha = \alpha_1 \times \nu$	Liver	$\alpha = \alpha_1 \times f$
Fat	$\alpha = \alpha_1 \times \nu$	Brain	$\alpha = \alpha_1 \times f$
Muscle		Kidney	$\alpha = \alpha_1 \times f$
(across fiber)	$\alpha = \alpha_1 \times \nu$	Spinal cord	$\alpha = \alpha_1 \times f$
Muscle		Water	$\alpha = \alpha_1 \times f^2$
(along fiber)	$\alpha = \alpha_1 \times \nu$	Castor oil	$\alpha = \alpha_1 \times f^2$
Aqueous and		Lucite	$\alpha = \alpha_1 \times f$
vitreous	$\alpha = \alpha_1 \times \nu$		
Lens of eye	$\alpha = \alpha_1 \times \nu$		
Skull bone	$\alpha = \alpha_1 \times \nu^2$		

medium than another because the ultrasound frequency may be near a relaxation frequency in one medium and far below a relaxation frequency in another. The effect of frequency on the attenuation of ultrasound in different media is described in Table 20-5.[8-11] Data in this table are reasonably good estimates of the influence of frequency on ultrasound absorption over the range of ultrasound frequencies used diagnostically. However, complicated structures such as tissue samples often exhibit a rather complex attenuation pattern for different frequencies, which probably reflects the existence of a variety of relaxation frequencies and other molecular energy absorption processes that are poorly understood at present. These complex attenuation patterns are reflected in the data in Figure 20-12.

The attenuation of ultrasound also varies strongly with the temperature of the medium. The influence of temperature is illustrated in Figure 20-13 for three frequencies of ultrasound traversing blood. Contrary to the data in Figure 20-13, other media may display an increase in attenuation at elevated temperatures.

The attenuation of ultrasound is about 50 times greater in lung than in most other tissues. This heightened attenuation may be caused by minute bubbles of air in lung tissue which absorb energy from an ultrasound beam and then radiate the energy as spherical wavelets in all directions. The effect of these small bubbles of air is termed *stable cavitation*. If an ultrasound beam is intense enough and of the right frequency, the ultrasound-induced mechanical disturbance of the medium can be so great that microscopic bubbles are produced in the medium. The bubbles are formed at foci, such as particles in the rarefaction zones, and may grow to a size of 1 cu mm. As the pressure in the rarefaction zone increases dur-

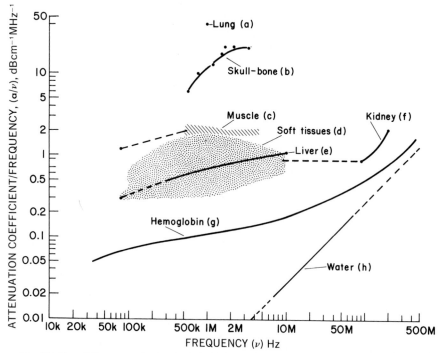

Fig 20-12. — Ultrasound attenuation coefficient as a function of frequency for various tissue samples. (Reprinted with permission from Wells, P. N. T.: Absorption and dispersion of ultrasound in biological tissue, Ultrasound Med. Biol. 1: 370, 1975.)

ing the next phase of the ultrasound cycle, the bubbles shrink to perhaps 10^{-2} cu mm and collapse, creating minute shock waves that seriously disturb the medium if produced in large quantities. This effect, termed *dynamic cavitation*, is introduced into a medium only at ultrasound intensities considerably above those used diagnostically. Dynamic cavita-

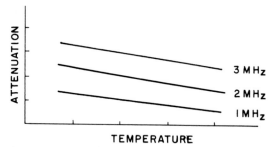

Fig 20-13. — Attenuation of ultrasound of three frequencies in blood as a function of temperature.

tion is most noticeable at frequencies around 30 – 100 kHz and is detectable only at exceptionally high intensities in the megahertz frequency range.

PROBLEMS
1. Explain what is meant by a longitudinal wave and describe how an ultrasound wave is propagated through a medium.
°2. For a disk-shaped 2-MHz (0.075 cm λ) transducer of radius 0.5 cm, compute the length of the Fresnel zone and the divergence angle of the Fraunhofer zone.
°3. An ultrasound beam is attenuated by a factor of 20 in passing through a medium. What is the attenuation of the medium in decibels?
°4. Determine the fraction of ultrasound energy transmitted and reflected at interfaces between: (a) fat and muscle, and (b) lens and the aqueous and vitreous humor of the eye.
°5. What is the angle of refraction for an ultrasound beam incident at an angle of 15 degrees from muscle into bone?
6. Explain why refraction contributes to resolution loss in ultrasound imaging.
°7. A region of tissue consists of 3 cm of fat, 2 cm of muscle (ultrasound propagated parallel to fibers) and 3 cm of liver. What is the approximate total energy loss of ultrasound in the tissue?

REFERENCES
1. Blitz, J.: *Fundamentals of Ultrasonics* (London: Butterworths, 1963).
2. Gooberman, G.: *Ultrasonics, Theory and Applications* (London: English University Press, 1968).
3. Buddemeyer, E.: The physics of diagnostic ultrasound, Radiol. Clin. North Am. 13:391, 1975.
4. Goldberg, B.: *Diagnostic Ultrasound in Clinical Medicine* (New York: Medcom Press, 1973).
5. McDicken, W.: *Diagnostic Ultrasonics* (New York: John Wiley & Sons, Inc., 1976).
6. Baker, D.: Physical and Technical Principles, in King, D. (ed.): *Diagnostic Ultrasound* (St. Louis: C. V. Mosby Co., 1974).
7. Chivers, R., and Hill, C.: Ultrasonic attenuation in human tissues, Ultrasound Med. Biol. 2:25, 1975.
8. Dunn, F., Edmonds, P., and Fry, W.: Absorption and Dispersion of Ultrasound in Biological Media, in Schwan, H. (ed.): *Biological Engineering* (New York: McGraw-Hill Book Co., 1969), p. 205.
9. Goldman, D., and Hueter, T.: Tabular data of the velocity and absorption of high-frequency sound in mammalian tissues, J. Acoust. Soc. Am. 28:35, 1956; errata J. Acoust. Soc. Am. 29:655, 1957.
10. Bhatia, A.: *Ultrasonic Absorption* (Oxford: Clarendon Press, 1967).
11. Kertzfield, K., and Litovitz, T.: *Absorption and Dispersion of Ultrasonic Waves* (New York: Academic Press, 1959).

°For those problems marked with an asterisk, answers are provided on the pages following the appendixes (see pp. 487 – 488).

21 / Ultrasound Transducers

A TRANSDUCER is any device that converts one form of energy into another. An ultrasound transducer converts electric energy into ultrasound energy, and vice versa. To accomplish this conversion, most ultrasound transducers use the piezoelectric effect, in which an electric signal is produced in response to ultrasound (pressure) waves incident on a transducer.[1-4] The same transducer is capable of generating pressure (ultrasound) waves when an electric signal is applied to the transducer.

PIEZOELECTRIC EFFECT

The piezoelectric effect is exhibited by certain crystals that, in response to applied pressure, develop a voltage across opposite surfaces of the crystal.[5] This effect is utilized in the production of an electric signal in response to incident ultrasound waves, where the magnitude of the electric signal varies with the wave pressure of the incident ultrasound. Similarly, application of a voltage across the crystal causes deformation of the crystal—either compression or extension depending upon the polarity of the voltage. This deforming effect, termed the *converse* piezoelectric effect, is used to produce an ultrasound beam from a transducer. Although a variety of crystals exhibit the piezoelectric effect at low temperatures, many are unsuitable as ultrasound transducers because their piezoelectric properties do not exist at temperatures near room temperature. The temperature above which a crystal's piezoelectric properties disappear is known as the *curie point* of the crystal.

For the generation of an ultrasound signal, a large deformation of the piezoelectric crystal is desirable when a given voltage is applied to the crystal. Deformation of the crystal is described as the strain S:

$$S = \frac{\text{Change in crystal thickness}}{\text{Original crystal thickness}}$$

The strain is related to the electric field intensity E by

$$S = dE$$

where d is the transmission coefficient of the crystal, and the electric field intensity E is the voltage across the crystal divided by the crystal thickness. Large transmission coefficients are desirable for a transmitting crystal.

TABLE 21-1.—PROPERTIES OF SELECTED PIEZOELECTRIC CRYSTALS

MATERIAL	TRANSMISSION COEFFICIENT d (m/V)	ELECTROMECHANICAL COUPLING COEFFICIENT k_c	CURIE POINT °C
Quartz	2.3×10^{-12}	0.11	550
Rochelle salt	27×10^{-12}	0.78	45
Barium titanate	$60-190 \times 10^{-12}$	0.30	120
Lead zirconate titanate (PET-4)	290×10^{-12}	0.70	328
Lead zirconate titanate (PET-5)	370×10^{-12}	0.70	365

For reception of ultrasound, the electric field intensity E produced by a wave pressure P applied to the crystal is described as

$$E = gP$$

where g is the reception coefficient of the crystal. Large reception coefficients are desirable for a receiving crystal.

A common definition of the efficiency of an ultrasound transducer is the fraction of applied energy that is converted to the desired energy mode. This definition of efficiency is described as the electromechanical coupling coefficient k_c of the transducer. If mechanical energy (i.e., pressure) is applied,

$$k_c^2 = \frac{\text{Mechanical energy converted to electric energy}}{\text{Applied mechanical energy}}$$

If electric energy is applied,

$$k_c^2 = \frac{\text{Electric energy converted to mechanical energy}}{\text{Applied electric energy}}$$

Values of d and k_c^2 for selected piezoelectric crystals are listed in Table 21-1.

Essentially all clinical diagnostic ultrasound units use piezoelectric crystals for the generation and detection of ultrasound. A number of piezoelectric crystals occur in nature [e.g., quartz, Rochelle salts, lithium sulfate tourmaline and ammonium dihydrogen phosphate (ADP)]. However, crystals used clinically are almost invariably manmade. The most common manmade crystals are barium titanate, lead metaniobate and lead zirconate titanate.

TRANSDUCER DESIGN

The piezoelectric crystal is the functional component of an ultrasound transducer. The crystal usually is designed as a circular disk with a thickness t equal to half the wavelength of the ultrasound desired from the transducer. A crystal of this thickness resonates at a frequency v:

$$v = \frac{c}{\lambda} \quad \text{where } \lambda = 2t$$
$$= \frac{c}{2t}$$

For a 1.5-mm-thick quartz disk (velocity of ultrasound in quartz = 5,740 m/sec):

$$v = \frac{5,740 \text{ m/sec}}{2(0.0015 \text{ m})}$$
$$= 1.91 \text{ MHz}$$

To establish electric contact with the piezoelectric crystal, faces of the crystal are coated with a thin conducting film and electric contacts are applied. The crystal is mounted at one end of a hollow metal or metal-lined plastic cylinder, with the front face of the crystal coated with protective plastic to provide efficient transfer of sound between the crystal and the body. The front face of the crystal is connected through the cylinder to ground potential. The remainder of the crystal is insulated electrically and acoustically from the cylinder.

With only air behind the crystal, ultrasound transmitted into the cylinder from the crystal is reflected from the cylinder's opposite end. The reflected ultrasound reinforces the ultrasound propagated in the forward direction from the transducer. This reverberation of ultrasound in the transducer contributes energy to the ultrasound beam and extends the time over which the ultrasound pulse is produced. Extension of the pulse-formation time is no problem in some clinical uses of ultrasound such as continuous-wave and pulsed-Doppler applications. For these purposes, ultrasound probes with air-backed crystals are used. However, most ultrasound imaging applications utilize short pulses of ultrasound, and suppression of ultrasound reverberation in the transducer usually is desirable. The suppression or "damping" of reverberation is accomplished by filling the transducer cylinder with a backing material such as tungsten powder embedded in epoxy resin. Sometimes rubber is added to the backing to increase the absorption of ultrasound. Often the rear surface of the backing material is sloped to prevent direct reflection of ultra-

Fig 21-1.—A typical ultrasound transducer.

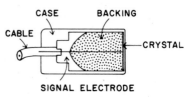

sound pulses back to the crystal. The construction of a typical ultrasound transducer is illustrated in Figure 21-1. The crystal may be flat, as shown in the drawing, or curved to focus the ultrasound beam. A crystal of this design can generate ultrasound signals as short as two to three cycles when stimulated with a momentary voltage pulse.

As a substitute for physical damping with selected materials placed behind the crystal, electronic damping appears promising. In certain special applications, including those that use small receiving transducers, a resistor connecting the two faces of an air-backed crystal may provide adequate damping. Another approach, termed *dynamic damping*, uses an initial electric pulse to stimulate the transducer, followed immediately by a voltage pulse of opposite polarity to suppress the continuation of transducer action.

FREQUENCY RESPONSE OF TRANSDUCER

An ultrasound transducer is designed to be maximally sensitive to ultrasound of a particular frequency, termed the *resonance frequency*, of the transducer. The resonance frequency is revealed by a curve of transducer response plotted as a function of ultrasound frequency. In Figure 21-2, the frequency response characteristics of two transducers are illustrated. The curve for the undamped transducer displays a sharp frequency response over a limited frequency range. Because of greater energy absorption in the damped transducer, the frequency response is much broader and not so sharply peaked at the transducer resonance frequency. On the curve for the undamped transducer, points f_1 and f_2 represent frequencies on either side of the resonance frequency where the response has diminished to half. These points are called the *half-power points*, and they encompass a range of frequencies termed the *bandwidth* of the transducer. The ratio of resonance frequency f_0 to the bandwidth $f_2 - f_1$ is termed the *Q value* of the transducer. The Q value describes the sharpness of the frequency response curve:

$$Q \text{ value} = \frac{f_0}{f_2 - f_1}$$

Transducers used in ultrasound imaging must furnish short ultrasound pulses and respond to returning echoes over a wide range of frequencies. For these reasons, heavily damped transducers with low Q values (e.g., 2-3) usually are desired. Since part of the damping is provided by the crystal itself, crystals such as PZT (lead zirconate titanate) or lead metaniobate with high internal damping and low Q values generally are preferred for imaging.

The efficiency of propagation of an ultrasound beam from a transducer into a medium depends on how well the transducer is coupled to the

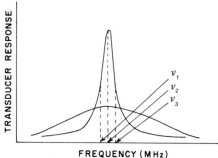

Fig 21-2. — Frequency response curves for undamped *(sharp curve)* and damped *(broad curve)* transducers.

medium. If the acoustic impedance of the coupling medium is not too different from that of either the transducer or the medium, and if the thickness of the coupling medium is much less than the ultrasound wavelength, then the ultrasound is transmitted into the medium with little energy loss. Transmission with almost no energy loss is accomplished, for example, with a thin layer of oil placed between transducer and skin during a diagnostic ultrasound examination. Transmission with minimum energy loss between transducer and medium occurs when the impedance of the coupling medium is intermediate between the impedances of the crystal and the medium. The ideal impedance of the coupling medium is

$$Z_{\substack{\text{coupling} \\ \text{medium}}} = \sqrt{Z_{\text{transducer}} \times Z_{\text{medium}}}$$

Also, the energy loss is minimized when the protective covering over the crystal is a quarter wave matching layer (i.e., the thickness of the protective covering is an odd multiple of quarter wavelengths of the transmitted ultrasound).

In a similar manner, coupling of the transducer to the transmitting medium affects the size of the electric signals generated by returning ultrasound pulses. These signals also are diminished by the cable between the transducer and associated electronics. For this reason, the cable should be as short as possible.

Two methods are commonly used to generate ultrasound beams. For continuous-wave beams, an oscillating voltage is applied with a frequency equal to that desired for the ultrasound beam. A similar voltage of prescribed duration is used to generate long pulses of ultrasound energy, as shown in Figure 21-3, *a*. For clinical ultrasound imaging, short pulses usually are preferred. These pulses are produced by shocking the crystal into mechanical oscillation by a momentary change in the voltage across the crystal. The oscillation is damped quickly by the methods described above to furnish ultrasound pulses as short as half a cycle. The duration

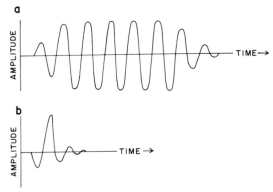

Fig 21-3. — Typical long *(a)* and short *(b)* ultrasound pulses.

of a pulse usually is defined as the number of half cycles in the pulse with an amplitude greater than one-fourth the peak amplitude. The effectiveness of damping is described by the pulse dynamic range, defined as the ratio of the peak amplitude of the pulse divided by the amplitude of ripples following the pulse. A typical ultrasound pulse of short duration is illustrated in Figure 21-3, *b*.

Because the transmission and reception patterns of an ultrasound transducer are affected by slight variations in the construction and manner of electric stimulation of the transducer, the exact shape of an ultrasound beam is difficult to predict. Consequently, beam shapes or profiles usually are measured and displayed for a particular transducer. One approach to the display of the characteristics of an ultrasound beam is with a set of pulse-echo response profiles. A profile is obtained by placing an ultrasound reflector some distance from the transducer and scanning the transducer in a direction perpendicular to the axis of the ultrasound beam. During the scan, the amplitude of the electric signal induced in the transducer by the reflected ultrasound is plotted as a function of the distance between the central axis of the ultrasound beam and the reflector. A pulse-echo response profile is shown in Figure 21-4, *A*, and a set of profiles obtained at different distances from the transducer is shown in Figure 21-4, *B*.

In Figure 21-4, *A*, the locations are indicated where the transducer response decreases to half (−6 dB) of the response when the transducer is aligned with the reflector. The distance between these locations is termed the *response width* of the transducer at the particular distance (range) from the transducer. If response widths are connected between profiles at different ranges (Fig 21-4, *C*), 6 dB response margins are obtained on each side of the ultrasound beam axis. Similarly, 20 dB re-

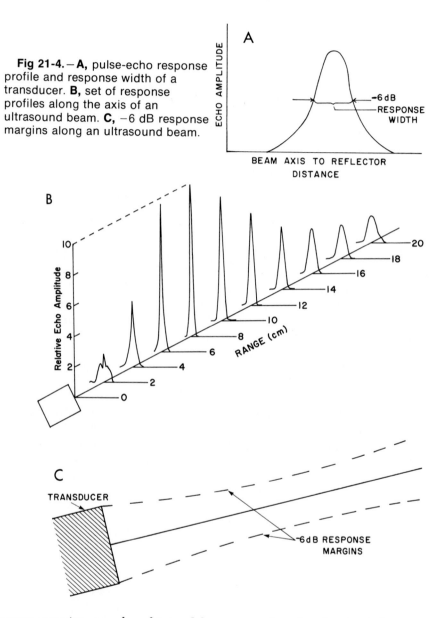

Fig 21-4.—**A,** pulse-echo response profile and response width of a transducer. **B,** set of response profiles along the axis of an ultrasound beam. **C,** −6 dB response margins along an ultrasound beam.

sponse margins may be obtained by connecting the ¹⁄₁₀ (−20 dB) response widths on each side of the beam axis.

Response profiles for a particular transducer are influenced by many factors, including the nature of the stimulating voltage applied to the transducer; the characteristics of the electronic circuitry of the receiver;

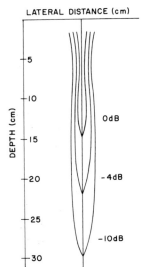

Fig 21-5.—Isoecho contours for a nonfocused transducer.

and the shape, size and character of the reflector. Usually, the reflector is a steel sphere or rod with a diameter of three to ten times the ultrasound wavelength. Response profiles may be distorted if the receiver electronics do not faithfully represent low-intensity signals. Most commercial ultrasound units cannot accurately display echo amplitudes much less than $\frac{1}{10}$ (-20 dB) of the largest echo recorded. These units are said to have limited dynamic range.

Another approach to describing the character of an ultrasound beam is with isoecho contours. Each contour depicts the locations of equal echo intensity for the ultrasound beam. At each of these locations, a reflecting object will be detected with equal sensitivity. The approach usually used to measure isoecho contours is to place a small steel ball at a variety of positions in the ultrasound beam, and to identify locations where the reflected echoes are equal. Connecting these locations with lines yields isoecho contours such as those in Figure 21-5. In this figure, the region

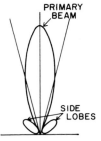

Fig 21-6.—Side lobes of an ultrasound beam.

of maximum sensitivity at a particular depth is labeled 0 dB, and isoecho contours of lesser intensity are labeled −4 dB, −10 dB, and so on. Iso-echo contours help depict the lateral resolution of a transducer, as well as variations in lateral resolution with depth and with changes in instrument settings such as beam intensity, detector amplifier gain and echo threshold.

Accompanying a primary ultrasound beam are small beams of greatly reduced intensity that are emitted at angles to the primary beam. These small beams are termed *side lobes* and are illustrated in Figure 21-6. Side lobes sometimes produce image artifacts in regions near the transducer.

The preceding discussion covers general-purpose, flat-surfaced transducers. For most ultrasound applications, transducers with special shapes are preferred. Among these special-purpose transducers are focused transducers, double-crystal transducers, ophthalmic probes, intravascular probes, esophageal probes, composite probes, variable-angle probes and transducer arrays.

FOCUSED TRANSDUCERS

A focused ultrasound beam is a beam that is narrower at some distance from the transducer face than its dimension at the face of the transducer.[6-9] In the region where the beam narrows (termed the *focal zone* of the ultrasound transducer), the ultrasound intensity may be heightened by 100 times or more compared with the intensity in front of or behind the focal zone. Because of this increased intensity, a much larger signal will be induced in a transducer if the reflector is positioned in the focal zone. The distance between the location for maximum echo in the focal zone and the element responsible for focusing the ultrasound beam is termed the *focal length* of the transducer.

Often, the focusing element is the piezoelectric crystal itself, which is shaped like a concave disk (Fig 21-7). An ultrasound beam also may be focused with refracting lenses or reflecting mirrors in a manner analogous to the effect of lenses and mirrors on visible light. Focusing lenses and mirrors are capable of increasing the intensity of an ultrasound beam by factors much greater than 100. Focusing and defocusing mirrors, usually constructed of tungsten-impregnated epoxy resin, are illustrated in Figure 21-8. Since the velocity of ultrasound generally is greater in a lens than in the surrounding medium, concave ultrasound lenses are

Fig 21-7.—Focused transducer.

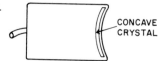

CONCAVE
CRYSTAL

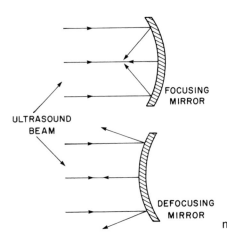

Fig 21-8. — Focusing and defocusing mirrors.

focusing and convex ultrasound lenses are defocusing, as shown in Figure 21-9. These effects are the opposite of those for the action of optical lenses on visible light. Ultrasound lenses usually are constructed of epoxy resins and plastics such as polystyrene.

Zone plates and zone lenses that cause diffraction and interference of ultrasound wavelets also can be used to focus an ultrasound beam (Fig 21-10). Zone lenses are particularly useful, because they furnish increases in intensity of 200 times or so. The main disadvantage of any zone lens is its restriction to ultrasound of a single frequency.

For an ultrasound beam with a circular cross section, focusing characteristics such as pulse-echo response width and relative sensitivity along the beam axis depend on the wavelength λ of the ultrasound, and on the

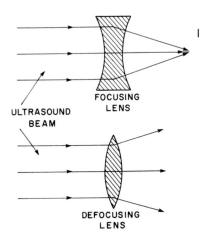

Fig 21-9. — Focusing and defocusing lenses.

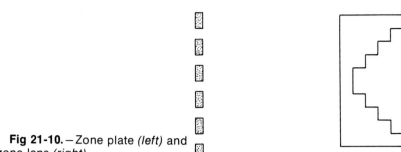

Fig 21-10.—Zone plate *(left)* and zone lens *(right)*.

focal length f and radius r of the transducer or other focusing element.* These variables may be used to distinguish the degree of focus of transducers by dividing the near field length r^2/λ by the focal length f (Table 21-2). For cupped transducer faces on all but weakly focused transducers, the focal length of the transducer is equal to or slightly shorter than the radius of curvature of the transducer face. If a plano-concave lens with radius of curvature r is attached to the transducer face, then the focal length f is

$$f = \frac{r}{1 - c_M/c_L}$$

where c_M and c_L are the velocities of ultrasound in the medium and lens, respectively.

The length of the focal zone of a particular ultrasound beam is the distance over which a reasonable focus and pulse-echo response are obtained. One estimate of focal zone length is

$$\text{Focal zone length} = 2 \lambda \left(\frac{f}{d}\right)^2$$

TABLE 21-2.—DEGREE OF FOCUS OF TRANSDUCERS EXPRESSED AS A RATIO OF THE NEAR FIELD LENGTH r^2/λ TO THE FOCAL LENGTH f

DEGREE OF FOCUS	NEAR FIELD LENGTH / FOCAL LENGTH
Weak	$r^2/\lambda f \leq 1.4$
Medium weak	$1.4 < r^2/\lambda f \leq 6$
Medium	$6 < r^2/\lambda f \leq 20$
Strong	$20 < r^2/\lambda f$

*The ratio f/d sometimes is described as the f-number of the transducer or other focusing element.

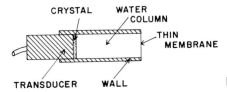

Fig 21-11. — Stand-off ophthalmic probe with a water column.

where $d = 2r$ = the diameter of the transducer. In ultrasound imaging, however, focal zone lengths usually are assumed to be three to seven times this length.

Transducers with slight focusing characteristics (i.e., weak and medium-weak focused transducers) are used commonly in contact ultrasound imaging units to improve the lateral resolution of the ultrasound beam at the depths of interest within the patient. Medium and strongly focused transducers are used with water paths to place the rather limited focal zone at the depth of interest within the patient. These transducers also are used for surgical applications of ultrasound where high ultrasound intensities in localized regions are needed for tissue destruction.

OPHTHALMIC PROBES

For ultrasound examinations of the eye, only a shallow depth of penetration of the ultrasound beam is required, and high-frequency (5–15 MHz) ultrasound may be used to improve the axial resolution of the ultrasound beam. The lateral resolution may be improved simultaneously by using small-diameter, focused transducers. To detect echoes from superficial structures in the eye, a water column often is interposed between the transducer and the cornea. A "stand-off" ophthalmic probe with a water column is illustrated in Figure 21-11.

INTRAVASCULAR PROBES

Very small ultrasound probes have been developed for intravascular work. Since the crystal diameter is small, the Fresnel zone is short and the beam diverges rapidly away from the transducer. Short pulses are difficult to obtain with these probes because little damping material is present.

DOPPLER PROBES

Doppler transducers consist of separate transmitting and receiving crystals, usually oriented at slight angles to each other so that the transmitting and receiving areas intersect at some distance in front of the transducer. Since a sharp frequency response is desired for a Doppler transducer, only a small amount of damping material is used. A typical Doppler transducer is shown in Figure 21-12.

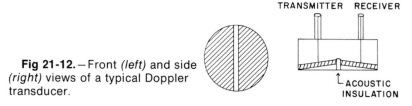

Fig 21-12. — Front *(left)* and side *(right)* views of a typical Doppler transducer.

TRANSDUCER ARRAYS

The assembly of a series of ultrasound transducers into a phased transducer array permits display of a continuous, complete ultrasound image to the observer. To obtain this "real-time" image, each transducer transmits an ultrasound pulse and then receives echoes from structures within the field of view of the transducer. The pulsing of the transducers is phased so that only one transducer is transmitting and receiving at any moment. In one commercial system, the transducer array is 8 cm long and contains 20 crystals, with each transducer pulsed 150 times per second.

TRANSDUCER DAMAGE

Ultrasound transducers can be damaged in many ways. The crystals are brittle and the wire contacts on the crystals are fragile; hence, transducers should be handled carefully. Excessive voltages to the crystal should be avoided, and only watertight probes should be immersed in water. A transducer should never be heated to a temperature exceeding the curie point of the piezoelectric crystal.

PROBLEMS

1. Explain what is meant by the piezoelectric effect and the converse piezoelectric effect.
°2. For a piezoelectric material with an ultrasound velocity of 6,000 m/sec, what thickness should a disk-shaped crystal have to provide an ultrasound beam with a frequency of 2.5 MHz?
3. What is meant by damping an ultrasound transducer and why is this necessary? What influence does damping have on the frequency response of the transducer?
°4. What is the estimated focal zone length for a 2-MHz (λ = 0.075 cm) focused ultrasound transducer with an *f*-number of 8?

REFERENCES

1. Posakony, G.: *Ultrasound Transducers*, Proceedings 1975 Ultrasonics Symposium, IEEE Cat. #75, CH0994-45u.

°For those problems marked with an asterisk, answers are provided on the pages following the appendixes (see pp. 487–488).

2. Eggleton, R.: State-of-the-art in single-transducer technology, Med. Phys. 3(5):303, 1976.
3. McDicken, W.: *Diagnostic Ultrasonics* (New York: John Wiley & Sons, Inc., 1976), p. 248.
4. Wells, P.: *Biomedical Ultrasonics* (New York: Academic Press, 1977), p. 45.
5. Mason, W.: *Piezoelectric Crystals and Their Application to Ultrasonics* (Princeton, N.J.: Van Nostrand, 1950).
6. Kossoff, G.: Improved techniques in ultrasonic echography, Ultrasonics 10:221, 1972.
7. Tarnoczy, T.: Sound focusing lenses and waveguides, Ultrasonics 3:115, 1965.
8. McElroy, J.: Focused ultrasonic beams, Int. J. Nondestructive Testing 3:27, 1971.
9. O'Neil, H.: Theory of focusing radiators, J. Acoust. Soc. Am. 21:516, 1949.

22 / The Doppler Effect

ULTRASOUND is used not only for display of static patient anatomy but also for identification of moving structures in the body. Approaches to the identification of moving structures include real-time pulse-echo imaging, motion mode (M mode) display of reflected ultrasound pulses and the Doppler-shift method. Discussed in this chapter are the basic principles of the Doppler-shift method. The Doppler method has a number of applications in clinical medicine, including detection of fetal heartbeat and multiple pregnancy, placenta localization, detection of air emboli, blood pressure monitoring, detection of blood flow and localization of blood vessel occlusions.[1, 2]

When there is relative motion between a source and a detector of ultrasound, the frequency of the detected ultrasound differs from that emitted by the source. The shift in frequency is illustrated in Figure 22-1. In Figure 22-1, A, an ultrasound source is moving with velocity v_s toward the detector. After time t following the production of any particular wavefront, the distance between the wavefront and the source is $(c - v_s)t$, where c is the velocity of ultrasound in the medium. The wavelength λ of the ultrasound in the direction of motion is shortened to

$$\lambda = \frac{c - v_s}{\nu_0}$$

where ν_0 is the frequency of ultrasound from the source. With the shortened wavelength, the ultrasound reaches the detector with an increased frequency ν:

$$\nu = \frac{c}{\lambda} = \frac{c}{(c - v_s)/\nu_0}$$
$$= \nu_0\left(\frac{c}{c - v_s}\right)$$

That is, the frequency of the detected ultrasound shifts to a higher value when the ultrasound source is moving toward the detector. The shift in frequency $\Delta\nu$ is

$$\Delta\nu = \nu - \nu_0 = \nu_0\left(\frac{c}{c - v_s}\right) - \nu_0$$
$$= \nu_0\left(\frac{v_s}{c - v_s}\right)$$

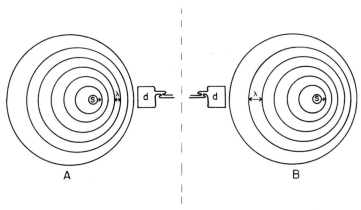

Fig 22-1. — Principles of Doppler ultrasound: **A,** source moving toward stationary detector *d*; **B,** source moving away from stationary detector *d*.

If the velocity c of ultrasound in the medium is much greater than the velocity v_s of the ultrasound source, $c - v_s \approx c$ and

$$\Delta\nu = \nu_0\left(\frac{v_s}{c}\right)$$

A similar expression is applicable to the case in which the ultrasound source is stationary and the detector is moving toward the source with velocity v_d. In this case the Doppler shift frequency is approximately

$$\Delta\nu = \nu_0\left(\frac{v_d}{c}\right)$$

where $c \gg v_d$.

If the ultrasound source is moving away from the detector (Fig 22-1, B), then the distance between the source and a wavefront is $ct + v_s t = (c + v_s)t$, where t is the time elapsed since the production of the wavefront. The wavelength λ of the ultrasound is

$$\lambda = \frac{c + v_s}{\nu_0}$$

and the apparent frequency ν is

$$\nu = \frac{c}{\lambda}$$

$$= \frac{c}{(c + v_s)/\nu_0}$$

$$= \nu_0\left(\frac{c}{c + v_s}\right)$$

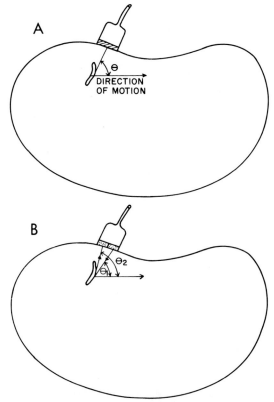

Fig 22-2. — **A,** angle θ between an incident ultrasound beam and the direction of motion of the object. **B,** for a dual probe with separate transmitting and receiving transducers, the angle θ is the average of the angles θ_1 and θ_2 that the transmitted and detected signals make with the direction of motion.

That is, the frequency shifts to a lower value when the ultrasound source is moving away from the detector. The shift in frequency $\Delta\nu$ is

$$\Delta\nu = \nu - \nu_0 = \nu_0\left(\frac{c}{c + v_s}\right) - \nu_0$$

$$= \nu_0\left(\frac{-v_s}{c + v_s}\right)$$

where the negative sign implies a reduction in frequency. If the velocity c of ultrasound is much greater than the velocity v_s of the source, $c + v_s \simeq c$ and $\Delta\nu = \nu_0(-v_s/c)$. A similar expression is applicable to the case where the ultrasound source is stationary and the detector is moving away from the source with velocity v_d.

$$\Delta\nu = \nu_0\left(\frac{-v_d}{c}\right)$$

when $c \gg v_d$.

If the source and detector are at the same location and ultrasound is reflected from an object moving toward the location with velocity v_0, the object acts first as a moving detector as it receives the ultrasound signal, and then as a moving source as it reflects the signal. As a result, the ultrasound signal received by the detector exhibits a frequency shift (when $c \gg v_0$)

$$\Delta\nu = 2\nu_0\frac{v_0}{c}$$

Similarly, for an object moving away from the source and detector, the shift in frequency $\Delta\nu$ is

$$\Delta\nu = 2\nu_0\left(\frac{-v_0}{c}\right)$$

where the negative sign indicates that the frequency of the detected ultrasound is lower than that emitted by the source.

The discussion above has assumed that the ultrasound beam is parallel to the motion of the object. For the more general case where the ultrasound beam strikes a moving object at an angle θ (Fig 22-2, A), the shift in frequency $\Delta\nu$ is

$$\Delta\nu = 2\nu_0\left(\frac{v_0}{c}\right)\cos\theta$$

A negative sign in this expression implies that the object is moving away from the ultrasound source and detector and that the frequency of detected ultrasound is shifted to a lower value. The angle θ is the angle between the ultrasound beam and the direction of motion of the object. If

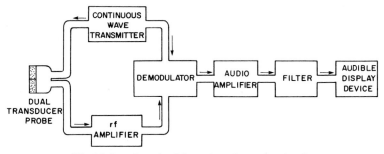

Fig 22-3. — A typical Doppler ultrasound unit.

the ultrasound source and detector are displaced slightly (Fig 22-2, *B*), then θ is the average of the angles that the transmitted and reflected beams make with the motion of the object. For the small displacement between ultrasound transmitter and detector commonly used in Doppler ultrasound units, this assumption contributes an error of only 2–3% in the estimated frequency shift.[3]

As an example of Doppler shift frequencies, 10-MHz ultrasound frequently is used for the detection of blood flow. For blood flowing at 15 cm/second toward the ultrasound source, the Doppler shift frequency is

$$\Delta\nu = 2\nu_0\left(\frac{v_0}{c}\right)$$
$$= (2)(10 \text{ MHz})\left(\frac{15 \text{ cm/sec}}{154,000 \text{ cm/sec}}\right)$$
$$= 1.9 \text{ kHz}$$

Ultrasound blood flow detectors usually are sensitive to Doppler shift frequencies up to about 6 kHz. For fetal heartbeat detectors, ultrasound frequencies of about 2 MHz usually are used, with the detector sensitive to Doppler shift frequencies up to 1 kHz. These Doppler shift frequencies are audible, and a loudspeaker, stethoscope or earphones can be used to detect the output signal from the Doppler unit.

A typical Doppler unit is diagramed in Figure 22-3. Characteristics of the Doppler probe, consisting of separate transmitting and receiving transducers, are discussed in Chapter 21. Application of a continuous electric signal to the transmitting transducer produces a continuous ultrasound beam at a prescribed frequency and at an intensity on the order of 30 mW/sq cm. As the beam enters the patient, it is reflected from stationary and moving surfaces, and the reflected signals are returned to the receiver. Suppose that two signals are received, one directly from the transmitting transducer and the other from a moving surface. These signals interfere with each other to produce a net signal with a "beat frequency" equal to the Doppler shift frequency. This Doppler shift signal is amplified in the rf (radiofrequency) amplifier with a gain of around 60 dB. The amplified signal is transmitted to the demodulator, where most of the signal is removed except the low-frequency beat signal. The beat signal is amplified in the audio amplifier and transmitted through the filter (where frequencies below the beat frequency are removed) to the loudspeaker or earphones for audible display. In practice, many moving interfaces reflect signals to the receiver, and many beat frequencies are produced. Differentiating among these frequencies to identify the signal of interest is one of the more difficult aspects of the clinical application of the Doppler effect. Instruments (sound spectrographs) to facilitate this differentiation and to furnish quantitative information about the amplitude of different beat frequency signals are used in a few institutions to extract more useful information about patients examined with Doppler units.[4]

At the present time, Doppler ultrasound units are used principally for two purposes. The first is detection of characteristic signals from the fetal heart and placenta.[5, 6] Obstetric Doppler units operate at about 2 MHz with a Doppler probe that exhibits maximum sensitivity 5 cm or so in front of the transducer. The second application of Doppler ultrasound is for determination of the presence or absence of blood flow in arteries and veins.[7, 8] For this application, detectors are operated at 5–10 MHz with a Doppler probe that exhibits a maximum sensitivity about 1 cm in front of the transducer. The reflected signals originate from blood corpuscles moving through the artery or vein being examined. Blood flow monitors have been used primarily to verify the presence or absence of blood flow in selected arteries and veins. However, units to provide quantitative estimates of blood flow are being developed, and their emergence into clinical use is expected in the near future. Although earlier Doppler units did not distinguish between blood flow toward and away from the transducer, newer directional Doppler units have this capability.

The use of Doppler units is accompanied by a number of difficulties. Voluntary and involuntary motions of the patient add large artifacts to a Doppler signal. In addition, stray signals not related to moving structures are a constant problem with Doppler units. The structure producing a particular Doppler signal often is difficult to identify, because reflected signals may originate within a rather large volume of tissue. Localization of a particular structure sometimes can be improved by obtaining reflected signals from a number of angles. The detection of Doppler shifts with pulsed ultrasound promises to yield better in-depth localization of moving structures as well as quantitative information about the rate of movement. Pulsed Doppler instruments have recently entered the commercial market.

Notwithstanding the problems described above, the use of Doppler ultrasound units is increasing rapidly in clinical medicine.

PROBLEMS

°1. Estimate the frequency shift for a 10-MHz ultrasound source moving toward a stationary detector in water (c = 1,540 m/second) at a speed of 5 cm/second.

Is the frequency shifted to a higher or lower value?

For those problems marked with an asterisk, answers are provided on the pages following the appendixes (see pp. 487–488).

°2. Estimate the frequency shift for an object moving at a speed of 10 cm/second away from a 10-MHz source and detector occupying the same location.

3. What is meant by a beat frequency?

4. Identify some of the major medical applications of Doppler systems.

REFERENCES

1. Reid, J., and Baker, D.: Physics and Electronics of the Ultrasonic Doppler Method, in Böck, J., and Ossoining, K. (eds.): *Ultrasonographia Medica*, Proc. First World Congress on Ultrasonics in Medicine and SIDUO III (Vienna: Verlag der Wiener Medizenischen Akademie/Vienna Academy of Medicine, 1971), vol. 1, p. 109.

2. McDicken, W.: *Diagnostic Ultrasonics* (New York: John Wiley & Sons, Inc., 1976), p. 219.

3. Wells, P.: The directivities of some ultrasonic Doppler peaks, Med. Biol. Eng. 8:241, 1970.

4. Licht, L.: A recording spectrograph for analysing Doppler blood velocity signals (particularly from aortic flow) in real time, J. Physiol. (Lond.) 207:42P, 1970.

5. Bishop, E.: Obstetric uses of the ultrasonic motion detector, Am. J. Obstet. Gynecol. 96:863, 1966.

6. Nelson, C., and Parkes, J.: Placental localisation using the Doppler portable ultrasonic apparatus, S. Afr. Med. J. 48:2393, 1974.

7. Fish, P.: Visualizing Blood Vessels by Ultrasound, in Roberts, C. (ed.): *Blood Flow Measurement* (London: Sector, 1972), p. 29.

8. Reneman, R. (ed.): *Cardiovascular Applications of Ultrasound* (Amsterdam: North-Holland Publishing Co., 1974).

23 / Ultrasound Display Systems

AN ULTRASOUND SIGNAL reflected from tissue is received as one or more pressure wavefronts impinging on the transducer. In response, the ultrasound transducer produces one or more voltage signals with amplitudes corresponding to the pressure of the returning ultrasound wavefront. These voltage pulses are processed and displayed usually in one of three presentation modes: A mode (amplitude modulation), B mode (brightness modulation) and M mode (motion modulation). Each of these modes of presentation has specific applications to medical diagnosis.

A MODE PRESENTATION

In the A mode presentation of pulse-echo images, a pulse generator applies a momentary high voltage (i.e., a few hundred volts for a few to a few hundred nanoseconds) to a 1–20 MHz ultrasound transducer. In response to this electric shock, the transducer vibrates and creates an ultrasound pulse of a microsecond or so duration corresponding to several pulse cycles. With proper coupling between the transducer and skin, this ultrasound pulse is transmitted into the body. Following the initial shock, the transducer remains quiescent for a millisecond or so to receive returning echoes from the body.

Echoes returning from the body induce voltage signals of a few millivolts across the crystal of the ultrasound transducer. These pulses are amplified in the first stage of the display device, termed the *rf (radiofrequency) amplifier* in Figure 23-1. An rf amplifier is required to handle frequencies without distortion in the megahertz frequency range. A preamplifier also may be used between the transducer and the rf amplifier. To compensate for the increased attenuation of ultrasound signals returning from greater depths in the body (i.e., at longer times after release of the ultrasound pulse from the transducer), the gain of the amplifier usually is increased with time after electrically shocking the transducer. This increasing gain is controlled by the swept gain generator in Figure 23-1 and is known by a variety of terms such as *swept gain, time gain compensation* (TGC) and *time varied gain* (TVG). The influence of the swept gain generator is illustrated in Figure 23-2.

After amplification of the voltage signals from millivolts to a few volts in the rf amplifier, the signals are transmitted to the demodulator where larger pulses are rectified and smoothed and smaller pulses are rejected.

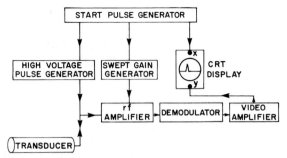

Fig 23-1. — Basic components of an A mode ultrasound unit.

From the demodulator the pulses are amplified by a factor of ten or so in the video amplifier and fed to the cathode-ray display tube where they are applied to the vertical deflection plates.

Immediately after the exciting voltage pulse is applied to the ultrasound transducer, a steadily increasing voltage is applied to the horizontal deflection plates of the cathode-ray tube (CRT) display device. This increasing voltage causes the electron beam to sweep from left to right at a constant rate across the phosphor screen of the display unit. Synchrony of the transducer exciting pulse, the swept gain generator and the CRT trace is maintained by the start pulse generator shown in Figure 23-1. Receipt of the echo voltage signal by the vertical deflection plates causes a sudden vertical deflection of the electron beam to produce a vertical spike on the electron beam trace. The position of this spike along the horizontal axis indicates the time of receipt of the echo. This time of receipt varies with the transit time of the transmitted and reflected ultrasound pulse to and from a reflecting interface in the body. That is, the transit time is an indication of the depth of the reflecting interface below the skin, and interfaces at greater depths below the skin are displayed on the CRT display as spikes at increasing displacements to the right. By varying the initial delay and sweep velocity of the electron beam in the horizontal direction, the positions at which returning echoes are displayed on the CRT display may be related to interfaces at specific depths below the skin. The height of the CRT spike indicates the fraction of

Fig 23-2. — Influence of the swept gain generator on the gain of the rf amplifier.

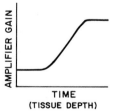

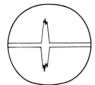 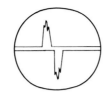

Fig 23-3. — Echoencephalo-graphic display without *(left)* and with *(right)* midline displacement.

wavefront pressure that is reflected at the interface and the degree to which the reflecting interface is perpendicular to the ultrasound beam. The propagation of the ultrasound pulse and the display of returning echoes are accomplished in a millisecond or less, and the entire process may then be repeated according to the pulse repetition frequency (PRF) of the instrument. For a permanent record, the phosphor screen of the CRT may be photographed with Polaroid or conventional photographic film.

By far the major applications of A mode presentations are in studies of the brain (echoencephalography) and the eye. A mode presentations are used also in setting the swept gain control for other presentation modes, and in distinguishing solid from cystic masses in the body. In echoencephalography, echoes from the head are studied to detect anomalies such as midline displacement, which may indicate the presence of a tumor or vascular abnormality. In this application, one transducer is placed against the right side of the skull and echoes reflected from midline structures of the brain are registered as an upward deflection on the CRT trace. A second transducer on the left side of the skull then repeats the process, except that the echo spike is deflected downward rather than upward in the CRT display. The appearance of the spikes at the same horizontal location on the CRT display indicates no midline displacement, whereas a horizontal displacement of the upward and downward spikes reveals a displacement of midline brain structures. A mode displays with and without midline displacement are shown in Figure 23-3.

In echoencephalography, little use is made of the amplitude of the voltage spike appearing on the CRT display, even though this variable provides information about the character of the reflecting interface. In other applications of A mode presentation, efforts have been directed toward the use of pulse amplitudes to gain information about the nature and orientation of the reflecting interfaces.[1-3]

B MODE PRESENTATION

In principle, a B mode presentation is simply an A mode display viewed from above. In this presentation mode, the location of a reflecting interface is indicated by the position of the echo dot on the CRT, and the reflected ultrasound pressure is revealed by the brightness of the

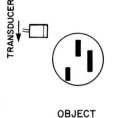

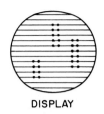

Fig 23-4. — Simple linear B mode image of the object on the left.

OBJECT   DISPLAY

echo dot rather than by the amplitude of an echo spike. In simple linear B scanning, the transducer is moved in a straight line along the edge of an object, as illustrated in Figure 23-4. As the transducer moves, a series of horizontal electron beam traces is initiated across the CRT display so that the position of each trace is synchronized with the location of the transducer at that moment. Along each trace, echoes are displayed as bright dots rather than as echo spikes. In the completed image, the dots form a composite image of structures in the object that produce the echoes (Fig 23-4).

Fig 23-5. — A classification of B mode scanning methods. (From McDicken, W.: *Diagnostic Ultrasonics: Principles and Use of Instruments* [London: Crosby Lockwood Staples Limited/Granada Publishing Limited, 1976], p. 143. Reprinted with permission.)

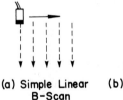

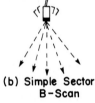

(a) Simple Linear B-Scan

(b) Simple Sector B-Scan

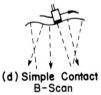

(c) Simple Radial B-Scan

(d) Simple Contact B-Scan

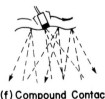

(e) Compound Linear B-Scan

(f) Compound Contact B-Scan

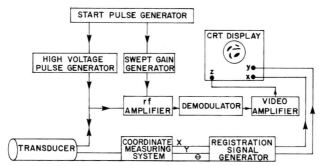

Fig 23-6. — Basic components of a B mode ultrasound unit.

If all interfaces in the object were perpendicular to the scanning ultrasound beam, then a simple linear B scan would furnish an acceptable ultrasound image of the boundaries of internal structures in the object. In anatomical objects, however, interfaces may be present at any angle, and those at angles greater than about 5 degrees from the perpendicular often will not reflect enough ultrasound energy toward the transducer to be displayed clearly in the image.

To improve the visualization of oblique interfaces, compound (sector) scanning often is preferred over simple linear scanning. In compound scanning, the orientation of the transducer is changed continuously during the scan so that the ultrasound beam is more likely to strike interfaces at a right angle during at least part of the scanning interval. Usually, changes in the transducer orientation are achieved by rocking the transducer from side to side as it is moved either in a straight line or over the surface of the patient. A combination of rocking and linear motion, termed *compound linear B scanning*, is used frequently when the scanning is performed in a water bath. For abdominal scanning, a water bath is seldom used, and the transducer is rocked and moved across the skin surface in a pattern referred to as *compound contact B scanning*. Different motions of the transducer can be achieved either manually or by the use of small motors. Various combinations of transducer orientation during the course of an ultrasound examination are depicted in Figure 23-5.

In a B scan image, the line of echoes on the display device must always be oriented in the same direction as the path of the ultrasound beam through the patient. To accomplish this synchronization, the horizontal and vertical coordinates of the transducer, as well as its angular orientation, must be monitored continuously during the examination. For this monitoring, potentiometers or other position encoders are used with characteristics that change with the position and angular orientation of the transducer. With these position sensors, signals are generated

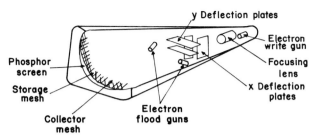

Fig 23-7. — A variable-persistence cathode-ray tube.

that change with transducer position and orientation. These signals are fed to the x and y deflection plates of the display device. In this manner, echoes can be portrayed at the proper locations on the display device.

Electronics for a B mode ultrasound scanner are similar to those for an A mode unit with the addition of the transducer coordinate and angular orientation components (Fig 23-6). In a number of B mode scanners, the display device also is similar and is essentially a cathode-ray tube with a few additional components termed the *electron flood guns*, the *collector mesh* and the *storage mesh*. The mesh components are positioned between the electron guns and the fluorescent screen (Fig 23-7). This modification of a conventional cathode-ray tube is termed a *storage* or *variable-persistence* cathode-ray tube. As the writing electron beam is moved across the fluorescent screen in response to position coordinate signals from the transducer sensors, the intensity (current) of the electron beam is altered in response to echo signals from the transducer. As electrons from the writing electron gun impinge on the storage mesh, they cause the ejection of electrons from this component. The ejected electrons are captured by the collector mesh. In this manner, the image is stored as regional variations in positive charge across the storage mesh, with the areas of greatest positive charge corresponding to the periods of highest intensity of the writing electron beam, and vice versa.

For display of the stored image, low-energy electrons are sprayed toward the storage mesh by the electron flood guns. As these electrons approach positive regions of the storage mesh, they are accelerated through the mesh and onto the fluorescent screen. Since the amount of light released by the fluorescent screen varies with the energy of the impinging electrons, an image is produced on the screen that reflects to a limited degree the distribution of positive charge across the storage mesh. Images may be stored for several minutes in a variable-persistence scope and for several hours if the electron flood guns are disabled. The major disadvantage of conventional cathode-ray tubes and variable-persistence scopes for display of B scan images is their limited gray scale

of hard-copy electrostatic printers. In Figure 23-9, a gray scale ultra-sound display obtained with a scan converter tube is compared with a black-and-white display of similar anatomy.

M MODE PRESENTATION

The M mode presentation of ultrasound images is designed specifical-ly for display of the motion of internal structures of the patient's anato-my. In the display, a trace of the position of each interface detected is presented as a function of time. The most frequent application of M mode scanning is echocardiography, in which the motion of various in-terfaces in the heart is depicted graphically on a CRT display or chart recording.

In a typical M mode visualization of motion, the structures of interest are located and portrayed as a series of dots (i.e., a B mode display) on the CRT display device. The position of the transducer is portrayed at the top of the display, and the depth of echo-producing structures is rep-resented by the vertical distance of the corresponding dot from the posi-tion of the transducer. With the transducer in a fixed position, a sweep voltage is applied to the CRT deflection plates, and in response the dots sweep to the right across the CRT screen. The speed of the horizontal sweep is controlled by the operator to capture the information desired. For stationary structures, the dots form horizontal lines in the image. Moving structures produce vertical fluctuations in the horizontal trace,

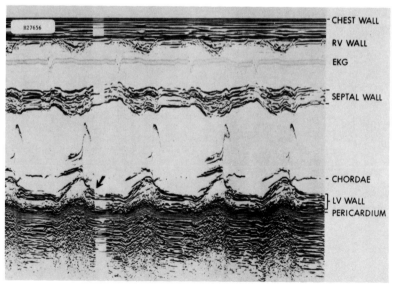

Fig 23-10. — A typical M mode echocardiographic tracing.

thereby depicting the motion of structures along one line through the object. The image may be displayed on a short-persistence cathode-ray tube or a storage scope, and may be recorded on film or, more frequently, a chart recorder. A typical M mode recording of the heart is shown in Figure 23-10.

FUTURE DEVELOPMENTS

Ultrasound imaging is destined to make significant advances in the near future. Just emerging into the commercial marketplace are multitransducer array B mode imaging devices that offer superior resolution and the possibility of real-time imaging of dynamic structures such as the heart. Computed tomography with transmitted ultrasound also is being explored to provide reconstruction images of the attenuation and velocity of ultrasound through selected planes of the patient's anatomy.[4, 5] The application of holographic imaging techniques to provide high-resolution, three-dimensional, real-time images is being explored, although initial efforts have been somewhat disappointing.[6, 7] Other methods for three-dimensional presentation of ultrasound images also are being pursued.[8] Pulsed Doppler systems are a promising technique under development to obtain information about specific moving structures in the body.[9]

PROBLEMS

1. Distinguish among A mode, B mode and M mode image presentation techniques.
2. Explain the purpose and operation of the swept gain generator.
3. Describe how the A mode presentation is used in echoencephalography, and how the images are obtained.
4. Explain how the composite dot image is compiled in a B mode presentation, and the different scanning techniques used to obtain B mode images.
5. Describe the operation of the scan converter image display device.
6. Outline the procedure for obtaining M mode images.

REFERENCES

1. Joyner, C., Herman, R., and Reid, J.: Reflected ultrasound in the detection and localization of pleural effusion, J.A.M.A. 200:399, 1967.
2. Ross, A., Genton, E., and Holmes, J.: Ultrasonic examination of the lung, J. Lab. Clin. Med. 72:556, 1968.
3. Mountford, R., and Wells, P.: Ultrasonic liver scanning: the A-scan in the normal and cirrhosis, Phys. Med. Biol. 17:261, 1972.
4. Johnson, S., et al.: Reconstruction of material characteristics from highly refraction distorted projections by ray tracing. *Image Processing for 2-D and 3-D Reconstruction from Projections: Theory and Practice in Medicine and the Physical Sciences.* A Digest of Technical Papers, August 4–7 (Stanford, Calif.: Institute of Electrical and Electronic Engineers, 1975), p. TUB2-1.

5. Carson, P., et al.: Initial Investigation of Computed Tomography for Breast Imaging with Focused Ultrasound Beams, in *Ultrasound in Medicine*, Proceedings of the American Institute of Ultrasound in Medicine (New York: Plenum Press, 1978), vol. 4, p. 319.

6. Holbrooke, D., McCurry, E., Richards, V., and Shibata, H.: Acoustical holography for surgical diagnosis, Ann. Surg. 178:547, 1973.

7. Redman, J., Watson, W., Fleming, J., and Hall, A.: Holographic display of data from ultrasonic scanning, Ultrasonics 7:26, 1969.

8. McDicken, W., Lindsay, M., and Robertson, D.: Three dimensional images using a fibre optic ultrasonic scanner, Br. J. Radiol. 45:70, 1972.

9. Wells, P.: A range-gated ultrasonic Doppler system, Med. Biol. Eng. 7:641, 1969.

24 / Protection from External Sources of Radiation

FOR A FEW YEARS after their discovery, x rays and radioactive materials were used with little regard for their biologic effects. After a few years, the consequences of careless handling and indiscriminate use of radiation sources became apparent. These consequences included severe burns and epilation and, later, leukemia and other forms of cancer in persons who received high exposures to radiation. Persons affected included many who pioneered the medical applications of ionizing radiation.

Since ionizing radiation had proved beneficial to humans in many ways, the question to be answered was: Can individuals in particular, and the human race in general, enjoy the benefits of ionizing radiation without suffering unacceptable consequences in current or future generations? This question often is described as the problem of *risk versus benefit*. To reduce the risk of using ionizing radiation, advisory groups were formed to establish upper limits for the exposure of individuals to radiation. The advisory groups have reduced the upper limits recommended for radiation exposure many times since the first limits were promulgated. These reductions reflect the use of ionizing radiation by a greater number of persons, the implications of new data concerning the sensitivity of biologic tissue to radiation and the improvements in the design of radiation devices and in the architecture of facilities where persons use radiation devices.

The philosophy underlying the control of radiation hazards is a *philosophy of risk*. With this philosophy advisory groups attempt to establish upper limits for radiation exposure that minimize the hazard to individuals and to the population but do not interfere greatly with the beneficial uses of radiation.[1] This philosophy of risk is depicted in Figure 24-1. The total biologic damage to a population is expressed as the sum of individual effects, such as reduced vitality, morbidity, shortened life span and genetic damage, which may result from receipt of some average dose rate over the lifetime of each individual in the population. The total biologic damage is assumed to increase gradually as the average dose rate increases to a value of perhaps 1 rem/week. Damage is assumed to increase more rapidly beyond a dose rate of about 1 rem/week. Although the exact shape is unknown for the curve of total biologic damage versus

440

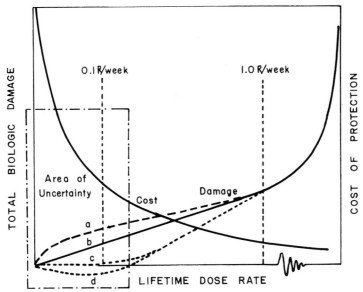

Fig 24-1.—Total biologic damage to a population, expressed as a function of the average dose rate to individuals in the population. The cost of protection is reduced as greater biologic damage is tolerated. (From Claus, W.: The Concept and Philosophy of Permissible Dose to Radiation, in Claus, W. [ed.]: *Radiation Biology and Medicine* [Reading, Mass.: Addison-Wesley Publishing Co., Inc., 1958].)

dose rate, the curve in Figure 24-1 probably is a reasonable estimate. The region of the curve enclosed within the rectangle labeled the Area of Uncertainty is the region of greatest interest to persons concerned with radiation protection; unfortunately, this part of the curve also is the region for which few data are available. As indicated by curve *c*, the damage may remain at zero for average dose rates below some threshold value. Conceivably, the curve for total biologic damage may fall below the axis near the origin (curve *d*), suggesting that very low dose rates are beneficial; however, few experimental data support this hypothesis. Perhaps the curve rises rapidly at the origin, as suggested in curve *a*. The data are meager for the biologic consequences of radiation exposure at low dose rates, and curve *b* usually is assumed to be correct. This curve suggests that the total biologic damage to a population is linearly proportional to the average dose rate down to a dose rate of zero for individuals in the population. This suggestion is referred to as the *linear hypothesis of radiation damage.*

Adequate data are not available for the area of uncertainty depicted in Figure 24-1. Consequently, the cost of radiation protection must be balanced against unknown biologic effects that might result if adequate protection were not provided. The cost of protecting individuals from ionizing radiation (e.g., by shielding, remote-control techniques, monitoring procedures and personnel restriction) is plotted as a function of the average dose rate acceptable to the population. The cost increases from almost zero with no restrictions on radiation exposure to a cost that approaches infinity if the population desires no exposure to radiation. Somewhere within the area of uncertainty, an upper limit must be accepted for the exposure of persons to radiation. This limit should be recognized as an upper limit for personnel radiation exposure that provides a risk acceptable to the population without depriving the population of benefits derived from the judicious use of ionizing radiation. In practice, the exposure of individuals to radiation should be kept as low as reasonably achievable.

MAXIMUM PERMISSIBLE DOSE

The responsibility for recommending limits for radiation exposure has been delegated to advisory groups composed of persons experienced in the use of ionizing radiation. In 1922, the American Roentgen Ray Society and the American Radium Society began a study of acceptable levels of radiation exposure. In 1928, the International Congress of Radiology formed the International Commission on Radiological Protection, referred to commonly as the ICRP. This organization is recognized as the international authority for the safe use of sources of ionizing radiation. The U.S. Advisory Committee on X-Ray and Radium Protection, known now as the National Council on Radiation Protection and Measurements (the NCRP), was formed in 1929 to interpret and implement recommendations of the ICRP for the United States.

Radiation Dose to Occupationally Exposed Persons

For the purpose of developing recommendations for the upper limits of exposure of personnel to ionizing radiation, the ICRP and NCRP assume that a population contains various groups of persons.[2, 3] For persons whose occupation requires exposure to radiation, recommendations concerning *maximum permissible doses* (MPD) are provided in Table 24-1. Maximum permissible doses such as these include contributions from radiation sources both inside and outside the body but exclude contributions from medical exposure and background radiation. The total dose in rems accumulated by an occupationally exposed person should not exceed $5(N - 18)$, where N is the age of the person in years. An area where a yearly whole body dose of 1.5 rem or more may be delivered to an individual should be considered a *controlled area* and should be supervised by a *radiation protection officer*. Persons working in a con-

TABLE 24-1.—MAXIMUM PERMISSIBLE DOSES FOR OCCUPATIONALLY EXPOSED PERSONS*

ANATOMICAL REGION	MAXIMUM QUARTERLY DOSE LIMIT (REM)	MAXIMUM YEARLY DOSE LIMIT (REM)
Whole body, gonads, eyes, red bone marrow	3 (see note 1)	5
Skin (other than hands and forearms)		15
Hands	25	75
Forearms	10	30
Other organs and organ systems	5 (see note 1)	15

*Data from NCRP report no. 39.

Notes: 1. It is assumed that generally a person will accumulate dose throughout the year in a random fashion and that the application of a maximum yearly dose limit is adequate. In cases where this is not true, e.g., in situations where an individual is likely to accumulate dose more or less uniformly from day to day at a rate that would allow the maximum yearly dose limit to be exceeded in a time interval less than one year, the application of maximum quarterly dose limits, or dose limits based on shorter time intervals, is advised.

2. The values in Table 24-1 may be modified according to the individual. For example, the pelvic dose limit for pregnant women is 0.5 rem throughout gestation.

3. The dose limits in Table 24-1 are to serve as guides for establishing responsible radiation protection procedures. To be consistent with the conservative philosophy of radiation protection, however, the NCRP recommends that every effort be made to hold the actual dose to an individual to as low a value as possible.

trolled area should carry one or more personal monitors for the measurement of radiation dose (e.g., a film badge, thermoluminescent dosimeter or pocket ionization chamber), and access to the area should be restricted.

Various problems arise when recommendations such as the foregoing are applied to particular individuals. For occupational exposures, some of these problems involve:

1. Persons with an unknown previous exposure. For the period of unknown exposure, the person is assumed to have received a maximum permissible dose for each year of age beyond 18.

2. Persons restricted by maximum permissible doses established in earlier years. Earlier MPD's were higher than those recommended now. Hence, these persons may have accumulated a dose greater than that given by the expression $5(N - 18)$. The yearly dose received by these persons should be reduced below 5 rem/yr until the total accumulated dose is reduced below $5(N - 18)$.

3. Persons beginning work at an age less than 18 years. For these persons, the dose-equivalent to the gonads, red bone marrow and whole body should not exceed 5 rem/yr and the dose accumulated by age 30 should not exceed 60 rem.

4. Women of reproductive capacity. These women should be employed only in situations where the dose to the abdomen is limited to 1.3 rem during any period of 13 weeks. Under this condition, the dose to an embryo should be considerably less than 1 rem during the first 2 months of organogenesis, the period during which the embryo is most sensitive to radiation.

5. Pregnant women. When a pregnancy has been determined, conditions of employment should be arranged to insure that the dose to the fetus is reduced below 0.5 rem during the entire gestation period.

Radiation Dose to Members of the Public

Personal monitors are not feasible for members of the public exposed occasionally to radiation. The effectiveness of protective measures for these persons is evaluated indirectly by sampling the air, water, soil and other elements of the environment. The expected dose for members of the public is computed from analyses of the environment and from knowledge of the living habits of the members. The *dose limit* for members of the public excludes the radiation dose contributed by background radiation and by medical exposure and is one tenth of the whole body maximum permissible dose for occupationally exposed persons. That is, the maximum permissible whole body dose is 0.5 rem/yr for members of the public.

Radiation Dose to a Population

The average radiation dose to an entire population is influenced not only by the radiation dose to individual members of the population but also by the total number of persons exposed in the population. Concern for the genetic effects of exposure to radiation underlies recommended limits for the exposure of a population to radiation. The *genetic dose* to a population is the radiation dose that, if received by each member of the population from conception to the mean age of childbearing (assumed to be 30 years of age), would provide a genetic burden to the entire population equal to the burden furnished by individuals in the population who actually are exposed to radiation. A *permissible genetic dose* is one that furnishes a genetic burden that is acceptable to the population. The genetic dose should be kept as low as possible and should not exceed 5 rem for all sources of radiation additional to background and medical exposure. Background contributes about 120 millirem/yr to the genetic dose. In most countries, medical procedures contribute about 1 rem to the

TABLE 24-2.—ESTIMATES OF AVERAGE RADIATION DOSE TO
GONADS FOR VARIOUS CLINICAL EXAMINATIONS*

| EXAMINATION | DOSE IN MILLIRADS | | AVERAGE NO. FILMS PER EXAMINATION |
	TESTICULAR	OVARIAN	
Skull	<1	4	3.7
Cervical spine	8	2	3.1
Upper extremity (excluding shoulder)	2	1	2.3
Lower extremity (excluding hip)	96	<1	2.4
Chest			
Roentgenography	5	8	1.4
Photofluorography	<1	8	
Fluoroscopy	1	71	
Thoracic spine	196	9	2.1
Shoulder	<1	<1	1.8
Upper gastrointestinal series			
Total†	137	558	
Roentgenography	130	360	4.4
Fluoroscopy	7	198	
Barium enema			
Total†	1,585	805	
Roentgenography	1,535	439	3.5
Fluoroscopy	50	366	
Cholecystography	2	193	3.7
Intravenous or retrograde pyelography	2,091	407	5.0
Abdomen	254	289	1.7
Lumbar spine	2,268	275	2.5
Pelvis	717	41	1.5
Hip	1,064	309	2.3

*From Penfil and Brown.[4]
†Totals were obtained by adding doses from roentgenography and fluoroscopy, because both fluoroscopy and one or more roentgenograms are included in most of these examinations.

genetic dose.[2] The average dose to the gonads is estimated in Table 24-2 for various clinical examinations in the United States.

The *genetically significant dose* to a population is the average annual gonadal dose to members of the population, adjusted for the expected number of children conceived by each individual after exposure to radiation. Factors influencing the genetically significant dose are the average annual gonadal dose and the age and sex of the individuals exposed. Contributions to the genetically significant dose are depicted in Figure 24-2 for various clinical examinations. The genetically significant dose contributed by medical procedures is estimated to be about 20 millirem for the populations of the United States and other medically advanced countries.[5]

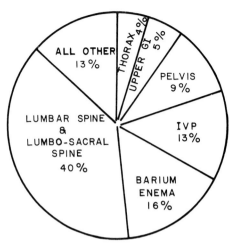

Fig 24-2.—Estimated contributions of various radiologic examinations to the genetically significant dose for the population of the United States in 1964. (From Penfil, R., and Brown, M.: Genetically significant dose to the United States population from diagnostic medical radiology, 1964, Radiology 90:209, 1968.)

RECOMMENDATIONS FOR SOURCES OF X AND γ RADIATION

Using recommendations of the ICRP for guidance, members of the NCRP have suggested a number of guidelines for evaluating the safety of x-ray equipment and sources of γ radiation. A complete description of these recommendations is available in Report 33 of the National Council on Radiation Protection.[6]

PROTECTIVE BARRIERS FOR RADIATION SOURCES

The walls, ceiling and floor of a room containing an x-ray machine or a radioactive source may be constructed to permit the use of adjacent rooms when the x-ray machine is energized or the radioactive source is exposed. With a MPD of 5 rem/yr for occupational exposure, the maximum permissible average dose-equivalent per week equals 0.1 rem. A dose of 0.1 rem/week (or less) is used when computing the thickness of radiation barriers required for controlled areas. For areas outside the supervision of a radiation safety officer, a value of 0.01 rem per week usually is used. Since the conversion from roentgens to rads is nearly 1 for x and γ rays, and since the quality factor also is 1 for these radiations, the maximum permissible exposure often is taken as 0.1 R/week or 0.01 R/week for computation of the barrier thicknesses for sources of x and γ rays. In a shielded room, *primary barriers* are designed to attenuate the primary (useful) beam from the radiation source and *secondary barriers* are designed to reduce scattered and leakage radiation from the source.

Protection from Small Sealed γ-Ray Sources

The exposure X in roentgens to an individual in the vicinity of a point source of radioactivity is

$$X = \frac{\Gamma_\infty At}{d^2}(B) \qquad (24\text{-}1)$$

where

> X = Exposure in roentgens.
> Γ = Exposure rate constant in (R-sq cm)/(hr-mCi) at 1 cm.
> A = Activity of source in millicuries.
> t = Time in hours spent in the vicinity of the source.
> d = Distance from the source in centimeters.
> B = Fraction of radiation transmitted by a protective barrier between the source and the individual.

The exposure may be reduced by: (1) increasing the distance d between the source and the individual: (2) decreasing the time t spent in the vicinity of the source and (3) reducing the transmission B of the protective barrier (Fig 24-3).

Example 24-1

What is the thickness of lead that reduces the exposure to 0.1 R/week for a person who sits at a distance of 1 m from 100 mg radium [0.5 mm Pt(Ir)] for 40 hr/week? The exposure rate constant Γ_∞ is 8.25 (R-sq cm)/(hr-mCi) for radium filtered by 0.5 mm Pt(Ir).

$$X = \frac{\Gamma_\infty At}{d^2}(B) \qquad (24\text{-}1)$$

$$B = \frac{Xd^2}{\Gamma_\infty At}$$

$$= \frac{(0.1)(100)^2}{(8.25)(100)(40)}$$

$$= 0.03$$

From Figure 24-3, about 7 cm of lead is required for the radiation barrier.

Primary Barriers for X-Ray Beams

For an individual some distance from an x-ray unit, the maximum expected exposure to radiation depends on:

1. The emission rate of radiation from the unit. As a general rule, a diagnostic x-ray unit furnishes an exposure rate of less than 1 R/min at 1 m for each milliampere of current flowing through the x-ray tube; that is, the exposure rate is ≤ 1 R/(mA-min) at 1 m.

2. The average tube current and the operating time of the x-ray unit per week. The product of these variables has units of mA-min/wk and is

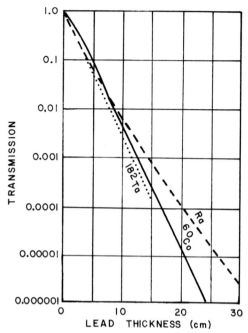

Fig 24-3.—Transmission through lead of γ rays from radium, ^{60}Co and ^{182}Ta. (Figures 24-3 and 24-4 from International Commission on Radiological Protection: *Report of Committee III on Protection against X Rays up to Energies of 3 MeV and Beta and Gamma Rays from Sealed Sources,* ICRP publ. 3 [New York: Pergamon Press, Inc., 1960].)

termed the *workload* W of the x-ray unit. Typical workloads for busy radiographic installations are described in Table 24-3.

3. The fraction of the operating time that the x-ray beam is directed toward the location of interest. This fraction is termed the *use factor U.* Typical use factors are listed in Table 24-4.

4. The fraction of the operating time that the location of interest is occupied by the individual. This fraction is termed the *occupancy factor T.* Typical occupancy factors are listed in Table 24-5. For controlled areas, the occupancy factor always is 1.

5. The distance d in meters from the x-ray unit to the location of interest, because the exposure decreases with $1/(\text{distance})^2$.

The maximum expected exposure to an individual at the location of interest may be estimated as

$$\text{Maximum expected exposure} = \frac{(1 \text{ R/mA-min at 1 m})(\text{mA-min/week})(\text{Use factor})(\text{Occupancy factor})}{(\text{Distance})^2}$$

TABLE 24-3.—TYPICAL WEEKLY WORKLOADS FOR BUSY INSTALLATIONS*

DIAGNOSTIC	DAILY PATIENT LOAD	WEEKLY WORKLOAD (W) MA-MIN† 100 kV or less	125 kV	150 kV
Admission chest (miniature, with phototiming grid)	100	100	—	—
Chest (14 × 17: 3 films per patient, no grid)	60	150	—	—
Cystoscopy	8	600	—	—
Fluoroscopy including spot filming	24	1,500	600	300
Fluoroscopy without spot filming	24	1,000	400	200
Fluoroscopy with image intensification including spot filming	24	750	300	150
General radiography	24	1,000	400	200
Special procedures	8	700	280	140

*From National Council on Radiation Protection and Measurements: *Structural Shielding Design and Evaluation for Medical Use of X Rays and Gamma Rays of Energies up to 10 MeV*. Recommendations of the NCRP, Report 49 (Washington, D.C., 1976).
†Peak pulsating x-ray tube potential.

TABLE 24-4.—USE FACTORS RECOMMENDED BY THE ICRP*

Full use $(U = 1)$	Floors of radiation rooms except dental installations, doors, walls and ceilings of radiation rooms exposed routinely to the primary beam
Partial use $(U = \frac{1}{4})$	Doors and walls of radiation rooms not exposed routinely to the primary beam; also, floors of dental installations
Occasional use $(U = \frac{1}{16})$	Ceilings of radiation rooms not exposed routinely to the primary beam. Because of the low use factor, shielding requirements for a ceiling usually are determined by secondary rather than primary beam considerations.

*Tables 24-4 and 24-5 from *Report of Committee III on Protection against X Rays up to Energies of 3 MeV and Beta and Gamma Rays from Sealed Sources*, ICRP publ. 3 (New York: Pergamon Press, Inc., 1960).

$$= \frac{WUT}{d^2} \qquad (24\text{-}2)$$

This exposure can be reduced to a maximum permissible level X_p (e.g., 0.1 or 0.01 R/week) by the introduction of an attenuation factor B into equation (24-2).

$$X_p = \frac{WUT}{d^2}(B)$$

TABLE 24-5.—OCCUPANCY FACTORS
RECOMMENDED BY THE ICRP

Full occupancy ($T = 1$)	Control spaces, offices, corridors and waiting spaces large enough to hold desks, darkrooms, workrooms and shops, nurse stations, rest and lounge rooms used routinely by occupationally exposed personnel, living quarters, children's play areas, occupied space in adjoining buildings
Partial occupancy ($T = \frac{1}{4}$)	Corridors too narrow for desks, utility rooms, rest and lounge rooms not used routinely by occupationally exposed personnel, wards and patients' rooms, elevators with operators, unattended parking lots
Occasional occupancy ($T = \frac{1}{16}$)	Closets too small for future occupancy, toilets not used routinely by occupationally exposed personnel, stairways, automatic elevators, pavements, streets

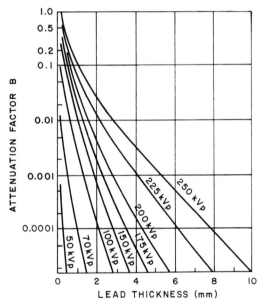

Fig 24-4.—Attenuation in lead of x rays generated at tube voltages from 50 to 250 kVp. The curves were obtained with a half-wave-rectified x-ray generator and with a 90-degree angle between the electron beam and the axis of the x-ray beam. The inherent filtration was 3 mm of aluminum for the 150 kVp to 250 kVp curves and 0.5 mm of aluminum for the other curves. X-ray beams generated with a constant tube voltage require barriers 10% thicker than those indicated by the curves.

TABLE 24-6.—THICKNESSES OF LEAD EQUIVALENT TO
THICKNESSES OF ORDINARY CONCRETE (DENSITY 2.2 GM/CC)
AT SELECTED TUBE VOLTAGES FOR BROAD X-RAY BEAMS°

| THICKNESS OF CONCRETE (CM) | LEAD EQUIVALENT (MM) FOR X RAYS GENERATED AT FOLLOWING VOLTAGES (KVP) | | | | | | | | | | |
	50	75	100	150	200	250	300	400	500	1,000	2,000
5	0.4	0.5	0.6	0.5	0.5	0.6	0.8	1.1	1.6	4.0	6
10	0.9	1.2	1.4	1.2	1.2	1.7	2.2	3.0	3.9	8.6	13
15	1.4	2.0	2.4	1.9	2.1	3.0	3.8	5.4	7.1	13	22
20	2.0	2.8	3.4	2.7	2.9	4.4	5.8	8.5	11	21	31
25	2.5	3.6	4.4	3.4	3.8	5.8	7.9	11	15	29	40
30	3.1	4.3	5.4	4.2	4.7	7.3	10	14	19	37	49
35	–	–	–	5.1	5.6	8.6	12	18	24	45	58
40	–	–	–	–	–	–	–	21	28	54	67
45	–	–	–	–	–	–	–	24	33	62	76
50	–	–	–	–	–	–	–	–	37	71	85
60	–	–	–	–	–	–	–	–	46	88	103
75	–	–	–	–	–	–	–	–	60	112	130
90	–	–	–	–	–	–	–	–	–	138	159

°From Appleton and Krishnamoorthy.[7]

The attenuation factor B is

$$B = \frac{X_p d^2}{WUT} \qquad (24\text{-}3)$$

With the attenuation factor B and the curves in Figure 24-4, the thickness of concrete or lead may be determined that reduces the exposure rate to an acceptable level. Listed in Table 24-6 are the thicknesses of lead that are equivalent to concrete walls of different thicknesses.

Example 24-2

A diagnostic x-ray generator has a busy workload of 1,000 mA-min/week at 100 kVp. The x-ray tube is positioned 4.5 m from a wall between the radiation room and a radiologist's office. The wall contains 3 cm of ordinary concrete. For a use factor of 0.5, what is the thickness of lead that must be added to the wall?

$$B = \frac{X_p d^2}{WUT} \qquad (24\text{-}3)$$

Since the radiologist's office is a controlled area for occupationally exposed persons, $X_p = 0.1$ R/week, $T = 1$ and

$$B = \frac{0.1 d^2}{WUT}$$
$$= \frac{(0.1)(4.5)^2}{(1,000)(0.5)(1)}$$
$$= 0.004$$

From the 100-kVp curve in Figure 24-4, the thickness of lead required is 1.0 mm. A 3-cm thickness of concrete is equivalent to 0.4 mm of lead (Table 24-6). Consequently, at least 0.6 mm (or $\frac{1}{32}$ in.) of lead should be added to the wall.

Secondary Barriers for Scattered X Radiation

Radiation may be scattered to a location that is not exposed to the primary x-ray beam. The amount of scattered radiation varies with the intensity of radiation incident upon the scatterer, the area of the x-ray beam at the scatterer, the distance between the scatterer and the location of interest and the angle of scattering of the x rays. For a scattering angle of 90 degrees with respect to a diagnostic x-ray beam 400 sq cm in cross-sectional area that is incident upon a scatterer, the exposure rate 1 m from the scatterer is 1/1,000 of the primary beam exposure rate at the scatterer (Fig 24-5). At other distances from the scatterer, the exposure rate varies as 1/(distance)^2.

Over a week, the exposure at the scatterer (the patient) is

$$\text{Exposure at scatterer} = \frac{WUT}{d^2}$$
$$= \frac{W}{d^2}$$

where U and T are 1, since the beam is always directed at the patient and a patient is always present. At some location a distance d' from and at right angles to the primary beam, the exposure due to scattered radiation is

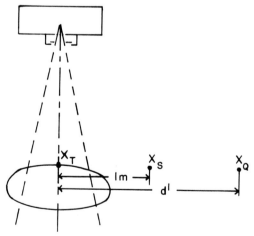

Fig 24-5. — Geometry for determining the radiation exposure X_Q at a distance d' from a scatterer where the exposure is X_T. The exposure X_S at a distance of 1 m from the scatterer is $1/1,000\, X_T$.

Exposure per week from scattered radiation $= \dfrac{(W/d^2)(1/1{,}000)(F/400)}{(d')^2}$

$$(24\text{-}4)$$

where $1/1{,}000$ is the ratio of scattered radiation at 1 m to primary radiation at the scatterer, F is the area of the x-ray beam at the scatterer, $F/400$ corrects the ratio $1/1{,}000$ for more or less scattered radiation from fields larger or smaller than 400 sq cm, and $(d')^2$ corrects the scattered radiation for the inverse square falloff of exposure with distance. The use factor always is 1 for scattered radiation. With insertion of an occupancy factor T for the location of interest, the exposure per week to an individual from scattered radiation may be estimated:

Exposure to individual due to scattered radiation (R/week) $= \dfrac{(W/d^2)(1/1{,}000)(F/400)(T)}{(d')^2}$ $\qquad$ (24-5)

To reduce the exposure to an acceptable level X_p, a secondary barrier may be interposed between the scatterer and the location of interest. The barrier introduces an attenuation factor B into equation (24-5).

$$X_p = \frac{(W/d^2)(1/1{,}000)(F/400)(T)}{(d')^2}(B)$$

The attenuation factor B is

$$B = \frac{X_p(d')^2}{(W/d^2)(1/1{,}000)(F/400)(T)} \qquad (24\text{-}6)$$

In diagnostic radiology, x-ray beams almost always are generated at tube voltages less than 500 kVp. Radiation scattered from these beams is almost as energetic as the primary radiation, and the barrier thickness for scattered radiation is determined from curves for the primary radiation.

Example 24-3

A diagnostic x-ray generator has a busy workload of 3,000 mA-min/week at 100 kVp and an average field size of 20×20 cm. The x-ray tube is positioned 1.5 m from a wall between the radiation room and a urology laboratory with uncontrolled access. The wall contains 3 cm of ordinary concrete. For an occupancy factor of 1, what thickness of lead should be added to the wall if the primary beam is not directed toward the wall?

$$B = \frac{X_p(d')^2}{(W/d^2)(1/1{,}000)(F/400)(T)} \qquad (24\text{-}6)$$

If the radiation scattered to the wall originates within a patient positioned 1 m below the x-ray tube, then

$$B = \frac{(0.01)(1.5)^2}{[3{,}000/(1)^2](1/1{,}000)(400/400)(1)}$$

where the maximum permissible exposure is 0.01 R/week for persons in the urology laboratory. From the 100-kVp curve in Figure 24-4 the thickness of lead required is 0.8 mm.

Secondary Barriers for Leakage Radiation

Radiation escaping in undesired directions through the x-ray tube housing is termed *leakage radiation*. According to the ICRP, this radiation should not exceed 0.1 R/hr at 1 m at the highest-rated kVp for the x-ray tube and at the highest mA permitted for continuous operation of the x-ray tube. To determine the maximum tube current for continuous operation, the anode thermal characteristics chart for the x-ray tube must be consulted (Fig 24-6). From this chart, it is possible to determine the maximum heat units per second that the x-ray tube can tolerate during continuous operation. By dividing this value by the maximum rated kVp for the x-ray tube, the maximum mA for continuous operation is computed. At this mA value, the exposure rate due to leakage radiation should not exceed 0.1 R/hr at 1 m from the x-ray tube.

To determine the maximum exposure per week at 1 m due to leakage radiation, the workload in mA-min/wk is divided by the maximum mA for continuous operation. The quotient is the effective operating time W' of the x-ray unit for purposes of computing the exposure due to leakage radiation. The exposure at a location of interest a distance d from the x-ray tube is

$$\text{Exposure due to leakage radiation} = \frac{(0.1)(W')}{60\ d^2}$$

where W' has units of minutes per week and 60 is a conversion from minutes to hours. The use factor for leakage radiation always is 1 because leakage radiation is emitted in all directions whenever the x-ray

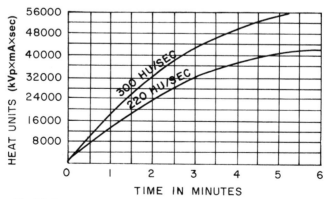

Fig 24-6. — A typical anode thermal characteristics chart.

tube is used. To determine the exposure to an individual due to leakage radiation, an occupancy factor T for the location of interest should be added to the equation

$$\text{Exposure to individual from leakage radiation} = \frac{0.1\,W'T}{60\,d^2} \qquad (24\text{-}7)$$

By adding an attenuation factor B to the equation, leakage radiation may be reduced to the permissible level X_p.

$$X_p = \frac{0.1\,W'T}{60\,d^2}(B)$$

The attenuation factor B is

$$B = \frac{60\,X_p d^2}{0.1\,W'T} \qquad (24\text{-}8)$$

Since leakage radiation is at least as energetic as the primary beam, the thickness of a barrier that provides the attenuation factor B is determined from curves in Figure 24-4 for the primary x-ray beam.

A barrier designed for primary radiation provides adequate protection against scattered and leakage radiation. For a barrier designed for scattered and leakage radiation only (i.e., a secondary barrier), the thickness is computed separately for each type of radiation. If the barrier thickness required for scattered radiation differs by more than three half-value layers from that required for leakage, the greater thickness is used for the barrier. If the thicknesses computed for scattered and leakage radiation differ by less than three half-value layers, then the thickness of the barrier is increased by adding one half-value layer to the greater of the two computed thicknesses. Half-value layers for diagnostic x-ray beams are listed in Table 24-7.

TABLE 24-7.—HALF-VALUE LAYERS IN MILLIMETERS OF LEAD AND IN CENTIMETERS AND INCHES OF CONCRETE FOR X-RAY BEAMS GENERATED AT DIFFERENT TUBE VOLTAGES°

ATTENUATING MATERIAL	HALF-VALUE LAYER						
	50 kVp	70 kVp	100 kVp	125 kVp	150 kVp	200 kVp	250 kVp
Lead (mm)	0.05	0.15	0.24	0.27	0.29	0.98	0.9
Concrete (in.)	0.17	0.33	0.6	0.8	0.88	1.0	1.1
Concrete (cm)	0.43	0.84	1.5	2.0	2.2	2.5	2.8

ATTENUATING MATERIAL	HALF-VALUE LAYER					
	300 kVp	400 kVp	500 kVp	1,000 kVp	2,000 kVp	3,000 kVp
Lead (mm)	1.4	2.2	3.6	7.9	12.7	14.7
Concrete (in.)	1.23	1.3	1.4	1.75	2.5	2.9
Concrete (cm)	3.1	3.3	3.6	4.4	6.4	7.4

° From National Council on Radiation Protection and Measurements, Report 34.[8]

Example 24-4

For the x-ray tube with a maximum rated kVp of 100 and the anode thermal characteristics chart shown in Fig 24-6, determine the maximum mA for continuous operation and the thickness of lead that should be added to the wall described in Example 24-3 to protect against both scattered and leakage radiation.

From Figure 24-6, the maximum anode thermal load that can be tolerated by the x-ray tube is 300 hu/sec.

$$\text{Maximum mA for continuous operation at maximum kVp} = \frac{300 \text{ hu/sec}}{100 \text{ kVp}} = 3 \text{ mA}$$

$$\text{Effective operating time } W' = \frac{3,000 \text{ mA-min/wk}}{3 \text{ mA}} = 1,000 \text{ min/wk}$$

$$B = \frac{60 \, X_p d^2}{0.1 \, W'T} \tag{24-8}$$
$$= \frac{60(0.01)(1.5)^2}{0.1 \, (1,000)(1)}$$
$$= 0.0135$$

From Figure 24-4, the thickness of lead required to protect against leakage radiation is 0.6 mm Pb. From Example 24-3, the thickness of lead required to protect against scattered radiation is 0.8 mm Pb. The difference between these thicknesses is less than three times the half-value layer of 0.24 mm Pb for a 100-kVp x-ray beam (see Table 24-6). Hence, the total thickness of lead required to shield against both scattered and leakage radiation is (0.8 + 0.24) = 1.04 mm Pb. The concrete in the wall provides shielding equivalent to 0.4 mm Pb, so 0.64 mm or $\frac{1}{32}$ in. of lead must be added to the wall.

Special Shielding Requirements for X-Ray Film

X-ray film is especially sensitive to radiation, and film storage areas and bins often must be shielded to a greater extent than areas occupied by individuals. For film storage areas, shielding computations are identical with those described above, except that maximum permissible exposures X_p must be reduced to much lower values. As a rule of thumb, the exposure should be limited to no more than 1 mR for the maximum storage time of the film (e.g., 2 weeks).

Estimation of Patient Dose in Diagnostic Radiology

The radiation dose delivered to a patient during a roentgenographic procedure may be estimated with reasonable accuracy with the rule of thumb of 1 R/mA-min at 1 m from a diagnostic x-ray unit. Frequently, this estimate is needed when a patient examined radiographically is discovered a short time later to have been in an early stage of pregnancy during the examination. In this case, an estimate of fetal dose is required. One procedure for estimating fetal dose is outlined in Example 24-5.

Example 24-5

A patient receives 2 minutes of fluoroscopy (80 kVp, 3 mA) and four spot films (80 kVp, 30 mAs) over the 20-cm-thick lower abdominal region. The x-ray tube-to-tabletop distance is 0.5 m for the x-ray unit used for the examination. A short time later it is determined that the patient was 3 weeks pregnant at the time of the examination. Estimate the dose to the fetus.

The rule of thumb of 1 R/mA-min yields [1 R/mA-min/(0.5)²] or 4 R/mA-min at a distance of 0.5 m. The exposure at the skin delivered during fluoroscopy is

$$\text{Fluoroscopic exposure} = \left(4 \frac{R}{mA\text{-}min}\right)(3 \text{ mA})(2 \text{ min})$$
$$= 24 \text{ R}$$

The exposure at the skin delivered by the spot films is

$$\text{Spot film exposure} = \frac{(4 \text{ R/mA-min})(30 \text{ mA-sec/film})(4 \text{ films})}{60 \text{ sec/min}}$$
$$= 8 \text{ R}$$

The total exposure at the skin is 24 R + 8 R = 32 R. For average-size patients, the transmission of the x-ray beam through the abdomen is roughly 0.1–0.5% of the incident exposure. With the assumption that the fetus is positioned midway in the abdomen, the exposure to the fetus may be approximated as the square root of the transmitted exposure, or 3–7%. With a conservative estimate of 7%, the exposure to the fetus is

$$\text{Exposure to fetus} = (32 \text{ R})(0.07)$$
$$= 2.2 \text{ R}$$

Since the exposure in roentgens is approximately equal numerically to the dose in rad, the absorbed dose to the fetus is roughly 2.2 rad.

AREA AND PERSONNEL MONITORING

The radiation exposure must be known for persons working with or near sources of ionizing radiation. This knowledge may be obtained by periodic measurements of exposure rates at locations accessible to the individuals. Furthermore, persons working with or near sources of ionizing radiation should be equipped with personnel monitors that reveal the amount of exposure the individuals have received. The monitor used most frequently is the film badge containing two or more small photographic films enclosed within a light-tight envelope. The badge is worn for a selected interval of time (1–4 weeks) at some convenient location on the clothing over the trunk of the body. During fluoroscopy, most persons wear the film badge under a lead apron to monitor the exposure to the trunk of the body. After the desired interval of time has elapsed, the film is processed and its optical density is compared with the optical density of similar films that have received known exposures. From this compari-

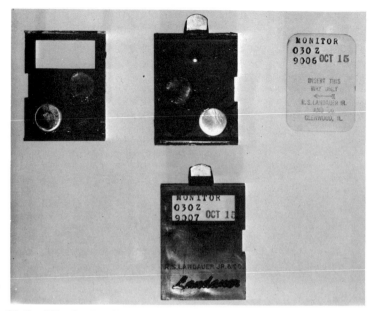

Fig 24-7.—Film badge for measuring the exposure of individuals to x and γ radiation and to high-energy β radiation. (Courtesy of R. S. Landauer, Jr., and Co.)

son, the radiation exposure may be determined for the film badge and, supposedly, for the individual wearing the film badge. Small metal filters mounted in the plastic holder for the film permit some differentiation between different types and energies of radiation that contribute to the exposure (Fig 24-7). Types of radiation that may be monitored with a film badge include x and γ rays, high-energy electrons and neutrons. Special holders have been designed for wrist badges and ring badges that are used to estimate the exposure to limited regions of the body. Although film badges furnish a convenient method for personnel monitoring, the difficulties of accurate dosimetry with photographic film limit the accuracy of measured exposures. Other methods for personnel dosimetry include pocket ionization chambers and thermoluminescent and photoluminescent dosimeters.

PROBLEMS
°1. What is the maximum permissible accumulated dose-equivalent for a 30-year-old occupationally exposed individual?
°2. A nuclear medicine technologist received an estimated 200 mrem whole

---

°For those problems marked with an asterisk, answers are provided on the pages following the appendixes (see pp. 487–488).

body dose-equivalent during the first 2 months of pregnancy. According to the NCRP, what is the maximum permissible dose equivalent over the remaining 7 months of pregnancy?

°3. The exposure rate constant Γ_∞ is 2.2 R-sq cm/hr-mCi for ^{131}I. What is the exposure over a 40-hr week at a distance of 2 m from 200 mCi of ^{131}I?

°4. For a workload of 750 mA-min/week for a dedicated 125-kVp chest roentgenographic unit, determine the shielding required behind the chest cassette at a distance of 6 ft from the x-ray tube if an office with uncontrolled access is behind the cassette.

°5. For the chest roentgenographic unit in Problem 4, determine the shielding required to protect against radiation scattered to a wall 2 m from and at right angles to the chest cassette, if the area behind the wall has uncontrolled access with an occupancy of 1.

°6. Repeat the computation in Problem 5 if film with a turnover time of 2 weeks is stored behind the wall.

°7. For the x-ray tube described by the anode thermal characteristics chart in Figure 24-6, determine the shielding required for leakage radiation at a wall 2 m from the x-ray tube, if the area behind the wall has uncontrolled access with an occupancy of 1. The x-ray tube is rated at 125 kVp maximum.

°8. For the wall in Problem 7, 1.0 mm of Pb is required to shield against scattered radiation. What thickness of shielding is required to protect against both scattered and radiation leakage?

REFERENCES

1. Claus, W.: The Concept and Philosophy of Permissible Dose to Radiation, in Claus, W. (ed.): *Radiation Biology and Medicine* (Reading, Mass.: Addison-Wesley Publishing Co., Inc., 1958), p. 389.

2. National Council on Radiation Protection and Measurements: *Basic Radiation Protection Criteria.* Recommendations of the NCRP, Report 39 (Washington, D.C., 1971).

3. International Commission on Radiological Protection: *Radiation Protection.* Recommendations of the ICRP, 1965, ICRP publ. 9 (New York: Pergamon Press, Inc., 1966).

4. Penfil, R., and Brown, M.: Genetically significant dose to the United States population from diagnostic medical roentgenology, 1964, Radiology 90:209, 1968.

5. *Population Exposure to X Rays:* US 1970, FDA report #73-8047, Public Health Service, U.S. Department of Health, Education and Welfare, Washington, D.C., 1973.

6. National Council on Radiation Protection: *Medical X-Ray and Gamma-Ray Protection for Energies up to 10 MeV.* Recommendations of the NCRP, Report 33 (Washington, D.C., 1968).

7. Appleton, G., and Krishnamoorthy, P.: *Safe Handling of Radioisotopes: Health Physics Addendum* (Vienna: International Atomic Energy Agency, 1960).

8. National Council on Radiation Protection and Measurements: *Medical X-Ray and Gamma-Ray Protection for Energies up to 10 MeV.* Recommendations of the NCRP, Report 34 (Washington, D.C., 1970).

25 / Protection from Internal Sources of Radiation

HAZARDS ASSOCIATED with radioactive nuclides deposited internally are controlled best by minimizing the absorption, inhalation and ingestion of radioactive materials into the body. The hazards of a radioactive nuclide deposited internally may be estimated by reference to the maximum permissible body burden for the nuclide.

BODY BURDENS AND CRITICAL ORGANS

The *body burden* of a particular radioactive nuclide in an individual is the activity of the nuclide that is present at some moment in the individual's body. The body burden is influenced by the rate of accumulation and physiologic elimination of the nuclide and by its rate of radioactive decay. The *maximum permissible body burden* is the constant activity of a particular radioactive nuclide that results in a maximum permissible dose to the whole body or to one or more organs in the body.[1] The maximum permissible body burden is computed with the assumption that the radioactive nuclide of interest is the only radioactive nuclide in the body. A nuclide retained in the body at a constant activity less than the maximum permissible body burden should cause macroscopic damage to the individual or to his progeny in only the rarest of instances.

The maximum permissible body burden for a radioactive nuclide of a bone-seeking element (e.g., strontium, calcium, radium or plutonium) is the number of microcuries required to deliver to bone a dose in rems equal to that provided by 0.1 μCi of ^{226}Ra in equilibrium with its decay products. This amount of radium distributed over the skeleton of an adult produces observable damage in only the rarest of instances. Body burdens for radioactive nuclides other than bone-seekers require the identification of "critical organs" for the nuclides. The selection of a critical organ or organs for a particular radioactive nuclide in a particular chemical form requires the evaluation of many factors, including (1) the concentration of the nuclide in different organs; (2) the sensitivity of different organs to ionizing radiation; (3) the importance of different organs to the health of the individual and (4) the radiation dose to the whole body and to the organs irradiated during intake and elimination of the nuclide. In most cases, the concentration of the nuclide in various organs is the dominant influence in the selection of a critical organ or organs.

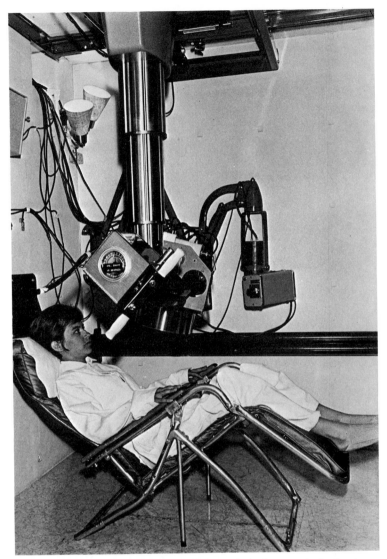

Fig 25-1.—Detector assembly and tilting chair for a whole body counter. (Courtesy of Colorado Department of Health.)

If a radioactive nuclide is distributed fairly uniformly throughout the body, then the whole body may be selected as the critical organ. For a nuclide with the whole body as the critical organ, the maximum permissible body burden for occupational exposure is the activity present continuously in the body that delivers a dose-equivalent of 5 rem/yr to the whole body. Radioactive nuclides (e.g., ^{35}S and ^{127m}Te in soluble form)

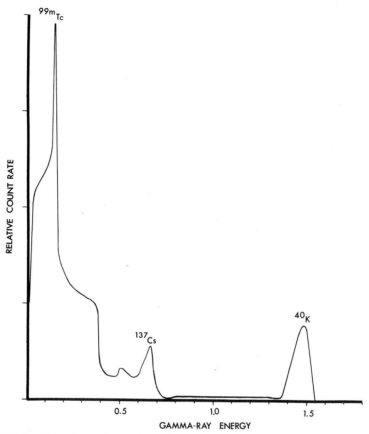

Fig 25-2.—Pulse height spectrum furnished by a whole body counter. (Courtesy of Colorado Department of Health.)

that concentrate in the testes are assigned maximum permissible body burdens for a dose of 5 rem/yr to the testes. Nuclides that concentrate in abdominal organs (e.g., liver, spleen, kidney, thyroid and gastrointestinal tract) are given limiting body burdens that provide 15 rem/yr to these organs.

Body burdens for gamma-emitting isotopes may be measured with a whole body counter.[2] Shown in Figure 25-1 is a whole body counter that includes a large NaI(Tl) crystal and a 512-channel analyzer. The person to be counted sits for a few minutes in a tilted chair directly under the crystal. The room is shielded heavily to reduce background radiation.

The pulse height spectrum in Figure 25-2 was obtained during a 40-min count of a nuclear medicine technologist. The percent abundance is 0.012 for ^{40}K in natural potassium, and a photopeak indicating the presence of this nuclide occurs in whole body pulse height spectra for all persons. The ^{137}Cs photopeak reflects the accumulation of this nuclide from radioactive fallout of nuclear explosions. The low-energy photopeak represents ^{99m}Tc, which probably was deposited internally as the technologist "milked" a ^{99m}Tc generator or worked with a ^{99m}Tc solution.

MAXIMUM PERMISSIBLE CONCENTRATION

Restricting the uptake of radioactive materials into the body is the most effective method for reducing hazards associated with radioactivity deposited internally. Restriction of the uptake of radioactive nuclides into the body may be achieved by controlling the concentration of radioactive nuclides in the air and water that persons breathe and drink. Maximum permissible concentrations in air and water have been established for exposures of 40 hr/week and 168 hr/week.[1] Concentrations in air and water less than the maximum permissible concentrations for a particular radioactive nuclide should provide a body burden for the nuclide that is less than the maximum permissible body burden.

TABLE 25-1.—MAXIMUM PERMISSIBLE BODY BURDENS AND MAXIMUM PERMISSIBLE CONCENTRATIONS FOR A FEW RADIOACTIVE NUCLIDES IN SOLUBLE AND INSOLUBLE FORM*

RADIOACTIVE NUCLIDE AND MODE OF DECAY	ORGAN OF REFERENCE†	MAXIMUM PERMISSIBLE BODY BURDEN (μCi)	MAXIMUM PERMISSIBLE CONCENTRATION (μCi/cc) 40-HR WEEK (MPC)$_w$	40-HR WEEK (MPC)$_a$	168-HR WEEK (MPC)$_w$	168-HR WEEK (MPC)$_a$
^{3}H(^{3}H$_2$O)(β^-) (sol.)	Body tissue	10^3	0.1	2×10^{-5}	0.03	5×10^{-6}
	Total body	2×10^3	0.2	2×10^{-5}	0.05	7×10^{-6}
^{3}H (immersion)	Skin			2×10^{-3}		4×10^{-4}
^{7}Be (ec,γ)	GI (LLI)‡		0.05	10^{-5}	0.02	4×10^{-6}
(sol.)	Total body	600	6	6×10^{-6}	2	2×10^{-6}
	Kidney	800	9	8×10^{-6}	3	3×10^{-6}
	Liver	800	9	8×10^{-6}	3	3×10^{-6}
	Bone	2×10^3	20	2×10^{-5}	7	6×10^{-6}
	Spleen	4×10^3	50	4×10^{-5}	20	2×10^{-5}
(insol.)	Lung			10^{-6}		4×10^{-7}
	GI (LLI)		0.05	9×10^{-6}	0.02	3×10^{-6}
^{35}S (β^-)	Testes	90	2×10^{-3}	3×10^{-7}	6×10^{-4}	9×10^{-8}
	Total body	400	7×10^{-3}	10^{-6}	3×10^{-3}	4×10^{-7}
(sol.)	Bone	800	0.02	2×10^{-6}	5×10^{-3}	8×10^{-7}
	Skin	3×10^3	0.07	10^{-5}	0.02	3×10^{-6}
	GI (LLI)		0.2	4×10^{-5}	0.05	10^{-5}
(insol.)	Lung			3×10^{-7}		9×10^{-8}
	GI (LLI)		8×10^{-3}	10^{-6}	3×10^{-3}	5×10^{-7}

*From National Bureau of Standards Handbook 69.[1]
†Critical organ shown in italic.
‡GI = gastrointestinal tract; LLI = lower large intestine.

A few maximum permissible body burdens and maximum permissible concentrations are listed in Table 25-1. Limits for each organ represent the estimated values necessary to provide a maximum permissible dose to the organ. Maximum permissible concentrations and maximum permissible body burdens are important for the estimation of the hazard to an individual following intake of one or more radioactive nuclides into the body.

EFFECTIVE HALF-LIVES

The concentration of a radioactive nuclide in a particular organ changes with time after intake of the nuclide into the body. The change in concentration reflects not only the radioactive decay of the nuclide, but also the influence of physiologic processes that move chemical substances into and out of various organs in the body. The effective half-life for uptake or for elimination of a nuclide in a particular organ is the time required for the nuclide to increase or decrease to half its maximum concentration in the organ. The *effective half-life for uptake* (T_{up}) of the radioactive nuclide is computed from the half-life T_1 for physiologic uptake, excluding radioactive decay, and the half-life $T_{1/2}$ for radioactive decay. The *effective half-life for elimination* (T_{eff}) of a radioactive nuclide from an organ is computed from the half-life T_b for physiologic elimination, excluding radioactive decay, and the half-life for radioactive decay. Expressions for the effective half-life for elimination and for uptake are stated in equations (25-1) and (25-2).

Decay constant for elimination of nuclide

$$= \text{Decay constant for physiologic elimination}$$
$$+ \text{Decay constant for radioactive decay}$$
$$\lambda_{eff} = \lambda_b + \lambda_{1/2}$$

The decay constant $\lambda_{1/2}$ equals $(0.693)/T_{1/2}$. Similarly, $\lambda_b = (0.693)/T_b$ and $\lambda_{eff} = (0.693)/T_{eff}$, where T_b is the half-life for physiologic elimination, excluding radioactive decay, and T_{eff} is the effective half-life for elimination.

$$\frac{0.693}{T_{eff}} = \frac{0.693}{T_b} + \frac{0.693}{T_{1/2}}$$
$$\frac{1}{T_{eff}} = \frac{1}{T_b} + \frac{1}{T_{1/2}}$$
$$T_{eff} = \frac{T_b T_{1/2}}{T_b + T_{1/2}} \tag{25-1}$$

An expression for the effective half-life T_{up} for uptake may be derived by procedure similar to that above.

$$T_{up} = \frac{T_1 T_{1/2}}{T_1 + T_{1/2}} \qquad (25\text{-}2)$$

where T_1 is the half-life for biologic uptake, excluding radioactive decay.

Example 25-1

[35]Sulfur in soluble form is eliminated from its critical organ, the testes, with a biologic half-life of 630 days. The half-life is 87 days for radioactive decay of [35]S. What is the effective half-life for elimination of this nuclide from the testes?

$$\begin{aligned} T_{eff} &= \frac{T_b T_{1/2}}{T_b + T_{1/2}} \\ &= \frac{(630 \text{ days})(87 \text{ days})}{(630 \text{ days}) + (87 \text{ days})} \\ &= 76 \text{ days} \end{aligned}$$

Example 25-2

[123]Iodine is absorbed into the thyroid with a half-life of 5 hr for physiologic uptake. The half-life for radioactive decay is 13 hr for [123]I. What is the effective half-life for uptake of ^{123}I into the thyroid?

$$\begin{aligned} T_{up} &= \frac{T_1 T_{1/2}}{T_1 + T_{1/2}} \\ &= \frac{(5 \text{ hr})(13 \text{ hr})}{(5 \text{ hr}) + (13 \text{ hr})} \\ &= 3.6 \text{ hr} \end{aligned}$$

RADIATION DOSE FROM INTERNAL RADIOACTIVITY

Occasionally, radioactive nuclides are inhaled, ingested or absorbed accidentally by individuals working with or near radioactive materials. Also, radioactive nuclides are administered orally and intravenously for the diagnosis and treatment of patient disorders. The radiation dose delivered to various organs in the body should be estimated for any person with a radioactive nuclide deposited internally.

Standard Man

To compute the radiation dose delivered to an organ by radioactivity deposited within the organ, the mass of the organ must be estimated. The ICRP has developed a "standard man," which includes estimates of the average mass of organs in the adult.[3] These estimates are included in Table 25-2.

TABLE 25-2. — AVERAGE MASS OF ORGANS
IN ADULT HUMAN BODY°

ORGAN	MASS (gm)	% OF TOTAL BODY†
Total body†	70,000	100
Muscle	30,000	43
Skin and subcutaneous tissue‡	6,100	8.7
Fat	10,000	14
Skeleton		
Without bone marrow	7,000	10
Red marrow	1,500	2.1
Yellow marrow	1,500	2.1
Blood	5,400	7.7
Gastrointestinal tract†	2,000	2.9
Contents of GI tract		
Lower large intestine	150	
Stomach	250	
Small intestine	1,100	
Upper large intestine	135	
Liver	1,700	2.4
Brain	1,500	2.1
Lungs (2)	1,000	1.4
Lymphoid tissue	700	1.0
Kidneys (2)	300	0.43
Heart	300	0.43
Spleen	150	0.21
Urinary bladder	150	0.21
Pancreas	70	0.10
Salivary glands (6)	50	0.071
Testes (2)	40	0.057
Spinal cord	30	0.043
Eyes (2)	30	0.043
Thyroid gland	20	0.029
Teeth	20	0.029
Prostate gland	20	0.029
Adrenal glands or suprarenal (2)	20	0.029
Thymus	10	0.014
Ovaries (2)	8	0.011
Hypophysis (pituitary)	0.6	8.6×10^{-6}
Pineal gland	0.2	2.9×10^{-6}
Parathyroids (4)	0.15	2.1×10^{-6}
Miscellaneous (blood vessels, cartilage, nerve, etc.)	390	0.56

°From International Commission on Radiological Protection: *Report of Committee II: Permissible Dose for Internal Radiation* (New York: Pergamon Press, Inc., 1969).
†Does not include contents of the gastrointestinal tract.
‡The mass of the skin alone is about 2,000 gm.

Internal Absorbed Dose

Consider a homogeneous mass of tissue containing a uniform distribution of a radioactive nuclide. The instantaneous dose rate to the tissue depends on three variables:

1. The concentration C in μCi/gm of the nuclide in the tissue.

2. The average energy $\overline{E}$ released per disintegration of the nuclide.
3. The fraction ϕ of the released energy that is absorbed in the tissue.

The average energy $\overline{E}$ released per disintegration may be estimated as:

$$\overline{E} = n_1E_1 + n_2E_2 + n_3E_3 + \ldots$$

where E_1, E_2, E_3, . . . are the energies of different radiations contributing to the absorbed dose, and n_1, n_2, n_3, . . . are the fractions of disintegrations in which the corresponding radiations are emitted. The average energy $\overline{E}_{abs}$ absorbed per disintegration is

$$\overline{E}_{abs} = n_1E_1\phi_1 + n_2E_2\phi_2 + n_3E_3\phi_3 + \ldots$$

where ϕ_1, ϕ_2, ϕ_3, . . . are the fractions of the emitted energies that are absorbed (i.e., the absorbed fractions). A shorthand notation for the addition process is

$$\overline{E}_{abs} = n_1E_1\phi_1 + n_2E_2\phi_2 + n_3E_3\phi_3 + \ldots$$
$$= \Sigma n_iE_i\phi_i$$

where Σ indicates the sum of the products $nE\phi$ for each radiation. The instantaneous dose rate R may be written as:

$$R(\text{rad/sec}) = C(\mu\text{Ci/gm})\overline{E}_{abs}(\text{MeV/disintegration})(3.7 \times 10^4 \text{ disintegrations/}$$
$$\text{sec-}\mu\text{Ci})(1.6 \times 10^{-6} \text{ erg/MeV})(0.01 \text{ rad/erg/gm})$$
$$= 5.92 \times 10^{-4} \, C\Sigma n_iE_i\phi_i \qquad (25\text{-}3)$$

The instantaneous dose rate may be expressed in units of rad per minute or rad per hour by multiplying equation (25-3) by 60 sec/min or 3.6×10^3 sec/hr:

$$R(\text{rad/min}) = 3.55 \times 10^{-2}C\Sigma n_iE_i\phi_i$$
$$R(\text{rad/hr}) = 2.13 \, C\Sigma n_iE_i\phi_i$$

By representing $2.13 \, n_iE_i$ by the symbol Δ_i, the last equation may be written

$$R(\text{rad/hr}) = C\Sigma\Delta_i\phi_i \qquad (25\text{-}4)$$

where Δ_i is termed the *absorbed dose constant* in units of gm-rad/μCi-hr.

Locally absorbed radiations are those that are absorbed within 1 cm of their origin. For these radiations, the absorbed fraction usually is taken as 1. Locally absorbed radiations include: (1) alphas, negatrons and positrons; (2) internal conversion electrons; (3) Auger electrons and (4) x and γ rays with energies less than 11.3 keV. Photons below this energy are absorbed in 1 cm of muscle with a probability exceeding 95%. Characteristic x rays considered to be locally absorbed radiations include: K-characteristic x rays from elements with $Z < 35$, L-characteristic x rays from elements with $Z < 85$ and M-characteristic x rays from all elements.

Radiations that are not absorbed locally have an absorbed fraction less

TABLE 25-3. — ABSORBED FRACTIONS FOR 140-keV
γ RAYS FROM ^{99m}Tc DEPOSITED IN VARIOUS
ORGANS OF THE STANDARD MAN[*]

SOURCE AND TARGET ORGAN	ABSORBED FRACTION	SOURCE AND TARGET ORGAN	ABSORBED FRACTION
Bladder	0.102	Lungs	0.421 E-01
Brain	0.139	Ovaries	0.181 E-01
Gastrointestinal tract (stomach)	0.863 E-01	Pancreas	0.379 E-01
Gastrointestinal tract (small intestine)	0.128	Spleen	0.660 E-01
Gastrointestinal tract (upper large intestine)	0.710 E-01	Testicles	0.389 E-01
Gastrointestinal tract (lower large intestine)	0.569 E-01	Thyroid	0.280 E-01
Kidneys	0.614 E-01	Total body	0.306
Liver	0.134		

[*]From Snyder, W., et al.: Estimates of absorbed fractions for monoenergetic photon sources uniformly distributed in various organs of a heterogeneous phantom, MIRD pamphlet 5, J. Nucl. Med. 10 (Suppl. 3), 1969.

than 1. Generally, these radiations are x and γ rays with energies $\geq$ 11.3 keV. Illustrated in Table 25-3 are absorbed fractions for 140-keV γ rays from ^{99m}Tc deposited in various organs of the standard man. More complete data on absorbed fractions, as well as extensive listings of absorbed dose constants, are available in publications of the Medical Internal Radiation Dose (MIRD) Committee of the Society of Nuclear Medicine.[*] Included in the MIRD compilations are absorbed fractions for organs at some distance from an accumulation of radioactivity. For these situations, the absorbed fraction is 0 for locally absorbed radiations and less than 1 for more penetrating radiations.

The instantaneous dose rate varies with changes in the concentration C of the nuclide in the mass of tissue. If the nuclide is eliminated exponentially,[†] then

$$C = C_{max}e^{-\lambda_{eff}t}$$
$$= C_{max}e^{-0.693t/T_{eff}}$$

where t is the time elapsed since the concentration was at its maximum value C_{max}. With exponential elimination

$$R(rad/hr) = C_{max}e^{-0.693t/T_{eff}} \Sigma\Delta_i\phi_i$$

For a finite interval of time t that begins at $t = 0$ when $C = C_{max}$, the cumulative absorbed dose D is

[*]Available from the Society of Nuclear Medicine, 475 Park Avenue South, New York, New York 10016.
[†]If the assumption of exponential elimination is too great a simplification, then the elimination of the nuclide from the tissue must be described by a more complex expression.

$$D(\text{rad}) = C_{\max}(1.44\ T_{\text{eff}})(1 - e^{-0.693t/T_{\text{eff}}})\ \Sigma\Delta_i\phi_i$$

with t and T_{eff} expressed in hours, and with $1.44\ T_{\text{eff}}$ termed the *average life* for elimination of the nuclide. More often, t and T_{eff} are expressed in days, and the equation becomes

$$D_{\text{rad}} = 34.6\ C_{\max}T_{\text{eff}}(1 - e^{-0.693t/T_{\text{eff}}})\Sigma\Delta_i\phi_i \tag{25-5}$$

The total absorbed dose during complete exponential elimination of the nuclide from the mass of tissue is obtained by setting $t = \infty$ in equation (25-5). The exponential term $e^{-0.693t/T_{\text{eff}}}$ approaches zero and

$$D(\text{rad}) = 34.6\ C_{\max}T_{\text{eff}}\Sigma\Delta_i\phi_i \tag{25-6}$$

That is, the total cumulative dose depends on the three variables that affect the dose rate (concentration, energy released per disintegration and fraction of the released energy that is absorbed), together with the time (represented by T_{eff}) that the nuclide is present in the tissue.

If the effective half-life for uptake of a radionuclide is short compared with the effective half-life for elimination, equation (25-6) may be used to estimate the total dose delivered from the moment the nuclide is distributed in a mass of tissue until the time it is eliminated completely. If the uptake of the nuclide must be considered, then it may be reasonably accurate to assume that the uptake is exponential. If elimination of the nuclide also is exponential, then the concentration C at some time t is

$$C = C_{\max}\ (e^{-0.093t/T_{\text{eff}}} - e^{-0.693t/T_{\text{up}}})$$

From this expression and equation (25-4), an expression may be derived for the total cumulative absorbed dose:

$$D(\text{rad}) = 34.6\ C_{\max}T_{\text{eff}}\left(1 - \frac{T_{\text{up}}}{T_{\text{eff}}}\right)\Sigma\Delta_i\phi_i \tag{25-7}$$

with T_{up} and T_{eff} expressed in days. If $T_{\text{eff}} \geq 20\ T_{\text{up}}$, the effective half-life T_{up} for uptake (i.e., the term $1 - T_{\text{up}}/T_{\text{eff}}$) may be neglected with an error no greater than 5% in the total cumulative absorbed dose.

Recently, a simplification of the MIRD approach to absorbed dose computations has been prepared for radionuclides absorbed in specific internal organs. In this approach, the quotient of $\Sigma\Delta_i\phi_i$ divided by the mass of the organ containing the radionuclide is recognized as having a specific value for a particular nuclide, source organ (organ containing the nuclide) and target organ (organ for which the absorbed dose is to be computed). This specific value is symbolized as S, and the absorbed dose may be computed as

$$D(\text{rad}) = \tilde{A}S \tag{25-8}$$

where $\tilde{A}$ is the cumulative activity in the organ. For exponential elimination and short uptake times, $\tilde{A}$ is simply $A_{\max}T_{\text{avg}}$, where $A_{\max}$ is the maximum activity in the organ and $T_{avg} = 1.44\ T_{eff}$. Further information on the "S method" of internal dose computation is available in MIRD pamphlet 11, available from the Society of Nuclear Medicine, 475 Park Avenue South, New York, New York 10016.

Example 25-3

One millicurie of $Na_2\ ^{35}SO_4$ is given orally to a 70-kg man. Approximately 0.5% of the activity is absorbed into the blood, and 50% of the absorbed activity is concentrated rapidly in the testes. What are the instantaneous dose rate, the dose delivered over the first week and the total dose delivered to the testes?

From Table 25-2, the mass of the testes is 40 gm in the standard man. For ^{35}S, only locally absorbed radiation is emitted, with an average energy of 0.049 MeV per disintegration. The total activity reaching the testes is $(1,000\ \mu Ci)(0.005)(0.5)$ $= 2.5\ \mu Ci$. The instantaneous dose rate R_β is

$$R_\beta = 5.92 \times 10^{-4}\ C\Sigma n_i E_i \phi_i \qquad (25\text{-}3)$$
$$= (5.92 \times 10^{-4})\left(\frac{2.5\ \mu Ci}{40\ gm}\right)(0.049\ MeV)$$
$$= 1.8\ \mu rad/sec$$

From Example 25-1, the effective half-life is 76 days for elimination of ^{35}S from the testes. Assuming rapid uptake and exponential elimination, the dose delivered over the first week is

$$D_\beta = 34.6\ C_{max} T_{eff}\ (1 - e^{-0.693 t/T_{eff}})\ \Sigma\Delta_i\phi_i \qquad (25\text{-}5)$$
$$= 34.6\ \left(\frac{2.5\ \mu Ci}{40\ gm}\right)(76\ days)(1 - e^{-0.693(7/76)})(2.13)(0.049\ MeV)$$
$$= 1.08\ rad\ over\ the\ first\ week$$

The total dose delivered to the testes during complete elimination of the nuclide is

$$D_\beta = 34.6\ C_{max} T_{eff}\ \Sigma\Delta_i\phi_i \qquad (25\text{-}6)$$
$$= 34.6\ \left(\frac{2.5\ \mu Ci}{40\ gm}\right)(76\ days)(2.13)(0.049\ MeV)$$
$$= 17.1\ rad$$

TABLE 25-4.—VALUES OF S FOR ^{99m}Tc
(source organ: liver)°

TARGET ORGAN	S
Liver	4.6 E-05
Ovaries	4.5 E-07
Spleen	9.2 E-07
Red bone marrow	1.6 E-06

°From Snyder, W., et al.: "S," *Absorbed Dose Per Unit Cumulated Activity for Selected Radionuclides and Organs*, MIRD pamphlet 11, Society of Nuclear Medicine, 475 Park Avenue South, New York, New York 10016.

Example 25-4

Estimate the absorbed dose to the liver, ovaries, spleen and bone marrow from the intravenous ingestion of 1 mCi of ^{99m}Tc-sulfur colloid that localizes uniformly and completely in the liver. Assume instantaneous uptake of the colloid in the liver and an infinite biologic half-life.

$$\tilde{A} = 1.44 \; T_{eff}A_{max}$$
$$= 1.44 \; (6 \text{ hr})(1{,}000 \; \mu\text{Ci})$$
$$= 8{,}600 \; \mu\text{Ci-hr}$$
$$D = \tilde{A}S$$
$$D_{LI} = (8{,}600 \; \mu\text{Ci-hr})(4.6 \times 10^{-5}) = 400 \text{ mrad}$$
$$D_{OV} = (8{,}600 \; \mu\text{Ci-hr})(4.5 \times 10^{-7}) = 3.9 \text{ mrad}$$
$$D_{SP} = (8{,}600 \; \mu\text{Ci-hr})(9.2 \times 10^{-7}) = 7.9 \text{ mrad}$$
$$D_{BM} = (8{,}600 \; \mu\text{Ci-hr})(1.6 \times 10^{-6}) = 14 \text{ mrad}$$

Example 25-5

Estimate the absorbed dose to the bone marrow from an intravenous injection of 1 mCi of ^{99m}Tc labeled to a compound that localizes 35% in bone ($\tilde{A} = 3{,}000$ μCi-hr) and 5% in the total body ($\tilde{A} = 400 \; \mu$Ci-hr), with the remaining activity excreted in the urine ($\tilde{A} = 600 \; \mu$Ci-hr for the bladder).

TABLE 25-5. — VALUES OF S FOR ^{99m}Tc[*]

| TARGET ORGAN | SOURCE ORGANS | | | |
	CORTICAL BONE	TRABECULAR BONE	TOTAL BODY	BLADDER
Red bone marrow	4.1 E-06	9.1 E-06	2.9 E-06	2.3 E-06

[*]From Snyder, W., et al.: "S," *Absorbed Dose Per Unit Cumulated Activity for Selected Radionuclides and Organs*, MIRD pamphlet 11, Society of Nuclear Medicine, 475 Park Avenue South, New York, New York 10016.

For the activity in bone, assume that half is in cortical bone and half is in trabecular bone.

$$D = \tilde{A}S$$
$$D_{BM} = 0.5 \; (3{,}000 \; \mu\text{Ci-hr})(4.1 \times 10^{-6}) = 6.2 \text{ mrad from activity}$$
in cortical bone
$$= 0.5 \; (3{,}000 \; \mu\text{Ci-hr})(9.1 \times 10^{-6}) = 13.7 \text{ mrad from activity}$$
in trabecular bone
$$= (400 \; \mu\text{Ci-hr})(2.9 \times 10^{-6}) = 1.2 \text{ mrad from activity in the}$$
total body
$$= (600 \; \mu\text{Ci-hr})(2.3 \times 10^{-6}) = 1.3 \text{ mrad from activity in the}$$
bladder

The total dose to the bone marrow is

$$(D_{BM})_{total} = (6.2 + 13.7 + 1.2 + 1.3) \text{ mrad}$$
$$= 22.4 \text{ mrad}$$

RECOMMENDATIONS FOR SAFE USE
OF RADIOACTIVE NUCLIDES

Persons working with unsealed radioactive sources must be protected not only from radiation emitted by the sources but also from ingestion, absorption or inhalation of radioactive material into the body. Procedures to minimize the intake of radioactive nuclides into the body depend on the facilities available within an institution and vary from one institution to another. A few guidelines for the safe use of radioactive materials are included in publications by individuals[4, 5] and by advisory groups such as the ICRP and NCRP.[6-13]

REFERENCES

1. National Committee on Radiation Protection: *Maximum Permissible Body Burdens and Maximum Permissible Concentrations of Radionuclides in Air and in Water for Occupational Exposure.* Recommendations of NCRP, National Bureau of Standards Handbook 69, 1959.
2. Hendee, W.: *Radioactive Isotopes in Biological Research* (New York: John Wiley & Sons, Inc., 1973).
3. International Commission on Radiological Protection: *Report of the Task Group on Reference Man*, ICRP publication 23 (New York: Pergamon Press, 1975).
4. Hendee, W., and Lohlein, S.: Handling radium in a hospital, Radiol. Technol. 39:221, 1968; Hendee, W., and Lohlein, S.: Handling therapeutic doses of radioactive nuclides in a hospital, Radiol. Technol. 40:81, 1968.
5. Moore, M., and Hendee, W.: *Radionuclide Handling and Radiopharmaceutical Quality Assurance*, Workshop Manual, Bureau of Radiological Health, USDHEW-FDA, 1977.
6. Shapiro, J.: *Radiation Protection* (Cambridge: Harvard University Press, 1972).
7. *Manual on Use of Radioisotopes in Hospitals* (Chicago: American Hospital Association, 1958).
8. International Atomic Energy Agency: Safety Series. No. 1: *Safe Handling of Radioisotopes*, 1963; No. 2: *Safe Handling of Radioisotopes — Health Physics Addendum*, 1960; No. 3: *Safe Handling of Radioisotopes — Medical Addendum*, 1960 (Vienna: IAEA).
9. International Commission on Radiological Protection: Report of Committee V (1953–62): *Handling and Disposal of Radioactive Materials in Hospitals and Medical Research Establishments*, ICRP publ. 5 (New York: Pergamon Press, 1964).
10. International Commission on Radiological Protection: *Protection of the Patient in Radionuclide Investigations*, ICRP publ. 17 (New York: Pergamon Press, 1971).
11. National Council on Radiation Protection and Measurements: *Precautions in the Management of Patients Who Have Received Therapeutic Amounts of Radionuclides.* Recommendations of the NCRP, Report No. 37, 1970.
12. National Committee on Radiation Protection: *Safe Handling of Radioactive*

Materials. Recommendations of NCRP, Report 30. National Bureau of·Standards Handbook 92, 1964.

13. National Council on Radiation Protection and Measurements: *Protection Against Radiation from Brachytherapy Sources.* Recommendations of the NCRP, Report No. 40, 1972.

Appendixes

REVIEW OF MATHEMATICS

1. Exponents

ALGEBRAIC NOTATION

NUMERICAL EXAMPLE

$x^0 = 1$

$4^0 = 1$

$x^1 = x$

$4^1 = 4$

$x^2 = (x)(x)$

$4^2 = (4)(4)$

$x^5 = (x)(x)(x)(x)(x)$

$4^5 = (4)(4)(4)(4)(4)$

$x^{a+b} = (x^a)(x^b)$

$4^5 = (4^2)(4^3)$ or $(4^1)(4^4)$, etc.

$x^{ab} = (x^a)^b$

$4^6 = (4^2)^3$ or $(4^1)^6$, etc.

$x^{-a} = \dfrac{1}{x^a}$

$4^{-2} = \dfrac{1}{4^2}$

$x^{a-b} = (x^a)(x^{-b}) = x^a/x^b$

$4^{-1} = 4^{2-3} = (4^2)(4^{-3}) = (4^2)/(4^3) = \dfrac{1}{4}$

$(x^a)^{-b} = x^{-ab}$

$(4^2)^{-3} = \dfrac{1}{(4^2)^3} = \dfrac{1}{4^6} = 4^{-6}$

$x^{1/2} = \sqrt{x}$

$4^{1/2} = \sqrt{4}$

$x^{2/5} = \sqrt[5]{x^2}$

$4^{2/5} = \sqrt[5]{4^2}$

$x^{-1/2} = \sqrt{\dfrac{1}{x}}$

$4^{-1/2} = \sqrt{\dfrac{1}{4}}$

$x^{-2/5} = \sqrt[5]{\dfrac{1}{x^2}}$

$4^{-2/5} = \sqrt[5]{\dfrac{1}{4^2}}$

$(x^{1/a})(x^{1/b}) = x^{1/a\ +\ 1/b}$

$(4^{1/2})(4^{1/3}) = 4^{1/2\ +\ 1/3} = 4^{5/6}$

2. Powers of Ten

$6 \times 10^4 = (6)(10^4) = 60{,}000$
$600 \times 10^4 = (600)(10^4) = 6{,}000{,}000$
$600 \times 10^{-4} = (600)(10^{-4}) = 0.06$
$6 \times 10^{-4} = (6)(10^{-4}) = 0.0006$

3. Logarithms

The logarithm y of a number x to a base a is the power to which the base a must be raised to yield the number x.

That is, if

$y = \log_a x$, then $a^y = x$

Common logarithms (denoted as log) are logarithms to the base 10.

$y = \log x$

$10^y = x$

Natural (Napierian) logarithms (denoted as ln) are logarithms to the base e ($e = 2.7183$).

$y = \ln x$

$e^y = x$

Common and natural logarithms are related by the constant 2.3026.

$\log (x) = (1/2.3026) \ln (x)$

$\ln (x) = 2.3026 \log (x)$

Logarithms are composed of two parts, a decimal fraction (the *mantissa*) which is always positive, and an integer (the characteristic) which may be positive or negative. In the example below, the characteristic is 1 and the mantissa is .699.

$\log (50) = 1.699$

The logarithm to the base 10 of a number x is positive if the number is greater than 1, and is negative if the number is less than 1. A few examples are shown below:

$\log (1) = 0$ because $10^0 = 1$

$\log (100) = 2$ because $10^2 = 100$

$\ln (e) = 1$ because $e^1 = e$

$\log (1.56) = 0.193$

$\log (15.6) = \log (1.56 \times 10^1) = \log (1.56) + \log (10^1) = 0.193 + 1 = 1.193$

$\log (156) = \log (1.56 \times 10^2) = \log (1.56) + \log (10^2) = 0.193 + 2 = 2.193$

$\log (0.156) = \log (1.56 \times 10^{-1}) = \log (1.56) + \log (10^{-1}) = 0.193 - 1 = -0.807$

$\log (0.0156) = \log (1.56 \times 10^{-2}) = \log (1.56) + \log (10^{-2}) = 0.193 - 2 = -1.807$

MULTIPLES

MULTIPLE	PREFIX	SYMBOL
10^9	giga	G
10^6	mega	M
10^3	kilo	k
10^{-1}	deci	d
10^{-2}	centi	c
10^{-3}	milli	m
10^{-6}	micro	μ
10^{-9}	nano	n
10^{-12}	pico	p

SELECTED ABBREVIATIONS OF UNITS

Å	angstrom
A (or amp)	ampere
amu	atomic mass unit
Ci	curie
CPM	counts per minute
CPS	counts per second
dpm	disintegrations per minute
dps	disintegrations per second
eV	electron volt
gm	gram
hu	heat unit
HVL	half-value layer
Hz	hertz
IP	ion pair
J	joule
LET	linear energy transfer
m	meter
mAs	milliampere second
MPC	maximum permissible concentration
MPD	maximum permissible dose
N	newton
C	Celsius
F	Fahrenheit
Ω	ohm
R	roentgen
RBE	relative biologic effectiveness
Rhm	roentgens per hour at 1 meter
V	volt
W	watt

MASSES IN ATOMIC MASS UNITS FOR NEUTRAL ATOMS OF STABLE NUCLIDES AND A FEW UNSTABLE NUCLIDES (DESIGNATED BY*)

ELEMENT	MASS NO.	ATOMIC MASS (AMU)	ELEMENT	MASS NO.	ATOMIC MASS (AMU)
$_0 n$	1*	1.008 665	$_{12}$Mg	23*	22.994 125
$_1$H	1	1.007 825		24	23.990 962
	2	2.014 102		25	24.989 955
	3*	3.016 050		26	25.991 740
$_2$He	3	3.016 030	$_{13}$Al	27	26.981 539
	4	4.002 603	$_{14}$Si	28	27.976 930
	6*	6.018 893		29	28.976 496
$_3$Li	6	6.015 125		30	29.973 763
	7	7.016 004	$_{15}$P	31	30.973 765
	8*	8.022 487	$_{16}$S	32	31.972 074
$_4$Be	7*	7.016 929		33	32.971 462
	9	9.012 186		34	33.967 865
	10*	10.013 534		36	35.967 090
$_5$B	8*	8.024 609	$_{17}$Cl	35	34.968 851
	10	10.012 939		36*	35.968 309
	11	11.009 305		37	36.965 898
	12*	12.014 354	$_{18}$Ar	36	35.967 544
$_6$C	10*	10.016 810		38	37.962 728
	11*	11.011 432		40	39.962 384
	12	12.000 000	$_{19}$K	39	38.963 710
	13	13.003 354		40*	39.964 000
	14*	14.003 242		41	40.961 832
	15*	15.010 599	$_{20}$Ca	40	39.962 589
$_7$N	12*	12.018 641		41*	40.962 275
	13*	13.005 738		42	41.958 625
	14	14.003 074		43	42.958 780
	15	15.000 108		44	43.955 490
	16*	16.006 103		46	45.953 689
	17*	17.008 450		48	47.952 531
$_8$O	14*	14.008 597	$_{21}$Sc	41*	40.969 247
	15*	15.003 070		45	44.955 919
	16	15.994 915	$_{22}$Ti	46	45.952 632
	17	16.999 133		47	46.951 769
	18	17.999 160		48	47.947 951
	19*	19.003 578		49	48.947 871
$_9$F	17*	17.002 095		50	49.944 786
	18*	18.000 937	$_{23}$V	48*	47.952 259
	19	18.998 405		50*	49.947 164
	20*	19.999 987		51	50.943 962
	21*	20.999 951	$_{24}$Cr	48*	47.953 760
$_{10}$Ne	18*	18.005 711		50	49.946 055

(Continued)

Source: Weidner, R., and Sells, R.: *Elementary Modern Physics* (2d ed.; Boston: Allyn & Bacon, Inc., 1968). Reprinted by permission of the publisher.

ELEMENT	MASS NO.	ATOMIC MASS (AMU)	ELEMENT	MASS NO.	ATOMIC MASS (AMU)
	19*	19.001 881		52	51.940 514
	20	19.992 440		53	52.940 653
	21	20.993 849		54	53.938 882
	22	21.991 385	25Mn	54*	53.940 362
	23*	22.994 473		55	54.938 051
11Na	22*	21.994 437	26Fe	54	53.939 617
	23	22.989 771		56	55.934 937
	57	56.935 398		95	94.905 839
	58	57.933 282		96	95.904 674
27Co	59	58.933 190		97	96.906 022
	60*	59.933 814		98	97.905 409
28Ni	58	57.935 342		100	99.907 475
	60	59.930 787	44Ru	96	95.907 598
	61	60.931 056		98	97.905 289
	62	61.928 342		99	98.905 936
	64	63.927 958		100	99.904 218
29Cu	63	62.929 592		101	100.905 577
	65	64.927 786		102	101.904 348
30Zn	64	63.929 145		104	103.905 430
	66	65.926 052	45Rh	103	102.905 511
	67	66.927 145	46Pd	102	101.905 609
	68	67.924 857		104	103.904 011
	70	69.925 334		105	104.905 064
31Ga	69	68.925 574		106	105.903 479
	71	70.924 706		108	107.903 891
32Ge	70	69.924 252		110	109.905 164
	72	71.922 082	47Ag	107	106.905 094
	73	72.923 463		109	108.904 756
	74	73.921 181	48Cd	106	105.906 463
	76	75.921 406		108	107.904 187
33As	75	74.921 597		110	109.903 012
34Se	74	73.922 476		111	110.904 189
	76	75.919 207		112	111.902 763
	77	76.919 911		113	112.904 409
	78	77.917 314		114	113.903 361
	80	79.916 528		116	115.904 762
	82	81.916 707	49In	113	112.904 089
35Br	79	78.918 330		115*	114.903 871
	81	80.916 292	50Sn	112	111.904 835
36Kr	78	77.920 403		114	113.902 773
	80	79.916 380		115	114.903 346
	82	81.913 482		116	115.901 745
	83	82.914 132		117	116.902 959
	84	83.911 504		118	117.901 606
	86	85.910 616		119	118.903 314
37Rb	85	84.911 800		120	119.902 199
	87*	86.909 187		122	121.903 442

ELEMENT	MASS NO.	ATOMIC MASS (AMU)	ELEMENT	MASS NO.	ATOMIC MASS (AMU)
$_{38}$Sr	84	83.913 431		124	123.905 272
	86	85.909 285	$_{51}$Sb	121	120.903 817
	87	86.908 893		123	122.904 213
	88	87.905 641	$_{52}$Te	120	119.904 023
$_{39}$Y	89	88.905 872		122	121.903 066
$_{40}$Zr	90	89.904 700		123	122.904 277
	91	90.905 642		124	123.902 842
	92	91.905 031		125	124.904 418
	94	93.906 314		126	125.903 322
	96	95.908 286		128	127.904 476
$_{41}$Nb	93	92.906 382		130	129.906 238
$_{42}$Mo	92	91.906 811	$_{53}$I	127	126.904 470
	94	93.905 091	$_{54}$Xe	124	123.906 120
	126	125.904 288		160	159.925 202
	128	127.903 540		161	160.926 945
	129	128.904 784		162	161.926 803
	130	129.903 509		163	162.928 755
	131	130.905 086		164	163.929 200
	132	131.904 161	$_{67}$Ho	165	164.930 421
	134	133.905 398	$_{68}$Er	162	161.928 740
	136	135.907 221		164	163.929 287
$_{55}$Cs	133	132.905 355		166	165.930 307
$_{56}$Ba	130	129.906 245		167	166.932 060
	132	131.905 120		168	167.932 383
	134	133.904 612		170	169.935 560
	135	134.905 550	$_{69}$Tm	169	168.934 245
	136	135.904 300	$_{70}$Yb	168	167.934 160
	137	136.905 500		170	169.935 020
	138	137.905 000		171	170.936 430
$_{57}$La	138*	137.906 910		172	171.936 360
	139	138.906 140		173	172.938 060
$_{58}$Ce	136	135.907 100		174	173.938 740
	138	137.905 830		176	175.942 680
	140	139.905 392	$_{71}$Lu	175	174.940 640
	142	141.909 140		176*	175.942 660
$_{59}$Pr	141	140.907 596	$_{72}$Hf	174	173.940 360
$_{60}$Nd	142	141.907 663		176	175.941 570
	143	142.909 779		177	176.943 400
	144*	143.910 039		178	177.943 880
	145	144.912 538		179	178.946 030
	146	145.913 086		180	179.946 820
	148	147.916 869	$_{73}$Ta	181	180.948 007
	150	149.920 915	$_{74}$W	180	179.947 000
$_{62}$Sm	144	143.911 989		182	181.948 301
	147*	146.914 867		183	182.950 324
	148	147.914 791		184	183.951 025
	149	148.917 180		186	185.954 440

(Continued)

ELEMENT	MASS NO.	ATOMIC MASS (AMU)	ELEMENT	MASS NO.	ATOMIC MASS (AMU)
	150	149.917 276	$_{75}$Re	185	184.953 059
	152	151.919 756		187*	186.955 833
	154	153.922 282	$_{76}$Os	184	183.952 750
$_{63}$Eu	151	150.919 838		186	185.953 870
	153	152.921 242		187	186.955 832
$_{64}$Gd	152	151.919 794		188	187.956 081
	154	153.920 929		189	188.958 300
	155	154.922 664		190	189.958 630
	156	155.922 175		192	191.961 450
	157	156.924 025	$_{77}$Ir	191	190.960 640
	158	157.924 178		193	192.963 012
	160	159.927 115	$_{78}$Pt	190*	189.959 950
$_{65}$Tb	159	158.925 351		192	191.961 150
$_{66}$Dy	156	155.923 930		194	193.962 725
	158	157.924 449		195	194.964 813
	196	195.964 967		205	204.974 442
	198	197.967 895	$_{82}$Pb	204	203.973 044
$_{79}$Au	197	196.966 541		206	205.974 468
$_{80}$Hg	196	195.965 820		207	206.975 903
	198	197.966 756		208	207.976 650
	199	198.968 279	$_{83}$Bi	209	208.981 082
	200	199.968 327	$_{90}$Th	232*	232.038 124
	201	200.970 308	$_{92}$U	234*	234.040 904
	202	201.970 642		235*	235.043 915
	204	203.973 495		238*	238.050 770
$_{81}$Tl	203	202.972 353			

NATURAL TRIGONOMETRIC FUNCTIONS

| ANGLE | | | | | ANGLE | | | | |
DEGREE	RADIAN	SINE	COSINE	TANGENT	DEGREE	RADIAN	SINE	COSINE	TANGENT
0	.000	0.000	1.000	0.000					
1	.017	.018	1.000	.018	46	0.803	0.719	0.695	1.036
2	.035	.035	0.999	.035	47	.820	.731	.682	1.072
3	.052	.052	.999	.052	48	.838	.743	.669	1.111
4	.070	.070	.998	.070	49	.855	.755	.656	1.150
5	.087	.087	.996	.088	50	.873	.766	.643	1.192
6	.105	.105	.995	.105	51	.890	.777	.629	1.235
7	.122	.122	.993	.123	52	.908	.788	.616	1.280
8	.140	.139	.990	.141	53	.925	.799	.602	1.327
9	.157	.156	.988	.158	54	.942	.809	.588	1.376
10	.175	.174	.985	.176	55	.960	.819	.574	1.428
11	.192	.191	.982	.194	56	.977	.829	.559	1.483
12	.209	.208	.978	.213	57	.995	.839	.545	1.540
13	.227	.225	.974	.231	58	1.012	.848	.530	1.600
14	.244	.242	.970	.249	59	1.030	.857	.515	1.664
15	.262	.259	.966	.268	60	1.047	.866	.500	1.732
16	.279	.276	.961	.287	61	1.065	.875	.485	1.804
17	.297	.292	.956	.306	62	1.082	.883	.470	1.881
18	.314	.309	.951	.325	63	1.100	.891	.454	1.963
19	.332	.326	.946	.344	64	1.117	.899	.438	2.050
20	.349	.342	.940	.364	65	1.134	.906	.423	2.145
21	.367	.358	.934	.384	66	1.152	.914	.407	2.246
22	.384	.375	.927	.404	67	1.169	.921	.391	2.356
23	.401	.391	.921	.425	68	1.187	.927	.375	2.475
24	.419	.407	.914	.445	69	1.204	.934	.358	2.605
25	.436	.423	.906	.466	70	1.222	.940	.342	2.747
26	.454	.438	.899	.488	71	1.239	.946	.326	2.904
27	.471	.454	.891	.510	72	1.257	.951	.309	3.078
28	.489	.470	.883	.532	73	1.274	.956	.292	3.271
29	.506	.485	.875	.554	74	1.292	.961	.276	3.487
30	.524	.500	.866	.577	75	1.309	.966	.259	3.732
31	.541	.515	.857	.601	76	1.326	.970	.242	4.011
32	.559	.530	.848	.625	77	1.344	.974	.225	4.331
33	.576	.545	.839	.649	78	1.361	.978	.208	4.705
34	.593	.559	.829	.675	79	1.379	.982	.191	5.145
35	.611	.574	.819	.700	80	1.396	.985	.174	5.671
36	.628	.588	.809	.727	81	1.414	.988	.156	6.314
37	.646	.602	.799	.754	82	1.431	.990	.139	7.115
38	.663	.616	.788	.781	83	1.449	.993	.122	8.144
39	.681	.629	.777	.810	84	1.466	.995	.105	9.514
40	.698	.643	.766	.839	85	1.484	.996	.087	11.43
41	.716	.658	.755	.869	86	1.501	.998	.070	14.30
42	.733	.669	.743	.900	87	1.518	.999	.052	19.08
43	.751	.682	.731	.933	88	1.536	.999	.035	28.64
44	.768	.695	.719	.966	89	1.553	1.000	.018	57.29
45	.785	.707	.707	1.000	90	1.571	1.000	.000	∞

COMMON LOGARITHMS

(To obtain Napierian [natural] logarithm of a number; multiply these logarithms by 2.3026.)

N	0	1	2	3	4	5	6	7	8	9
0	....	0000	3010	4771	6021	6990	7782	8451	9031	9542
1	0000	0414	0792	1139	1461	1761	2041	2304	2553	2788
2	3010	3222	3424	3617	3802	3979	4150	4314	4472	4624
3	4771	4914	5051	5185	5315	5441	5563	5682	5798	5911
4	6021	6128	6232	6335	6435	6532	6628	6721	6812	6902
5	6990	7076	7160	7243	7324	7404	7482	7559	7634	7709
6	7782	7853	7924	7993	8062	8129	8195	8261	8325	8388
7	8451	8513	8573	8633	8692	8751	8808	8865	8921	8976
8	9031	9085	9138	9191	9243	9294	9345	9395	9445	9494
9	9542	9590	9638	9685	9731	9777	9823	9868	9912	9956
10	0000	0043	0086	0128	0170	0212	0253	0294	0334	0374
11	0414	0453	0492	0531	0569	0607	0645	0682	0719	0755
12	0792	0828	0864	0899	0934	0969	1004	1038	1072	1106
13	1139	1173	1206	1239	1271	1303	1335	1367	1399	1430
14	1461	1492	1523	1553	1584	1614	1644	1673	1703	1732
15	1761	1790	1818	1847	1875	1903	1931	1959	1987	2014
16	2041	2068	2095	2122	2148	2175	2201	2227	2253	2279
17	2304	2330	2355	2380	2405	2430	2455	2480	2504	2529
18	2553	2577	2601	2625	2648	2672	2695	2718	2742	2765
19	2788	2810	2833	2856	2878	2900	2923	2945	2967	2989
20	3010	3032	3054	3075	3096	3118	3139	3160	3181	3201
21	3222	3243	3263	3284	3304	3324	3345	3365	3385	3404
22	3424	3444	3464	3483	3502	3522	3541	3560	3579	3598
23	3617	3636	3655	3674	3692	3711	3729	3747	3766	3784
24	3802	3820	3838	3856	3874	3892	3909	3927	3945	3962
25	3979	3997	4014	4031	4048	4065	4082	4099	4116	4133
26	4150	4166	4183	4200	4216	4232	4249	4265	4281	4298
27	4314	4330	4346	4362	4378	4393	4409	4425	4440	4456
28	4472	4487	4502	4518	4533	4548	4564	4579	4594	4609
29	4624	4639	4654	4669	4683	4698	4713	4728	4742	4757
30	4771	4786	4800	4814	4829	4843	4857	4871	4886	4900
31	4914	4928	4942	4955	4969	4983	4997	5011	5024	5038
32	5051	5065	5079	5092	5105	5119	5132	5145	5159	5172
33	5185	5198	5211	5224	5237	5250	5263	5276	5289	5302
34	5315	5328	5340	5353	5366	5378	5391	5403	5416	5428
35	5441	5453	5465	5478	5490	5502	5514	5527	5539	5551
36	5563	5575	5587	5599	5611	5623	5635	5647	5658	5670
37	5682	5694	5705	5717	5729	5740	5752	5763	5775	5786
38	5798	5809	5821	5832	5843	5855	5866	5877	5888	5899
39	5911	5922	5933	5944	5955	5966	5977	5988	5999	6010
40	6021	6031	6042	6053	6064	6075	6085	6096	6107	6117

N	0	1	2	3	4	5	6	7	8	9
0	. . . .	0000	3010	4771	6021	6990	7782	8451	9031	9542
41	6128	6138	6149	6160	6170	6180	6191	6201	6212	6222
42	6232	6243	6253	6263	6274	6284	6294	6304	6314	6325
43	6335	6345	6355	6365	6375	6385	6395	6405	6415	6425
44	6435	6444	6454	6464	6474	6484	6493	6503	6513	6522
45	6532	6542	6551	6561	6571	6580	6590	6599	6609	6618
46	6628	6637	6646	6656	6665	6675	6684	6693	6702	6712
47	6721	6730	6739	6749	6758	6767	6776	6785	6794	6803
48	6812	6821	6830	6839	6848	6857	6866	6875	6884	6893
49	6902	6911	6920	6928	6937	6946	6955	6964	6972	6981
50	6990	6998	7007	7016	7024	7033	7042	7050	7059	7067
51	7076	7084	7093	7101	7110	7118	7126	7135	7143	7152
52	7160	7168	7177	7185	7193	7202	7210	7218	7226	7235
53	7243	7251	7259	7267	7275	7284	7292	7300	7308	7316
54	7324	7332	7340	7348	7356	7364	7372	7380	7388	7396
55	7404	7412	7419	7427	7435	7443	7451	7459	7466	7474
56	7482	7490	7497	7505	7513	7520	7528	7536	7543	7551
57	7559	7566	7574	7582	7589	7597	7604	7612	7619	7627
58	7634	7642	7649	7657	7664	7672	7679	7686	7694	7701
59	7709	7716	7723	7731	7738	7745	7752	7760	7767	7774
60	7782	7789	7796	7803	7810	7818	7825	7832	7839	7846
61	7853	7860	7868	7875	7882	7889	7896	7903	7910	7917
62	7924	7931	7938	7945	7952	7959	7966	7973	7980	7987
63	7993	8000	8007	8014	8021	8028	8035	8041	8048	8055
64	8062	8069	8075	8082	8089	8096	8102	8109	8116	8122
65	8129	8136	8142	8149	8156	8162	8169	8176	8182	8189
66	8195	8202	8209	8215	8222	8228	8235	8241	8248	8254
67	8261	8267	8274	8280	8287	8293	8299	8306	8312	8319
68	8325	8331	8338	8344	8351	8357	8363	8370	8376	8382
69	8388	8395	8401	8407	8414	8420	8426	8432	8439	8445
70	8451	8457	8463	8470	8476	8482	8488	8494	8500	8506
71	8513	8519	8525	8531	8537	8543	8549	8555	8561	8567
72	8573	8579	8585	8591	8597	8603	8609	8615	8621	8627
73	8633	8639	8645	8651	8657	8663	8669	8675	8681	8686
74	8692	8698	8704	8710	8716	8722	8727	8733	8739	8745
75	8751	8756	8762	8768	8774	8779	8785	8791	8797	8802
76	8808	8814	8820	8825	8831	8837	8842	8848	8854	8859
77	8865	8871	8876	8882	8887	8893	8899	8904	8910	8915
78	8921	8927	8932	8938	8943	8949	8954	8960	8965	8971
79	8976	8982	8987	8993	8998	9004	9009	9015	9020	9025
80	9031	9036	9042	9047	9053	9058	9063	9069	9074	9079
81	9085	9090	9096	9101	9106	9112	9117	9122	9128	9133
82	9138	9143	9149	9154	9159	9165	9170	9175	9180	9186

(Continued)

N	0	1	2	3	4	5	6	7	8	9
0	. . . .	0000	3010	4771	6021	6990	7782	8451	9031	9542
83	9191	9196	9201	9206	9212	9217	9222	9227	9232	9238
84	9243	9248	9253	9258	9263	9269	9274	9279	9284	9289
85	9294	9299	9304	9309	9315	9320	9325	9330	9335	9340
86	9345	9350	9355	9360	9365	9370	9375	9380	9385	9390
87	9395	9400	9405	9410	9415	9420	9425	9430	9435	9440
88	9445	9450	9455	9460	9465	9469	9474	9479	9484	9489
89	9494	9499	9504	9509	9513	9518	9523	9528	9533	9538
90	9542	9547	9552	9557	9562	9566	9571	9576	9581	9586
91	9590	9595	9600	9605	9609	9614	9619	9624	9628	9633
92	9638	9643	9647	9652	9657	9661	9666	9671	9675	9680
93	9685	9689	9694	9699	9703	9708	9713	9717	9722	9727
94	9731	9736	9741	9745	9750	9754	9759	9763	9768	9773
95	9777	9782	9786	9791	9795	9800	9805	9809	9814	9818
96	9823	9827	9832	9836	9841	9845	9850	9854	9859	9863
97	9868	9872	9877	9881	9886	9890	9894	9899	9903	9908
98	9912	9917	9921	9926	9930	9934	9939	9943	9948	9952
99	9956	9961	9965	9969	9974	9978	9983	9987	9991	9996
100	0000	0004	0009	0013	0017	0022	0026	0030	0035	0039
N	0	1	2	3	4	5	6	7	8	9

EXPONENTIAL QUANTITY e RAISED TO SELECTED NEGATIVE POWERS (e^{-x})

χ		0.00	0.01	0.02	0.03	0.04	0.05	0.06	0.07	0.08	0.09
0.0		1.0000	0.9900	0.9802	0.9704	0.9608	0.9512	0.9418	0.9324	0.9231	0.9139
0.1		.9048	.8958	.8869	.8781	.8694	.8607	.8521	.8437	.8353	.8270
0.2		.8187	.8106	.8025	.7945	.7866	.7788	.7711	.7634	.7558	.7483
0.3		.7408	.7334	.7261	.7189	.7118	.7047	.6977	.6907	.6839	.6771
0.4		.6703	.6637	.6570	.6505	.6440	.6376	.6313	.6250	.6188	.6126
0.5		.6065	.6005	.5945	.5886	.5827	.5769	.5712	.5655	.5599	.5543
0.6		.5488	.5434	.5379	.5326	.5273	.5220	.5169	.5117	.5066	.5016
0.7		.4966	.4916	.4868	.4819	.4771	.4724	.4677	.4630	.4584	.4538
0.8		.4493	.4449	.4404	.4360	.4317	.4274	.4232	.4190	.4148	.4107
0.9		.4066	.4025	.3985	.3946	.3906	.3867	.3829	.3791	.3753	.3716
1.0		.3679	.3642	.3606	.3570	.3535	.3499	.3465	.3430	.3396	.3362
1.1		.3329	.3296	.3263	.3230	.3198	.3166	.3135	.3104	.3073	.3042
1.2		.3012	.2982	.2952	.2923	.2894	.2865	.2837	.2808	.2780	.2753
1.3		.2725	.2698	.2671	.2645	.2618	.2592	.2567	.2541	.2516	.2491
1.4		.2466	.2441	.2417	.2393	.2369	.2346	.2322	.2299	.2276	.2254
1.5		.2231	.2209	.2187	.2165	.2144	.2122	.2101	.2080	.2060	.2039
1.6		.2019	.1999	.1979	.1959	.1940	.1920	.1901	.1882	.1864	.1845
1.7		.1827	.1809	.1791	.1773	.1755	.1738	.1720	.1703	.1686	.1670
1.8		.1653	.1637	.1620	.1604	.1588	.1572	.1557	.1541	.1526	.1511
1.9		.1496	.1481	.1466	.1451	.1437	.1423	.1409	.1395	.1381	.1367
2.0		.1353	.1340	.1327	.1313	.1300	.1287	.1275	.1262	.1249	.1237
2.1		.1225	.1212	.1200	.1188	.1177	.1165	.1153	.1142	.1130	.1119
2.2		.1108	.1097	.1086	.1075	.1065	.1054	.1043	.1033	.1023	.1013
2.3		.1003	*9926	*9827	*9730	*9633	*9537	*9442	*9348	*9255	*9163
2.4	0.0	9072	8982	8892	8804	8716	8629	8544	8458	8374	8291
2.5	0.0	8208	8127	8046	7966	7887	7808	7730	7654	7577	7502
2.6	0.0	7427	7353	7280	7208	7136	7065	6995	6925	6856	6788
2.7	0.0	6721	6654	6587	6522	6457	6393	6329	6266	6204	6142
2.8	0.0	6081	6020	5961	5901	5843	5784	5727	5670	5613	5558
2.9	0.0	5502	5448	5393	5340	5287	5234	5182	5130	5079	5029
3.0	0.0	4979	4929	4880	4832	4783	4736	4689	4642	4596	4550
3.1	0.0	4505	4460	4416	4372	4328	4285	4243	4200	4159	4117
3.2	0.0	4076	4036	3996	3956	3916	3877	3839	3801	3763	3725
3.3	0.0	3688	3652	3615	3579	3544	3508	3474	3439	3405	3371
3.4	0.0	3337	3304	3271	3239	3206	3175	3143	3112	3081	3050

χ		0.0	0.1	0.2	0.3	0.4	0.5	0.6	0.7	0.8	0.9
3	0.0	4979	4505	4076	3688	3337	3020	2732	2472	2237	2024
4	0.0	1832	1657	1500	1357	1228	1111	1005	*9095	*8230	*7447
5	0.00	6738	6097	5517	4992	4517	4087	3698	3346	3028	2739
6	0.00	2479	2243	2029	1836	1662	1503	1360	1231	1114	1008
7	0.000	9119	8251	7466	6755	6112	5531	5004	4528	4097	3707
8	0.000	3355	3035	2747	2485	2249	2035	1841	1666	1507	1364
9	0.000	1234	1117	1010	*9142	*8272	*7485	*6773	*6128	*5545	*5017
10	0.0000	4540	4108	3717	3363	3043	2754	2492	2254	2040	1846

°Each number denoted by an asterisk should be considered as being preceded by 0.0 (e.g., °9926 is 0.09926).

EXPONENTIAL QUANTITY e RAISED TO SELECTED POSITIVE POWERS (e^x)

χ	0.00	0.01	0.02	0.03	0.04	0.05	0.06	0.07	0.08	0.09
0.0	1.000	1.010	1.020	1.031	1.041	1.051	1.062	1.073	1.083	1.094
0.1	1.105	1.116	1.127	1.139	1.150	1.162	1.174	1.185	1.197	1.209
0.2	1.221	1.234	1.246	1.259	1.271	1.284	1.297	1.310	1.323	1.336
0.3	1.350	1.363	1.377	1.391	1.405	1.419	1.433	1.448	1.462	1.477
0.4	1.492	1.507	1.522	1.537	1.553	1.568	1.584	1.600	1.616	1.632
0.5	1.649	1.665	1.682	1.699	1.716	1.733	1.751	1.768	1.786	1.804
0.6	1.822	1.840	1.859	1.878	1.896	1.916	1.935	1.954	1.974	1.994
0.7	2.014	2.034	2.054	2.075	2.096	2.117	2.138	2.160	2.181	2.203
0.8	2.226	2.248	2.270	2.293	2.316	2.340	2.363	2.387	2.411	2.435
0.9	2.460	2.484	2.509	2.535	2.560	2.586	2.612	2.638	2.664	2.691
1.0	2.718	2.746	2.773	2.801	2.829	2.858	2.886	2.915	2.945	2.974
1.1	3.004	3.034	3.065	3.096	3.127	3.158	3.190	3.222	3.254	3.287
1.2	3.320	3.353	3.387	3.421	3.456	3.490	3.525	3.561	3.597	3.633
1.3	3.669	3.706	3.743	3.781	3.819	3.857	3.896	3.935	3.975	4.015
1.4	4.055	4.096	4.137	4.179	4.221	4.263	4.306	4.349	4.393	4.437
1.5	4.482	4.527	4.572	4.618	4.665	4.712	4.759	4.807	4.855	4.904
1.6	4.953	5.003	5.053	5.104	5.155	5.207	5.259	5.312	5.366	5.419
1.7	5.474	5.529	5.585	5.641	5.697	5.755	5.812	5.871	5.930	5.989
1.8	6.050	6.110	6.172	6.234	6.297	6.360	6.424	6.488	6.554	6.619
1.9	6.686	6.753	6.821	6.890	6.959	7.029	7.099	7.171	7.243	7.316
2.0	7.389	7.463	7.538	7.614	7.691	7.768	7.846	7.925	8.004	8.085
2.1	8.166	8.248	8.331	8.415	8.499	8.585	8.671	8.758	8.846	8.935
2.2	9.025	9.116	9.207	9.300	9.393	9.488	9.583	9.679	9.777	9.875
2.3	9.974	10.07	10.18	10.28	10.38	10.49	10.59	10.70	10.80	10.91
2.4	11.02	11.13	11.25	11.36	11.47	11.59	11.70	11.82	11.94	12.06
2.5	12.18	12.30	12.43	12.55	12.68	12.81	12.94	13.07	13.20	13.33
2.6	13.46	13.60	13.74	13.87	14.01	14.15	14.30	14.44	14.59	14.73
2.7	14.88	15.03	15.18	15.33	15.49	15.64	15.80	15.96	16.12	16.28
2.8	16.44	16.61	16.78	16.95	17.12	17.29	17.46	17.64	17.81	17.99
2.9	18.17	18.36	18.54	18.73	18.92	19.11	19.30	19.49	19.69	19.89
3.0	20.09	20.29	20.49	20.70	20.91	21.12	21.33	21.54	21.76	21.98
3.1	22.20	22.42	22.65	22.87	23.10	23.34	23.57	23.81	24.05	24.29
3.2	24.53	24.78	25.03	25.28	25.53	25.79	26.05	26.31	26.58	26.84
3.3	27.11	27.39	27.66	27.94	28.22	28.50	28.79	29.08	29.37	29.67
3.4	29.96	30.27	30.57	30.88	31.19	31.50	31.82	32.14	32.46	32.79

χ	0.0	0.1	0.2	0.3	0.4	0.5	0.6	0.7	0.8	0.9
3	20.09	22.20	24.53	27.11	29.96	33.12	36.60	40.45	44.70	49.40
4	54.60	60.34	66.69	73.70	81.45	90.02	99.48	109.9	121.5	134.3
5	148.4	164.0	181.3	200.3	221.4	244.7	270.4	298.9	330.3	365.0
6	403.4	445.9	492.7	544.6	601.8	665.1	735.1	812.4	897.8	992.3
7	1097	1212	1339	1480	1636	1808	1998	2208	2441	2697
8	2981	3295	3641	4024	4447	4915	5432	6003	6634	7332
9	8103	8955	9897	10938	12088	13360	14765	16318	18034	19930

Answers to Selected Problems

CHAPTER 1
1. 8; 16; 0.1369 amu; 127.5 MeV; 8.0 MeV/nucleon
2. 15.999 amu
4. Tungsten, 58,220 eV; hydrogen, 10.1 eV
5. 0.51 MeV
6. 2.37×10^{24}
7. 15.2×10^{15} J; 3.63×10^{12} k-cal

CHAPTER 2
1. 4.6 hr; 6.9 hr; 156 hr
2. 3.5×10^{-7}; 6.6×10^{15}; 1.8×10^{-6}
4. 36.7%
6. 2.4×10^{19} sec^{-1}; 0.124 Å
8. 3.14 hr
10. 6.15×10^{14}; 9.2×10^{-8} gm
11. 30.3 mCi
12. 1.09 days; 4,100 Ci; 16.4 Ci
13. ^{74}As, positron decay and/or electron capture; ^{76}As, negatron decay
14. 80

CHAPTER 3
1. 2.02 keV/cm
2. 51,900 IP/cm
3. 0.018

CHAPTER 4
2. 3.12×10^{17}; 5,000 J/sec
4. 11.5 degrees
5. No; yes
6. No; 1 should be eliminated
7. 2 per min
8. 250 keV; 0.023; 0.05 Å
9. 2 mm
10. 9.6 mm

CHAPTER 5
1. 100 kV
2. 133 V
4. 6
6. 220 V
7. None

CHAPTER 6
2. 0.59
3. 0.94 cm
5. 12 keV; 35 keV
7. 138 keV; 12 keV; decreased
8. 865 keV

CHAPTER 7
1. 1.06×10^9 MeV/(sq m-sec); 1.06×10^{10} MeV/sq m
2. 0.65 J/kg
3. 310 J/sq m; 1.94×10^{15} photons/sq m
4. 2.1×10^{11}
5. 7.4
6. 1.53×10^{-10} A
7. 52 pF
8. 270 R

CHAPTER 8
1. 10^{-4} J; 10^{-3} J
2. 0.85
3. 1,500 mrem
4. 0.014 C
5. 1.44×10^{18}

CHAPTER 9
1. (a) 1.5 mm Al; (b) 2.15 mm Al; (c) 0.7
2. 75 kVp
3. 76.2 kVp

CHAPTER 11
1. (a) No; (b) yes; yes; (c) yes
2. No

4. 4.25×10^6

5. $0.6 \, \text{mV}$

CHAPTER 12

1. (a) 6 CPM, 1.67%; (b) ~ 5 CPM, 3.56%; (c) 8 CPM, 5.8%

2. 3.6×10^{10}

3. 10,500; 2,000

4. 1.60; 60%

7. (a) 75 mCi/ml; (b) 0.064

8. 5.56 sec

9. t-value = 2.31; $p = 0.022$

10. Figure of merit (1:2) = 0.67; system 2 preferred

11. (a) 12.3%; (b) 3.9%

CHAPTER 13

2. 2.76 MeV = photopeak; 2.25 MeV = single-escape peak; 1.74 MeV = double-escape peak; 1.38 MeV = photopeak; 0.87 MeV = single-escape peak; 0.51 MeV = annihilation peak; 0.20 MeV = back-scatter peak

4. About 580

7. 220 mCi

8. 3,400 yr

9. $2.84 = 10^5 \, \text{Ci/gm}$

CHAPTER 14

1. 59%

2. 5,500 ml

4. 43%

5. (a) ^{241}Am; (b) ^{197}Hg

10. 100 cm/min

CHAPTER 15

1. 10% and 3%

2. 125 mR

CHAPTER 16

1. 3,240

3. Yes

4. 9 MHz

CHAPTER 20

2. 3.33 cm, 5.2 degrees

3. $-13 \, \text{dB}$

4. (a) $\alpha_T = 0.989; \alpha_R = 0.011$
   (b) $\alpha_T = 0.99; \alpha_R = 0.011$

5. 33.5 degrees

7. 6.9 dB

CHAPTER 21

2. 1.2 mm

4. 9.6 cm

CHAPTER 22

1. 325 Hz; higher

2. 1.3 kHz

CHAPTER 24

1. 60 rem

2. 300 mrem

3. 440 mR

4. 2.0 mm Pb

5. None

6. 0.4 mm Pb

7. 0.7 mm Pb

8. 1.27 mm Pb

Index